Social Reform Movements to Protect
America's Vulnerable 1830–1940

WOMEN &
CHILDREN
First

Edited by David J. Rothman and
Sheila M. Rothman

A Garland Series

MATERNAL MORTALITY IN NEW YORK CITY AND PHILADELPHIA, 1931–1933

Edited by David J. Rothman
and Sheila M. Rothman

Garland Publishing, Inc.
New York & London
1987

For a complete list of the titles in this series
see the final pages of this volume.

The facsimile of *Maternal Mortality in New York City* has been made from a copy
in the Yale Medical School; that of *Maternal Mortality in Philadelphia* is from
the Library of Congress.

Library of Congress Cataloging-in-Publication Data
Maternal mortality in New York City and Philadelphia, 1931–1933.

(Women & children first)
Reprint (1st work). Originally published: Maternal mortality in New York
City / New York Academy of Medicine, Committee on Public Health Relations.
New York : Commonwealth Fund, 1933.
Reprint (2nd work). Originally published: Maternal mortality in Philadelphia,
1931–1933 / Committee on Maternal Welfare, Philadelphia County / Medical
Society. Philadelphia : Philadelphia County Medical Society, 1934.
Bibliography: p.
Includes index.
1. Mothers—New York (City)—Mortality—History—20th century.
2. Pregnancy, Complications of—New York (City)—History—20th century.
3. Maternal health services—New York (City)—History—20th century.
4. Mothers—Pennsylvania—Philadelphia—Mortality—History—20th
century.   5. Pregnancy, Complications of—Pennsylvania—Philadelphia—
History—20th century.   6. Maternal health services—Pennsylvania—
Philadelphia—History—20th century.   7. New York (City)—Statistics,
Medical.   8. Philadelphia (Pa.)—Statistics, Medical.   9. New York (City)—
Statistics, Vital.   10. Philadelphia (Pa.)—Statistics, Vital.   I. Rothman,
David J.   II. Rothman, Sheila M.   III. New York Academy of Medicine.
Committee on Public Health. Maternal mortality in New York City.   1987.
IV. Philadelphia County Medical Society. Committee on Maternal Welfare.
Maternal mortality in Philadelphia, 1931–1933.   1987.
RG530.3.U52N476   1987   614.5′992   87-21144
ISBN 0-8240-7688-5 (alk. paper)

The volumes in this series are printed on
acid-free, 250-year-life paper.

Printed in the United States of America

Maternal Mortality in New York City
A Study of All Puerperal Deaths
1930–1932
New York Academy of Medicine
Committee on Public Health Relations

Maternal Mortality in Philadelphia
1931–1933
Philadelphia County Medical Society

Editors' Note

The dramatic decline of infant mortality in the first decades of the 20th century was not matched by a similar decline in maternal mortality. These investigations by the medical profession are an effort to discover why the maternal mortality rate remained high. They explore conditions in hospitals and delivery rooms in two large cities and their controversial recommendations include better training of doctors, separate delivery rooms for childbirth, and the exclusion of midwives from obstetrics.

D.J.R.
S.M.R.

MATERNAL MORTALITY
IN NEW YORK CITY

MATERNAL MORTALITY
IN NEW YORK CITY

A STUDY OF ALL PUERPERAL DEATHS
1930–1932

BY THE NEW YORK ACADEMY OF MEDICINE
COMMITTEE ON PUBLIC HEALTH RELATIONS

RANSOM S. HOOKER, M.D., F.A.C.S.
Director of the Study

NEW YORK
THE COMMONWEALTH FUND
LONDON · HUMPHREY MILFORD
OXFORD UNIVERSITY PRESS
1933

PRINTED BY E. L. HILDRETH & COMPANY, INC., BRATTLEBORO, VERMONT

FOREWORD

IT has often been stated during the last few years that the maternal mortality rate in this country is high, and unnecessarily high. These statements have never been backed by carefully collected and studied statistics.

In 1930 the Public Health Relations Committee of the New York Academy of Medicine undertook to make such a study in New York City covering a period of three years. The facts are presented in the following pages. They are presented honestly and frankly. No attempt has been made to hide facts. It is worth emphasizing that every death was investigated by personal interview, often by several interviews, with those connected with the case. The evidence was analyzed and was carefully studied by experienced obstetricians.

The findings and conclusions are submitted to the members of the medical profession for their information and action. They are urged to study this report carefully and dispassionately.

JAMES ALEXANDER MILLER, M.D.,
Chairman

PREFACE

AS far back as 1917, the Public Health Relations Committee of the New York Academy of Medicine began to interest itself in the problem of puerperal mortality. In November of that year, Dr. George W. Kosmak stated before the Committee that, while the death rates from other preventable causes had been steadily declining, the deaths from puerperal causes had remained stationary. He emphasized the fact that there were then no satisfactory statistical data on the subject of puerperal deaths in the city of New York, and, particularly, on puerperal septicaemia. At his suggestion, a sub-committee of the Public Health Relations Committee was appointed to undertake a comprehensive study of the entire subject.

This Committee prepared a questionnaire which was submitted to a number of the hospitals in which a large proportion of institutional deliveries took place, hoping by this means to obtain all facts relevant to the puerperal deaths of the five previous years. When, however, the material was assembled and studied, it became apparent that the records obtained in this way were not only incomplete but, in many instances, inaccurate, and any conclusions arising from them would be valueless. Accordingly, the material was not used and the study not completed.

It was, then, not until 1923 that interest in the subject again became active. At that time Dr. W. W. Keene of Philadelphia requested the Academy of Medicine to undertake a thorough study of puerperal infections in collaboration with the Philadelphia College of Surgeons and County Medical

Society. This was considered, but the idea was finally abandoned because it was felt that studies should be undertaken independently in the two cities.

In 1927, another attempt was made to collect data on puerperal deaths in New York, this time by a study of the facts and figures available in the Registrar's Office in the Bureau of Vital Statistics, with the assistance of Dr. Leon Jules Blumenthal of the Department of Health. The data thus collected yielded nothing of significance, and that effort was also abandoned.

Finally, in 1928, the Committee on Public Health Relations requested Dr. Ralph W. Lobenstine and Dr. George W. Kosmak to submit to them plans for a "study of the phases of the public health problems of obstetrics as they affect New York City."

Dr. Lobenstine and Dr. Kosmak recommended that a study of the maternity situation in New York City be undertaken immediately, with special reference to the following:

1. Puerperal deaths as related to hospitals, private doctors, midwives, environment, operative interference, etc.

2. Survey of facilities for confinements in hospitals and clinics.

3. Development of suggestions for the average standards of obstetrical care.

4. Thorough examination of the midwife situation.

The Committee on Public Health Relations appointed a sub-committee consisting of Dr. Frederic E. Sondern, Chairman, and Drs. Philip Van Ingen, Benjamin P. Watson, and Ransom S. Hooker.

This sub-committee decided to undertake an examination patterned somewhat on the lines of the similar survey being made by Dr. Fred L. Adair and his associates, with the co-operation of the Children's Bureau at Washington—the so-called "Fifteen States Study"'—and to adopt their question-naire, in order that satisfactory comparisons might be made with the results of the study of conditions in the fifteen states, exclusive of New York. The Committee further decided that a detailed study should be started on the first of January, 1930, to continue for three years. It was felt that the investi-gation, to be of the most value, should run concurrently with the deaths, and the committee was able to enlist the coopera-tion of the Department of Health in obtaining weekly reports of the deaths from puerperal causes occurring during the pre-vious week, thus making it possible to obtain the material for the questionnaires while the cases were still fresh in the minds of the attendants.

The Committee requested Drs. Benjamin P. Watson, John O. Polak, George W. Kosmak, and Harry Aranow to act as an Obstetrical Advisory Committee. Dr. Ransom S. Hooker was appointed director of the study. The work of gathering and tabulating the material was done by Dr. Mary-nia Farnham (on full time) and Dr. Elizabeth Arnstein (on part time), a statistical clerk and her assistant, Miss Mabel Seaman and Miss Margaret Streib (both registered nurses). Miss Dorothy Jones, also a registered nurse, volunteered her services to interview all midwives and, in addition, did a great deal of valuable work in assembling the material for the dis-cussion of the midwife situation. Mrs. M. S. Thompson and Mrs. Paul C. Colonna also gave their services in collecting bibliography. A considerable part of the writing of the report was done by Dr. Farnham, who also was of assistance in cor-relating the various factors.

The Obstetrical Society of New York provided a loan to

start the work, as planned, and the funds to carry out the full study were most generously supplied by the Commonwealth Fund, to which we wish to express our appreciation for the interest which made the work possible.

Throughout the period of the study, all our efforts have been greatly forwarded by the unqualified cooperation given by everyone involved. Dr. Shirley W. Wynne, Commissioner of Health, Dr. Charles Bolduan and the Bureau of Vital Statistics of the Board of Health, particularly Mr. Louis Weiner and Miss Florence Swenson, have never failed to help us in every way possible. To those who have so generously given time and effort, we wish to say that without them our work could not have been accomplished. Dr. Lowell J. Reed, Professor of Biostatistics at Johns Hopkins University, very kindly examined a part of the tabulated material and offered his advice as to the validity of many of the findings. Miss Marjorie Bellows, statistician for the Westchester County Department of Health, very generously assisted in the preparation and correction of a large number of the tabulations presented, but the Committee assumes full responsibility for the deductions drawn from the data, as these have not always been submitted to Dr. Reed or Miss Bellows.

The members of the Obstetrical Advisory Committee have always given their time in coming to the monthly meetings, and their advice and assistance have been of incalculable value. The death of Dr. Polak deprived the Committee of a most able and enthusiastic member. Dr. Charles A. Gordon has most efficiently taken Dr. Polak's place.

The Committee would like to express its appreciation of the attitude of all the doctors interviewed by the investigators. In every instance the physician met the investigator cordially and gave active cooperation and assistance. One of the most vital factors, if not the crucial one, in a study of this kind is the attitude of those who are in possession of the facts which the investigator wishes to discover. The medical profession has more than met this challenge, and to their disinterested and active cooperation is due a large measure of the value of this report.

The hospital authorities have given assistance in every way possible, making their records available for study and answering the questionnaires we have sent to them from time to time.

R. S. H.

June 30, 1933

CONTENTS

LIST OF TABLES

LIST OF CHARTS

I

STATEMENT OF THE PROBLEM

THE problems surrounding the mortality among women from causes directly or indirectly associated with child-bearing have long been a matter of concern to the medical profession. It is frequently asserted, and with justice, that the death rate from these causes in the United States is higher than that in most countries of our civilized status. The statement is equally true of New York City, where the puerperal mortality rate per 1,000 live births is only slightly lower than the rate for the country as a whole (or that portion of it in the Registration Area). The facts of the situation in New York City are revealed annually in the report of the Bureau of Vital Statistics of the Department of Health. These figures are necessarily crude; they are unavoidably subject to error; they tell the story merely as it appears in numbers without any possibility of exposing what may lie behind those numbers, but they indicate, beyond question, the presence of a situation disturbing in the extreme. These are the deaths of an isolated and socially significant class—women in the active, childbearing years—and as such they must be of searching concern to the medical profession and equally to society in general. The social problems arising out of this situation are too obvious to require restatement here.

The spectacular progress of the last years in the reductions of many death rates has not been paralleled by any drop in the rate of death from puerperal causes. Communicable diseases have shown steadily declining incidence and fatality rates with the wide application of the increasing methods for prophylaxis; infant mortality has been steadily declining, but puerperal mortality has remained stationary. This failure to show any improvement is the more significant when it is realized that, during this time, modern obstetrics has evolved from a neglected and relatively insignificant department of medical practice to a highly specialized one, demanding the attention of the best skill of the medical profession. Great progress has been made in the understanding and treatment of the more serious abnormalities of pregnancy and delivery. These advances have failed to produce a decrease in the deaths. The conviction has been growing that this group of diseases, if subjected to intensive study and investigation, would yield the information which could be utilized to produce an improvement comparable to that in other fields of preventive medicine.

The problem presents strictly technical, medical, and laboratory aspects which we have attempted to examine and analyze: the conditions of hospital equipment as to amount, distribution, and quality; the ability of the doctors and midwives charged with the conduct of pregnancy and delivery; the medical knowledge of the causes, means of prevention, and proper treatment of the various complications and abnormalities of pregnancy and delivery. These are of primary importance and have been carefully scrutinized. In addition, however, the problem of puerperal mortality, more, perhaps, than any other, has extensive social aspects which are equally important with the medical in assuring a happy outcome: the social and economic position of the woman, the type of conditions under which she must live, her ignorance or intelligence.

These social problems are so closely interwoven with the medical ones that a careful examination of them, also, would be required to give a complete picture of the situation. Their magnitude is so overwhelming and their ramifications so extensive that separate and intensive study would be required to give a thorough and satisfactory representation of the situation in those aspects. So far as our time and facilities have allowed, we have attempted to gain information on this element of the whole. The results of the far too cursory examination will be given in their proper place.

The technique of the performance and presentation of such a survey divided itself into three major aspects: first, the amassing of the material—that is, the discovery and detailed study, at first hand, of every death associated with, or directly caused by, pregnancy or childbirth; second, the analysis, classification, and correlation of these facts; and last, the determination of the conclusions to be drawn therefrom, together with the recommendations seeming to arise out of these conclusions. To find the true facts behind each case, the actual cause of each death, and which was the faulty link in each long, involved chain of circumstances; to analyze all the facts together for the significant trends that seemed to lie in them; and to point out, if possible, where remedies might be applied to the amelioration of the conditions, have been the objectives to which we have directed our efforts. The results of such an examination of the puerperal deaths in New York City during the years 1930, 1931, and 1932 are offered in the succeeding pages.

COMPARATIVE DATA

THE problem of this investigation has been specifically stated to be the study of the maternal mortality situation in New York City. In any study such as this, interest is naturally aroused in the situation elsewhere. Comparisons with other countries and cities in other parts of this country may well be thought to lie within the scope of this report, and their omission requires explanation.

Comparisons may be extraordinarily important and of great significance, but they must be comparisons based upon entirely similar situations. Obviously, figures and data on the situations in foreign countries, where there are mixed rural and urban elements and a consequent diversity of conditions, are not properly comparable to those of New York City. Moreover, New York is unique among the great cities of the world in its wide variety of racial strains, with all that means in social habitudes and environmental maladjustments. There are, moreover, wide variations in the methods of calculating rates and percentages as well as differences in coding deaths. To give one example: In New York City the puerperal death rate is calculated per 1,000 live births, while in New York

TABLE 1

BIRTH AND DEATH RATES FOR THE UNITED STATES REGISTRATION AREA*

YEAR	PER 1,000 POPULATION		PER 1,000 LIVE BIRTHS			
	Birth rate	General death rate	Infant mortality	Total maternal mortality	Puerperal septi-caemia	Other puerperal causes
1920	23.7	13.0	85.8	8.0	2.7	5.3
1921	24.2	11.6	75.6	6.8	2.7	4.1
1922	22.3	11.7	76.2	6.6	2.4	4.2
1923	22.2	12.2	77.1	6.7	2.5	4.1
1924	22.4	11.7	70.8	6.6	2.4	4.1
1925	21.5	11.8	71.7	6.5	2.4	4.0
1926	20.7	12.3	73.3	6.6	2.4	4.1
1927	20.6	11.4	64.6	6.5	2.5	4.0
1928	19.8	12.1	68.7	6.9	2.5	4.4
1929	18.9	11.9	67.6	7.0	2.6	4.3
1930	18.9	11.3	64.6	6.7	2.4	4.3
1931	18.0	11.1	61.6	6.6	2.5	4.1
1932†	—	—	—	—	—	—

*Figures taken from the mortality statistics of the Bureau of the Census.
†Data for 1932 not available.

State the calculation is made per 1,000 births, live and still. The variations exist in every set of figures that are to be considered, and as they vitiate any comparisons which might be made, we have felt that there were no valid deductions to be derived from comparative data, and have accordingly omitted any discussion of them.

It is, however, of great interest to compare the figures for successive years from the same source. These figures show no decrease in the puerperal death rate over a period of ten years in the country, the state, or the city of New York, as is shown by Tables 1, 2, and 3A.

TABLE 2

BIRTH AND DEATH RATES FOR NEW YORK STATE
EXCLUSIVE OF NEW YORK CITY*

YEAR	PER 1,000 POPULATION		PER 1,000 LIVE BIRTHS	PER 1,000 BIRTHS‡		
	Birth rate	General death rate	Infant mortality	Total maternal mortality	Puerperal septi-caemia	Other puerperal causes
1920	21.3	14.8	87.6	6.72	1.97	4.75
1921	21.6	13.4	80.4	5.91	2.19	3.72
1922	20.3	13.8	80.4	6.11	1.90	4.21
1923	19.9	14.0	79.2	6.09	1.87	4.22
1924	19.9	13.3	71.0	5.78	1.98	3.78
1925	19.2	13.3	71.0	5.90	2.25	3.65
1926	18.3	14.0	73.6	5.87	1.98	3.89
1927	18.2	13.0	63.4	6.05	2.03	4.02
1928	17.5	13.3	64.5	6.25	1.98	4.27
1929	16.6	13.7	63.3	5.84	1.95	3.89
1930	16.5	12.8	59.8	5.71	2.09	3.62
1931	15.7	12.5	59.6	5.91	2.18	3.73
1932†	15.1	12.5	55.2	5.88	2.11	3.78

*Figures obtained from the Division of Vital Statistics of the New York State Department of Health.
†Provisional figures.
‡Including stillbirths.

Comparison of Tables 3A and 3B shows the difference in maternal mortality rates for the past three years between the New York City Department of Health figures and those of our study.

The variation in the general maternal mortality rate is due, in part, to the fact that the investigators were able to discover a considerable number of cases which the Registrar's Office had not been able to classify as puerperal, because the death certificate bore no mention of pregnancy. The puerperal sepsis rate varies from that of the Department of Health because septicaemia following caesarean section is included not in this group but in other puerperal causes, and because of the frequent omission from the certificate of any mention of a septicaemia.

CONDITIONS IN NEW YORK CITY

In order that what follows may be understood fully, it will be necessary to give a very brief exposition of the physical, social, and racial characteristics of the New York City metropolitan area.

New York City is divided into five boroughs: the Bronx, lying on the mainland just to the north of the island of Manhattan, taking in an area of 42.74 square miles and a population of 1,265,258 in 1930; Manhattan, an island of 22.2 square miles area and a population of 1,867,312; Brooklyn, lying on the western end of Long Island, comprising an area of 74.14 square miles and a population of 2,560,401; Queens, lying north and east of Brooklyn on Long Island with an area of 109.88 square miles and a population of 1,079,129; and Richmond, on Staten Island, with an area of 59.99 square miles and a population of 158,346. A glance at the relative areas and populations of the five boroughs will give some idea of the great variations of population densities

TABLE 3A

BIRTH AND DEATH RATES FOR NEW YORK CITY*

YEAR	PER 1,000 POPULATION		PER 1,000 LIVE BIRTHS			
	Birth rate	General death rate	Infant mortality	Total maternal mortality	Puerperal septi-caemia‡	Other puerperal causes
1920	23.4	12.9	85.4	5.33	1.31	4.02
1921	23.1	11.1	71.1	5.56	1.27	4.29
1922	21.8	11.7	74.5	5.39	1.17	4.22
1923	21.3	11.4	66.4	4.82	0.89	3.93
1924	21.1	11.5	67.6	5.20	0.98	4.22
1925	20.4	11.4	64.6	5.41	1.08	4.33
1926	19.5	11.8	67.8	4.74	0.95	3.79
1927	19.6	10.7	55.9	5.38	1.38	4.00
1928	18.8	11.6	65.5	5.29	1.17	4.12
1929	18.2	11.3	58.5	5.05	0.93	4.12
1930	17.6	10.8	57.2	5.19	0.88	4.31
1931	16.3	10.9	55.6	5.76	1.58	4.18
1932†	15.2	10.3	50.9	5.69	1.54	4.16

*Figures obtained from the New York City Department of Health. As the rates for New York City are not computed on the same basis as the New York State or the Census Bureau figures, comparison between them must not be made.
†Provisional figures.
‡Septicaemia following caesarean section is not included with puerperal septicaemia as the New York City Department of Health codes these deaths with "Other accidents of childbirth" (code number 149).

TABLE 3B

PUERPERAL MORTALITY RATES AS ESTABLISHED BY THIS SURVEY

YEAR	PER 1,000 LIVE BIRTHS		
	Total maternal mortality	Puerperal septicaemia	Other puerperal causes
1930	5.49	2.15	3.34
1931	6.12	2.36	3.76
1932	5.98	2.44	3.54

and their correlative factors. Manhattan shows the greatest density of any of the boroughs with 650 persons to the acre in its lower east side. In the upper east side, in a district bounded on the east by First Avenue, on the west by Third Avenue, and on the north and south by East 104th Street and 99th Street respectively, there are 565 persons to the acre. Brooklyn's maximum density is 445 persons to the acre. This is found in an area at the terminal of the Williamsburg Bridge, which links Brooklyn and Manhattan. The remaining boroughs have no congestion comparable to that found in these sections of Manhattan and Brooklyn.

As the boroughs vary in density of population, they vary also in the living conditions attendant upon congestion. Manhattan is almost entirely a closely packed apartment and tenement city with the open areas confined to the parks, squares, and playgrounds. The street is the normal gathering place of its inhabitants, both child and adult, of the lower economic strata. The Bronx may be thought of as a somewhat thinned-out version of Manhattan, wholly lacking in Manhattan's slums, but made up of large closely built apartments with a tendency in its more distant parts to the separate dwellings characteristic of a city of moderate size. Housing in Brooklyn is more varied, ranging from extremely congested tenements to separate homes. Queens and Richmond present a different picture. Here the congestion is much less, there are several model housing projects, the slum is unknown, and the picture is more typical of the moderate-sized city.

The density of population is reflected to some extent in the quality of the housing. This is not unqualifiedly true because of the so-called "super-slum" or the very high apartment building which increases the density of the population without depressing the standard of living. Such buildings are characteristic, indeed, of the housing chosen by the highest economic groups. But for the most part, extreme density of population means a correspondingly degraded housing condition. In 1932 "old-law tenements," which were so appalling in 1901 that an investigation into their conditions gave rise to the then "new tenement law" of that date, were still housing 1,800,000 people, or between a quarter and a third of the population of the city. It is a safe estimate that there are 150,000 rooms in the city without any window admitting outside air. It is not debatable that such structures, with their inevitable overcrowding, filth, and destruction of human decency and dignity, are unfit for human habitation. In 1901, the Health Department had demonstrated that there was a distinctly higher death rate in these areas. The Aberdeen report on the relation between slum housing conditions and maternal mortality, especially septicaemia,[2] however, failed to demonstrate any distinct relationship. We have been able to make only the most superficial examination into this element of the subject and will present those results in the section devoted to the study of the various economic areas of the city (Chapter V, page 148).

New York, moreover, has the most widely varied racial distribution of any city in the world. Practically every race on earth has its representation here. When these racial and national groups attain any considerable size, they have a tendency to live in compact districts, retaining, to a striking degree, many of their distinctive habitudes of speech, dress, diet, and social adjustment. These national traits are reflected no more strongly in any direction than in the attitudes and customs surrounding family constitution, marriage, and childbearing.

The Negro population of New York City is estimated at 248,000, living mostly in the Harlem district in Manhattan, between 116th Street and 150th Street and Fifth Avenue on the east and St. Nicholas Avenue on the west. Here is the center of Negro life and activity, so set apart that the word

"Harlem" has come to mean the Negro quarter. The Italians are equally set apart, living largely in the lower east side and the lower part generally of the island of Manhattan. Here they have brought into being a life that is, in its essence, national. The streets, in these districts, are eloquent of it, both literally and pictorially. This is no less true of the Chinese, whose Chinatown in lower Manhattan, one of the city's show places, maintains, to a striking degree, the character and customs of the race. The Jewish population, now centered in Brooklyn, is greater than that of any other city in the world, numbering upwards of 1,700,000. These are the major national groups. Others are smaller in numbers and thus of less importance.

The integrity of racial units tends to augment the problems of medical care and public health. Education to induce such racial groups to abandon long-cherished social habits is slow; methods must be adapted to each group. Added to the purely cultural and social problem of trying to unify disparate and unassimilated groups, are the strictly medical and reflected public health problems of physical change set up by the transplantation of races to new climates and environments. The Negro in the north comes immediately to mind with the possible effect of the change in climate on the incidence of rickets. These effects are not accurately known or understood, but that they do play a part in the health problem of New York City is an admitted fact.

It is to be regretted that time and facilities in this study have not sufficed to allow any but the most cursory examination of the role of race and racial origin in the problem before us, more especially as New York is the obviously ideal community for the study of such a problem. However, a few figures on native and foreign-born mothers will be presented later.

II

METHODS OF THE STUDY

COLLECTING AND COMPILING THE DATA

W E have felt that it was of the greatest importance to have the investigation of the deaths in question follow their occurrence as closely as possible. So much of the material is a matter of the memory of the individual who must supply the information, that unless he is seen while the case is still fresh in mind a great deal will be forgotten or only vaguely remembered, and the details of each case will not be accurately recorded.

The cooperation of the Department of Health made it possible for us to do this. Each week there was forwarded to us from the Registrar's Office a photostatic copy of every death certificate which carried a puerperal condition, whether primary or contributory, as cause of death, or which merely stated the existence of pregnancy. By this method we received notification of deaths from one to two weeks after their occurrence, and the investigation took place within a month.

In getting the information required, we first sought the physician who signed the death certificate. In those instances where the patient had been delivered by one physician and cared for by another during the subsequent period preceding her death, we visited and interviewed the accoucheur, also, for the full details of the pregnancy and delivery. It has been the usual practice to see personally all those who were in attendance upon the patients at any time during pregnancy, delivery, or the puerperium. By thus obtaining all information at first hand, we have hoped to reduce to a minimum the inescapable margin of error.

All cases which had any stay in a hospital were subjected to further study. The hospital record was examined directly. Through the Department of Health the field investigators were given the authority of officers of the Department, which permitted direct access to the hospital records. It is the opinion of the investigators that the written record, including as it does history and written report of the physical examination with reports of operative procedures, laboratory examinations, temperature chart, and most valuable of all, perhaps, the nurse's record of the patient's condition from hour to hour, will yield the most complete, accurate, and satisfactory view of the case possible. Often, the picture provided by the nurse's record will serve to establish a diagnosis that has not been recorded. For example, a case of ruptured ectopic pregnancy was designated as a death from embolus, while on reading the nurse's notes regarding the increasing dyspnoea, restlessness, and thirst, it became evident that the death was almost surely due to secondary hemorrhage.

In the cases in the city hospitals or those hospitals maintaining large ward services with complete records, the hospital chart has usually sufficed, and the questionnaire* could be filled out directly from the detailed record of the patient. In such cases the attending physician was not always visited. When the information was obtained in an interview with the attendant, the investigator relied on notes made immediately after the conversation, as it was felt that taking notes directly from the attendant might be confusing and might yield less significant results than the more informal method.

After the questionnaire had been filled in, the investigator wrote a summary in which she included all details omitted from the questionnaire.

The information on the completed history was then trans-

* For copy, see Appendix, page 257.

ferred to a chart on which all the cases for each month were recorded, each column of the chart corresponding to one question on the blank.

When all the cases for a month had been completed, and all the information transferred to the charts, a meeting of the Advisory Committee was called to examine the cases and decide upon the actual cause of death and the preventability. The director and the two field investigators were also present at these meetings. The investigators were able to answer questions and clarify any points which were not entirely clear and also to learn what further information the Committee desired on any given case.

From this basic material, which is presented in the Appendix, our correlations have been made. The card punch system has been used for the major part of these. Since, however, that could not be used until all the data had been collected, we made a practice of drawing up basic tables, charts, and correlations from month to month as the completed data were made available. Thus the determination of fundamental trends could be kept practically parallel with the gathering of material.

In this way, the decision as to the proper and possibly useful correlations was greatly simplified and many errors and omissions were avoided. We have by this method been able to accumulate a very large amount of material for examination and study. Our time has so limited us that we are able to present in this report only the salient and outstanding features of the material. It is to be hoped that the opportunity may be presented, at a later time, for completing the analysis and correlation.

Our rates and percentages have been drawn from the numerical summaries in the usual manner accepted for the handling of vital statistics.

ALLOCATING CASES TO CAUSE OF DEATH

IN classifying the cases according to the cause of death, we have followed as closely as seemed to us proper, in the interests of accuracy, the *Internatonal List of Causes of Death,* using the 1929 edition. This revision, in the sections devoted to puerperal causes, represents a marked improvement over the 1920 revision, but in the process of condensation it has seemed to us to sacrifice the detailed accuracy with which we wished to present our findings. This is particularly true in the general titles *Other accidents of pregnancy* (Number 143) and *Other toxemias of pregnancy* (Number 147).

In the following paragraphs, it will be simplest if we indicate where and in what way we have altered the classifications as they appeared in the *International List.*

Number 140, *Abortion with septic conditions,* we have followed unaltered.

Number 141, *Abortion without mention of septic conditions, including hemorrhage,* we have further subdivided into the underlying causes and have presented the figures for therapeutic abortions separately.

Number 142, *Ectopic gestation,* we have used unchanged.

Number 143, *Other accidents of pregnancy, except hemorrhage,* is a loose classification to include any death occurring during pregnancy which is not included in the more definite classifications. In every instance, we have determined the true cause of death, most often toxaemia or extra-puerperal conditions, and placed the case under the code number corresponding to that cause.

Number 144, *Hemorrhage,* has been followed as stated.

Number 145, *Puerperal septicaemia,* is unchanged.

Number 146, *Albuminuria and eclampsia,* is sufficiently definite to answer our needs.

Number 147, *Other toxemias of pregnancy.* Since all our cases falling into this category have been pernicious vomiting of pregnancy, we have so named this section.

Number 148, *Puerperal phlegmasia alba dolens, embolus, and sudden death,* has seemed to us to require no alteration.

Number 149, *Other accidents of childbirth.* In this section are included deaths from shock, whether due to operative interference or attendant upon spontaneous delivery or accidents of labor such as rupture and inversion of the uterus, and we have so classified our cases.

Number 150, *Other and unspecified conditions of the puerperal state,* we have called *Accidents of the puerperium,* and in this section have placed all the deaths from puerperal psychosis and mastitis.

The *Manual of Joint Causes of Death* was designed to insure uniformity in the ascribing of primary causes of death. It is particularly addressed to the registrars who have access only to the statements on the death certificate. Because of the greatly detailed knowledge we have had access to, we have at times felt justified in varying from the order of precedence laid down by the manual. For instance, where puerperal sepsis has been mentioned, which mention would make it mandatory on the registrar to ascribe that death to sepsis, we have found that sepsis could not have caused the death in question. Case No. 1941 clearly illustrates this point. The patient developed a very mild sepsis before delivery and very soon afterward died from a ruptured uterus and attendant hemorrhage. In every case where sepsis has been present in a case terminated by embolus, we have ascribed the case to sepsis. Thus it is evident that our variations from the order of priority of the *Manual* have been only when there has been absolutely clear justification for setting aside this order.

DISPARITIES BETWEEN ACTUAL AND RECORDED
CAUSE OF DEATH

THE establishment of the true cause of death, being prerequisite to the further study of the mortality, has been our first consideration. In this task we have, of course, had the data given on the death certificates, but such information has been taken as our point of departure, to be accepted or not as our study of the individual case warranted. Thus in many instances our investigation has yielded information which established as the cause of death some condition which could not be established from an examination of the death certificate. In a considerable number of cases, we have established diagnoses which differed from those of the registrar's office.

TABLE 4

ERRORS ON DEATH CERTIFICATES PREVENTING
CORRECT CODING

CAUSE OF DEATH AS DETERMINED BY ADVISORY COMMITTEE	TOTAL DEATHS	ERRORS ON DEATH CERTIFICATES					
		TOTAL		NO MENTION OF TRUE CAUSE OF DEATH		CONDITION GIVEN AS CAUSE OF DEATH FOUND TO BE NON-EXISTENT	
		Number	Per cent	Number	Per cent	Number	Per cent
Total	2041	364	*17.8*	324	*15.9*	40	*2.0*
Septic abortion	262	24	*9.2*	23	*8.8*	1	*.4*
Abortion	95	33	*34.7*	33	*34.7*	—	—
Ectopic gestation	120	13	*10.8*	12	*10.0*	1	*.8*
Hemorrhage	197	35	*17.8*	22	*11.2*	13	*6.6*
Puerperal septicaemia	510	149	*29.2*	146	*28.6*	3	*.6*
Albuminuria and eclampsia	231	31	*13.4*	15	*6.5*	16	*6.9*
Pernicious vomiting	14	4	*28.6*	2	*14.3*	2	*14.3*
Phlegmasia alba dolens and embolus	89	10	*11.2*	8	*9.0*	2	*2.2*
Accidents of labor	171	28	*16.4*	27	*15.8*	1	*.6*
Accidents of puerperium	8	2	*25.0*	1	*12.5*	1	*12.5*
Extra-puerperal causes	344	35	*10.2*	35	*10.2*	—	—

The reason for this lies in the fact that in many, if not most, of these certificates, there was either careless or deliberate omission of any mention of the actual cause of death, such as those certificates where cardiac failure or broncho-pneumonia has been given as the cause, when in reality there was a puerperal sepsis. Occasionally there has been a totally erroneous cause of death given on the certificate.

Table 4 gives the number of instances in which such disparity between stated and actual cause of death occurs.

In the column headed "No mention of true cause of death" we have indicated the number of cases in which the actual cause of death as determined by investigation was not mentioned on the death certificate either as primary or contributory cause—a total of 15.9 per cent. In these cases, terms such as "cardiac failure," "shock," "ileus," "puerperal toxaemia," "embolism," and "broncho-pneumonia" were particularly common, where septicaemia was, in fact, the true cause.

In the column headed "Condition given as cause of death found to be non-existent" we have shown the number of other cases in which a condition given on the certificate was found not to have existed. In these instances, the registrars would of necessity have erroneously assigned the recorded condition as the cause of death.

The "Total" column shows the total number and percentage of instances in which incorrect coding must have resulted. For the entire series, the total percentage of error was 17.8. In the diagnosis of abortion, this rose to 34.7, the next highest being 29.2 per cent of error in the death certificates where the cause of death was septicaemia. There was a noticeable tendency to ascribe the death to the latest phenomenon, as in the cases of pernicious vomiting where the death was often ascribed to shock or cardiac failure attendant upon the operation.

The figures in the preceding paragraphs offer fresh evidence of the futility of making comparisons based on relative data. When so large a percentage of error can be definitely shown to exist, it is evident that, with a greater number of persons handling the certificates, the variation between countries and even different localities of the same country will be of such dimensions that useful comparisons are impossible.

III

PREVENTABILITY OF DEATH

THE reduction of mortality and morbidity in all branches of medical practice has been shown to lie increasingly in the field of prevention, and obstetrical practice is no exception to this general rule. We have felt that a determination of the proportion of the deaths in this series which could have been avoided was one of the most valuable objectives of the study. In judging whether or not the death was inevitable, the criterion has always been that of the best possible skill, both in diagnosis and treatment, which the community could make available. Furthermore, in forming the decision, determination was made of the place where responsibility for such a preventable death should be lodged: on the attendant, whether physician or midwife, or on the patient herself. All the cases were assigned to either preventable or non-preventable groups.

It was realized that, with our present knowledge, it was impossible to arrive at a scientifically correct determination of preventability. Moreover, it was felt that accuracy would be best served by a careful study of each case individually. It will, therefore, be necessary for the reader to have some information as to how the decisions were reached. The criteria following represent not an attempt to formulate a definite set of standards, but rather a more or less flexible system which was used as a guide to give uniformity to the findings.

All the data available were assembled (as given on the questionnaire reproduced in the Appendix, page 257) for each death. This information was supplemented by a summary of the case by the physician who did the investigation. Each case was reviewed and analyzed by a committee of four obstetricians at a meeting attended also by the director of the study and the workers who had investigated the cases. In examining the cases, the Advisory Committee attempted to base its judgment on the facts presented without prior knowledge of the identity of the attendant. At these meetings, a decision was reached as to the true cause of death and the preventability in each case.

GENERAL CRITERIA

In forming a decision, all the relevant factors were considered, as follows:

Prenatal Care

Was there prenatal care? Was it adequate from the point of view of regularity and frequency of the visits? Was the examination thorough and sufficient for the determination of pulmonary, cardiac, and renal efficiency and for the detection of constitutional disease, such as tuberculosis and syphilis, and if such were present, were they properly treated? Was the pelvis correctly measured and a presumably accurate prognosis of labor made? Was abnormal position diagnosed? If complications arose, were they promptly recognized and properly treated?

The Conduct of Labor and Delivery

Was the hospital or sanitarium properly equipped for obstetrical work by provision of a delivery room separate from the operating room used for general surgery? Was the aseptic and antiseptic preparation for labor and delivery (the equipment, the patient, and the attendant) satisfactory? In the case of delivery in the home, was there proper provision for delivery? Did the attendant have the assistance required if the delivery was abnormal? Were the deliveries done in the home confined to those which could be properly conducted there? Was the delivery spontaneous? If so, was it unduly prolonged? What anaesthetic was used and was it properly selected and skilfully administered? If the delivery was operative, was the labor allowed to progress too long before undertaking the operative termination? Was an obstructed labor promptly recognized? Was the method of delivery a judicious one, carried out at the right time and skilfully performed? Particularly in the case of major obstetrical operations, such as version and extraction and caesarean section, was careful consideration given to the adequacy of the indications?

The Puerperium

Was there properly conducted isolation? Was there sufficient rest in bed? Was there adequate and satisfactory nursing care? Were complications promptly recognized and properly treated?

ILLUSTRATIVE CASES

In order to clarify these general principles, a more specific discussion of how they were applied in the study of deaths from the various puerperal causes is given in the following paragraphs. The cases cited in illustration were chosen because they were most nearly "average," care being taken to avoid those which were extreme in either direction.

Ectopic Gestation

In the case of a death resulting from a ruptured ectopic gestation, if the attendant failed to recognize the condition, or to safeguard the patient by a transfusion if there was indication for it, the case would be counted preventable and the responsibility placed upon the physician. The same would be true in any case dying of peritonitis following an operation for ectopic gestation.

If the patient neglected to consult a physician at the onset of abnormal symptoms, such as pain or vaginal bleeding, the death would again be classed as preventable, but the patient herself would be held responsible.

A death following prompt recognition of the condition and a properly safeguarded operation would be considered not preventable.

Hemorrhage

If a woman died from hemorrhage, either accidental or from a placenta praevia or premature separation of the placenta, the death would be classed as preventable if it appeared that there had been improper choice of the method of delivery or if the attendant had delayed or failed entirely to secure, or attempt to secure, a transfusion. The responsibility, in such a case, would rest upon the physician. This would also be the case if the choice of procedure were improper: if intervention were delayed where the indications were evident or if the intervention undertaken had been injudiciously decided upon. Particular mention may be made of the tendency to hasten the extraction after a podalic version had been performed to control the hemorrhage from a placenta praevia.

Case No. 706. A primigravida entered the hospital after a normal pregnancy, during which she had had no prenatal care. At admission she was in labor and was bleeding fairly profusely from a marginal placenta praevia. Manual dilatation and version and extraction were immediately done. Postpartum, the bleeding persisted. Pituitrin and massage of the fundus were the only measures resorted to. She died very soon after delivery.

In this case the attendant failed properly to safeguard the patient before undertaking a hazardous operation for which the indications were doubtful and omitted to pack the uterus or to administer a transfusion when the bleeding persisted postpartum. For these reasons this case was considered preventable and the responsibility placed upon the attendant.

If a patient had had repeated hemorrhages during her pregnancy, and had failed to seek medical care until her condition had become critical, her death would be considered preventable, but the blame would attach to her.

This was true of Case No. 129: A gravida four neglected to consult a physician in spite of recurrent vaginal bleeding beginning in the fourth month of her pregnancy. She was received into a hospital after an alarming hemorrhage at the onset of labor. The hemorrhage was controlled by a version, and an extraction was done when dilatation was complete. Her death, which followed, was classed as preventable but the responsibility rested upon the patient herself.

When, however, every possible precaution was taken by both patient and attendant, and delivery properly carried out, the death was classed as non-preventable.

Such a case is No. 1157. A primigravida entered the hospital in labor after a normal pregnancy. Labor was of ten hours' duration terminated by craniotomy on a hydrocephalic foetus. Postpartum, the uterus failed to contract satisfactorily. Secondary hemorrhage began an hour after delivery. The uterus was immediately packed, she was given pituitrin and ergot and continuous clyses, while arrangements were being made for a transfusion which could not be performed before she died.

Puerperal Septicaemia

When we come to the group of patients dying of septicaemia, the problem of classifying the death as preventable or
non-preventable becomes much more difficult. In theory, any
death from sepsis in a patient who has no existing septic focus
either in the genital tract or elsewhere in the body is preventable. In practice this is not so. A woman who has had no vaginal examinations, who delivers spontaneously and suffers no
trauma, may become infected and die of sepsis. It is impossible to be certain in any given case that there has not been a
breach in the aseptic technique or that one of the attendants
has not an infection which was transmitted to the patient. We
have presumed, in cases of the type mentioned above, when
the delivery occurred in a hospital and under circumstances
which, in theory, could be considered satisfactory, that the
case was not preventable. This is not a reliable guide, but in
light of the limited knowledge as to the origin of puerperal
septicaemia it has seemed to be the one which would result in
the most just evaluation of the situation. If, however, a series
of deaths from septicaemia occurred in one institution within
a short period of time, the cases would be classed as preventable—the presumption being either that there was a carrier
among those in attendance upon the maternity patients or
that the aseptic technique was faulty—and the institution
would be blamed.

As with the other deaths, each one was analyzed separately
with all the circumstances surrounding it, but certain general
principles were used in deciding the preventability of each
case, as follows:

When there had been any artificial interference whatever
preceding a death from septicaemia, that death has usually
been classified as preventable and the responsibility ascribed
to the doctor.

Those cases of septicaemia which followed a spontaneous

labor and an entirely uninterfered-with delivery, properly conducted, were classified as non-preventable.

Failure of the patient to follow the advice of the attendant threw that case into the preventable class, the responsibility lying with the patient.

Whenever a midwife had failed to call a physician promptly in the course of a difficult or abnormal labor, the case was considered preventable and the blame placed on the midwife.

The following cases may be cited in illustration of the foregoing:

Case No. 1206. A primigravida had been under the care of her physician during pregnancy, but he failed to observe the presence of a contracted pelvis. He then allowed her to remain in labor five days, doing repeated vaginal examinations, before calling consultation. The consultant found the pelvic deformity and was forced to deliver an already dead foetus by craniotomy.

It is obvious that the carelessness and incapacity of the first attendant must be held entirely responsible for the patient's death from septicaemia two days after delivery.

Case No. 853. A gravida three went into labor spontaneously after a normal pregnancy. Labor was of seven hours' duration and delivery was spontaneous without injury to the perineum. Nevertheless, two days later she developed a typical sepsis and died on the eighth day after delivery.

In this case, it was impossible to discover any evidence of failure on the part of the attendant to give entirely satisfactory care. The case was, therefore, classified as not preventable.

Case No. 682. A secundigravida, with a previous non-viable stillbirth, had satisfactory prenatal care. When she was seen by her attendant at the onset of labor, position was posterior and, as he anticipated a difficult labor, he advised her to go to a hospital. She repeatedly refused to enter a hospital during a protracted and difficult labor. The physician finally had to deliver her by mid forceps at home. She developed septicaemia and died three weeks later.

Obviously the attendant cannot be held responsible for the death of a patient who refuses to follow his advice.

Case No. 981. A primigravida had a normal pregnancy under the care of a midwife. She went into labor at term. Labor was prolonged and progress was slow. After seventy-two hours the midwife ruptured the membranes and when this failed to accelerate progress, she called a physician. He sent the patient to a hospital where she was found to have a flat pelvis, making delivery impossible. Accordingly a low flap caesarean section was done but she died of septicaemia a short time thereafter.

In this case the midwife was blamed because she neglected to call a physician in the presence of an obviously obstructed labor.

Toxaemia

If a patient died of eclampsia or other pregnancy toxaemia and had not consulted a doctor until the onset of acute symptoms, the death would be classed as preventable and the blame placed on the patient. Case No. 1213 illustrates this situation. A primigravida came to the prenatal clinic for care. She went into the hospital in the thirtieth week because of a mild toxaemia. After her discharge, she failed to cooperate further, refusing second hospitalization, and finally neglecting her clinic visits. She was ultimately admitted in a critical condition and died in spite of treatment.

If a patient under the care of a physician or clinic showed evidences of a toxaemia and the doctor failed to prescribe the proper treatments or to make a medical follow-up to see that those treatments were being carried out, the death would be counted preventable and the responsibility placed on the physician, as in the following case, No. 901. A gravida four, having come to the clinic for prenatal care early in her pregnancy and attended the clinic regularly, began to have albuminuria and vomiting in the thirty-sixth week. A diagnosis of gall stone colic was made. Five hours later total blindness had supervened. She was then rushed to the hospital where an immediate classical section was done. She died within an hour.

If, however, the condition was promptly recognized and properly treated, the death would be classified as not preventable. In Case No. 899 a primigravida had careful observation at frequent intervals and showed no signs of toxaemia until the thirty-second week, when there was a slight trace of albumin and a rise of pressure to 150 systolic. She was put to bed on a restricted diet. One week later her symptoms were greatly aggravated and she was promptly hospitalized. Convulsions began and all treatment failed. She died within ten hours of the first convulsion without going into labor. In this case the treatment of the patient, although entirely satisfactory, was unavailing, and the death was accordingly judged non-preventable.

Accidents of Labor

Deaths occurring during the course of, or closely following, operative interference, such as version and extraction, forceps delivery, or caesarean section, have in most instances been classed as preventable, and the responsibility placed on the physician. These deaths were almost always due to the anaesthesia, to hemorrhage from severe lacerations of the cervix or rupture of the uterus, or to the shock attendant upon prolonged and maladroit operative procedures.

In the following case, No. 268, the attendant failed to recognize an obstructed labor and subjected the patient to the exhaustion attendant upon a greatly prolonged labor, plus the trauma of attempted operative delivery, and was, therefore, held responsible for the fatal outcome. A primigravida sought prenatal care early in her pregnancy, which was normal. A large sacral promontory had been noted, but it was not felt that it would obstruct a normal delivery. After seventy-two hours of labor, three futile attempts were made to apply forceps to the floating head. She was then removed to a second hospital where a caesarean section had to be performed.

If, from the data, it was clear that there was no injury and the death could quite certainly be ascribed to true postpartum shock, it was considered non-preventable.

Case No. 269 seemed definitely one of this class and was accordingly considered not preventable. A gravida nine had excellent prenatal care. Her pregnancy was entirely normal. Labor was induced at term because of premature rupture of the membranes. After four hours she was delivered spontaneously and without laceration. There was no hemorrhage but she went into shock immediately and died within an hour, in spite of vigorous anti-shock treatment.

Deaths during or immediately following caesarean section were nearly always blamed on the operator unless the woman came under his care after a long or obstructed labor. In such a case the death was accounted preventable and the liability for the outcome was placed on the woman herself. If she had been under the care of another physician or a midwife, the case would be classed as preventable and the previous attendant held accountable, provided the second operator selected, and skilfully performed, the proper operation. Whenever the classical type of section was performed under such circumstances and sepsis resulted, the death would be classed as preventable and the operator held responsible. For example, in Case No. 265 a primigravida consulted her physician early in her pregnancy, which was normal except for a generally contracted pelvis which the physician did not correctly measure. She went into labor spontaneously and after eighty-two hours, when it was evident that she could not be delivered from below, he did a classical section. She had signs of infection at the time of operation and grew rapidly worse, dying three days after delivery.

Cardiac Disease

If a patient suffering from heart disease did not consult a physician until late in pregnancy or until driven to do so by broken compensation, the death has been called preventable and the responsibility ascribed to the patient. In Case No. 721, a secundigravida with a very severe mitral lesion refused a therapeutic abortion and failed to follow the advice given her by her physician. At term she was decompensated and after a mid-forceps delivery failure grew more pronounced and she died two hours later.

If a patient were under the care of a physician and he failed to recognize the condition or, after recognizing it, failed to take proper safeguards such as prolonged rest in bed, digitalization, and proper type of delivery, the death would be classed as preventable and the responsibility placed upon the physician.

Case No. 1106. A gravida three had had two previous caesarean sections because of a severe cardiac condition and a contracted pelvis. She came to the prenatal clinic and was watched there but no special precautions were taken. When failure threatened she was hospitalized and a caesarean section was immediately performed. Post operative, her heart failed completely and she died within three days.

CRITICAL FACTORS IN PREVENTABILITY

ALL the cases which had been classified as preventable, and in which the responsibility for the death had been designated according to the plan given in the preceding paragraphs, were further studied to ascertain where, in the course of the patient's treatment, occurred the error which, in the opinion of the Committee, was primarily responsible for the fatal outcome. It was found that the errors in those cases in which the attendant, either physician or midwife, had been held responsible, fell naturally into two groups:

1. Those cases in which there had been an error in judgment, in which class were included instances of poor judgment in the recognition or treatment of complications of pregnancy; improper choice of anaesthesia; the wrong choice of operation for delivery, such as the performance of a classical caesarean section on a potentially infected patient; the performance of the proper operation but without proper safeguards such as transfusion in the case of patients bleeding from a ruptured ectopic pregnancy or placenta praevia; the failure of the attendant to recognize his own limitations either in omitting to call a consultant or in performing an operation for which, in the opinion of the Committee, his training and experience did not qualify him.

2. Those cases in which there had been an error in technique, which group includes all cases in which the attendant was unable properly to perform the operation which was the correct choice, or in which there was an obvious breach in his aseptic technique or that of his assistants, as evidenced by the development of sepsis in a presumably uninfected patient. This has been presumed to be the case in caesarean sections performed on patients with intact membranes, not in labor, and having had no internal examinations. Also included in this group were those cases in which improper administration or choice of anaesthetic had been the actual cause of the fatal result, as well as those in which faulty blood matching resulted in death directly from transfusion.

In many of the cases, the two factors were combined to produce the fatal outcome; where this was so the deaths have been classed in the group which includes the predominant element.

Cases in which the patient has been held responsible showed two types of failure to meet the requirements for proper care, and were so grouped:

1. Those cases where the patient failed to obtain medical advice, in which group we include the cases in which either from ignorance or neglect the patient failed to obtain proper care during the prenatal period or to call an attendant at the onset of labor or the development of strikingly abnormal symptoms.

2. Those cases in which the patient failed to cooperate with her attendant by neglecting or refusing to follow his advice for the proper regime during pregnancy, the treatment of abnormalities, or the management of delivery or the puerperium, such as neglect of diet or bed rest in the treatment of toxaemia, refusal to go to hospital when so advised, and lack of cooperation in getting a sufficiently long period of rest in the puerperal period.

It must be borne in mind that in many, if not most, instances where the patient has been held responsible, we recognize that she is, in fact, helpless by reason of circumstances which are not of her making and lie outside of her control. She may be, and very often is, the victim of poverty or ignorance and, in such eventualities, it is manifestly the failure of society to provide proper and effective education, assistance, and care, which have forced her, unwittingly and surely unwillingly, to become the deciding factor in her own death. Clearly, it is only those patients who have wilfully failed to obtain care and follow the advice given by their attendants, who can justly be held responsible for the outcome.

EXTENT OF PREVENTABILITY AND LOCUS OF RESPONSIBILITY

THE results of the analysis and examination of the entire series of cases to determine preventability and responsibility
are given in Tables 5A and 5B for the series as a whole and
separately for each cause of death.

TABLE 5A

CLASSIFICATION OF DEATHS BY PREVENTABILITY

CAUSE OF DEATH	TOTAL		NOT PREVENTABLE		PREVENTABLE	
	Num-ber	Per cent	Num-ber	Per cent	Num-ber	Per cent
Total deaths	2,041	*100*	698	*34.2*	1,343	*65.8*
Abortion	310	*100*	71	*22.9*	239	*77.1*
Therapeutic abortion	47	*100*	15	*31.9*	32	*68.1*
Ectopic gestation	120	*100*	31	*25.8*	89	*74.2*
Hemorrhage	197	*100*	47	*23.9*	150	*76.1*
Puerperal septicaemia	510	*100*	127	*24.9*	383	*75.1*
Albuminuria and eclampsia	231	*100*	63	*27.3*	168	*72.7*
Pernicious vomiting	14	*100*	6	*42.9*	8	*57.1*
Phlegmasia alba dolens and embolus	89	*100*	81	*91.0*	8	*9.0*
Accidents of labor	171	*100*	22	*12.9*	149	*87.1*
Accidents of puerperium	8	*100*	8	*100.0*	—	—
Extra-puerperal causes	344	*100*	227	*66.0*	117	*34.0*

Out of all the deaths, 2,041 in number, 1,343 were, in
the judgment of the Advisory Committee, preventable. That
number of women, if they had had proper treatment and care,
could and should have been brought safely through parturition. In this connection, it is significant to note that this is regarded by the Advisory Committee as a conservative figure
for preventable deaths.

The decisions regarding preventability are dependent upon
judgments made with the advantage of a full knowledge of
all the elements in the case and an absence of the difficulties
attendant upon the necessity for immediate action. The Com-

TABLE 5B

CLASSIFICATION OF PREVENTABLE DEATHS BY RESPONSIBILITY

CAUSE OF DEATH	TOTAL		ASCRIBED TO PHYSICIAN		ASCRIBED TO PATIENT		ASCRIBED TO MIDWIFE	
	Number	Per cent	Number	Per cent	Number	Per cent	Number	Per cent
Total preventable deaths	1,343	100	820	61.1	493	36.7	30	2.2
Abortion	239	100	41	17.1	197	82.4	1	.4
Therapeutic abortion	32	100	28	87.5	4	12.5	—	—
Ectopic gestation	89	100	73	82.0	16	18.0	—	—
Hemorrhage	150	100	115	76.7	27	18.0	8	5.3
Puerperal septicaemia	383	100	313	81.7	56	14.6	14	3.7
Albuminuria and eclampsia	168	100	49	29.2	116	69.0	3	1.8
Pernicious vomiting	8	100	2	25.0	6	75.0	—	—
Phlegmasia alba dolens and embolus	8	100	5	62.5	3	37.5	—	—
Accidents of labor	149	100	134	89.9	11	7.4	4	2.7
Accidents of puerperium	—	—	—	—	—	—	—	—
Extra-puerperal causes	117	100	60	51.2	57	48.7	—	—

mittee has wished, therefore, to avoid *obiter dicta*, attempting to arrive at the decisions which could and should have been made, under the circumstances demanding them, by properly qualified attendants. Wherever there was doubt or disagreement, or where complete data on any given case were lacking, the judgment was "not preventable." This may be particularly emphasized in regard to puerperal septicaemia. The difficulties surrounding the forming of considered and just decisions regarding the preventability in this situation are perplexing in the extreme. It was impossible to have assurance that the technique had been faulty in the case of a spontaneous delivery, so, lacking the accurate information which could only have been obtained by actual observation of the delivery, the Committee has, as stated above, invariably classified these cases as non-preventable.

About two-thirds of all deaths were preventable. Further analysis of the causes of death as related to preventability shows that deaths due to abortions, with the exception of therapeutic abortions, were 77.1 per cent preventable, a figure quite in accordance with *a priori* judgments, since these are frequently self-induced or illegally obtained. In 82.4 per cent of the cases the responsibility was considered to be the patient's. True responsibility in the induced cases rests with the individual who performed the induction but that information, inevitably, is unobtainable and the only possible alternative is the one chosen. In the case of therapeutic abortions, 68.1 per cent were adjudged preventable, and the physician was held responsible in 87.5 per cent of these cases. Wherever septicaemia followed a therapeutic abortion, it was inevitably preventable, and the high percentage of preventability in this series was further contributed to by the tendency of the attendants to postpone the abortion until the fatal outcome could not be averted.

In the judgment of the Advisory Committee, 74.2 per

cent of the deaths from ectopic gestation could have been avoided. In 82.0 per cent of these the responsibility was ascribed to the physician. Failure to operate and, even more often, failure to replace the loss of blood to support the patient properly, and, where peritonitis supervened, fault at operation were among the reasons for regarding these deaths as preventable. In 18.0 per cent of the cases, the patient failed to realize the gravity of her symptoms and to seek medical care promptly and was, therefore, judged responsible.

Deaths from the results of hemorrhage were classed as preventable in 76.1 per cent of the cases, 76.7 per cent of which were ascribable to the physician, 18.0 per cent to the patient, and 5.3 per cent to the midwife. The failure to utilize all methods for the control of the hemorrhage, such as proper tamponade of the uterus, combined with the oxytocic drugs, as well as tardiness in combating the effects of hemorrhage by transfusion of blood and infusions of fluids, accounts for the high percentage of preventable cases in this group. The patients, in the instances where they were held responsible for the outcome, had failed to obtain suitable care or had minimized the gravity of their symptoms and had allowed a critical situation to supervene. The cases in which the midwife was held responsible were due to her failure to evaluate the gravity of hemorrhage and to procure the prompt assistance which might have saved the patient's life.

Of the deaths from septicaemia 75.1 per cent were judged preventable. Responsibility for 81.7 per cent of these was ascribed to the physician, 14.6 per cent to the patient, and 3.7 per cent to the midwife. The large number of caesarean operations of the classical type performed on previously infected patients, undue prolongation of labors inevitably demanding operative termination, repeated internal examinations preceding operative deliveries, all contributed to the large preventable percentage in which the responsibility was judged to lie with the physician. The Committee felt that many of the preventable deaths for which the midwife was judged responsible were due to the fact that the particular midwife concerned had failed to maintain proper asepsis.

Albuminuria and eclampsia was classified as preventable in 72.7 per cent of the cases. It is not surprising to find that of this number 69.0 per cent were considered the patient's responsibility. The studies of these cases revealed a surprising tendency to disregard manifest danger signals, very many of the women being first brought under observation at the time of the first convulsion. In 29.2 per cent, the physician was judged responsible for the outcome. These cases were the ones in which there had been neglect or carelessness in handling the early stages of the toxaemia or improper institution of operative procedures. The repeated use of the caesarean operation as the method of treatment in the convulsive stages of toxaemia has also influenced the result. In 1.8 per cent of these preventable cases, the responsibility has been assigned to the midwife. This is due, in large measure, to the midwife's neglect in sending the patient to a physician when the progress of the pregnancy was not entirely normal.

Those deaths ascribed to phlegmasia alba dolens and embolism were found to be preventable in 8 of the 89 cases (9.0 per cent). The physician was held responsible for 5 of these 8 deaths and the patient for the other 3. That any of these should have been regarded as preventable is due to the consideration that the physician neglected to safeguard the patient with phlegmasia alba dolens by prolonging the period of inactivity, or that the patient disregarded the physician's advice under similar circumstances.

Accidents of labor, embracing as they do all the types of operative shock, ruptured uterus, severe traumata to the birth canal, which result in death very soon after delivery, are almost all preventable—87.1 per cent being so classified, with the physician considered responsible in 89.9 per cent, the patient in 7.4 per cent, and the midwife in 2.7 per cent of the preventable cases. Many of these cases represent instances of incompetence: repeated futile operative attempts; gross mishandling of delivery; inability to perform the operations without the infliction of severe and dangerous trauma to the birth canal; failure to recognize manifest obstructions; and allowing labor to continue until the patient's condition was so critical that any operative procedure would tax her strength beyond its limit.

In the cases where death was due to extra-puerperal causes, 34.0 per cent were classed as preventable, the responsibility being nearly equally divided between the physician and the patient. Many of the patients had cardiac disease. The improper management of pregnancy and failure of the patient to accord proper cooperation to her attendant account for the great proportion of these deaths.

In Table 6 we show the preventable deaths for which the physician was responsible divided into those which, in the

TABLE 6

ANALYSIS OF PREVENTABLE DEATHS FOR WHICH RESPONSIBILITY WAS ASCRIBED TO PHYSICIAN

(*Exclusive of deaths following abortion*)

CAUSE OF DEATH	TOTAL		ERROR OF JUDGMENT		ERROR IN TECHNIQUE	
	Number	Per cent	Number	Per cent	Number	Per cent
Total	751	*100*	369	*49.1*	382	*50.9*
Ectopic gestation	73	*100*	37	*50.7*	36	*49.3*
Hemorrhage	115	*100*	72	*62.6*	43	*37.4*
Puerperal septicaemia	313	*100*	108	*34.5*	205	*65.5*
Albuminuria and eclampsia	49	*100*	49	*100.0*	—	—
Pernicious vomiting	2	*100*	2	*100.0*	—	—
Phlegmasia alba dolens and embolus	5	*100*	2	*40.0*	3	*60.0*
Accidents of labor	134	*100*	58	*43.3*	76	*56.7*
Extra-puerperal causes	60	*100*	41	*68.3*	19	*31.7*

opinion of the Advisory Committee, were due to error in judgment and those due to error in technique. Faulty judgment included all those cases where the attendant had failed properly to evaluate abnormalities of pregnancy, and had thus allowed a situation, which in its early stages was susceptible of correction, to develop to a point where treatment was useless; where there was an error in the choice of operation, such as the use of the caesarean operation in the convulsive stages of a pregnancy toxaemia; or where the operation was performed at a time which rendered it hazardous. Faulty technique is self-descriptive and includes those instances where, in light of the facts which were revealed by the investigation, it was evident that the attendant was really incompetent to perform the procedure which was required.

The figures for the total number of cases where the responsibility was ascribed to the physician show an almost equal division between faults of judgment and faults of technique, 49.1 per cent and 50.9 per cent respectively. This appears to reveal a surprisingly high degree of actual technical incompetence. These cases show a tendency on the part of the attendants to underrate the seriousness of obstetrical operations. The Advisory Committee is of the opinion that the obstetrical operative procedures are not to be undertaken unless the attendant is unquestionably competent, since many of them require a high degree of skill. They are of the opinion that this lack of respect for operative undertakings is a grave source of danger to the patient.

When the total series is similarly divided for each cause of death, the components reveal how the two errors are distributed. In cases of ectopic gestation, judgment and technique are of equal importance. There must be accurate and prompt diagnosis and proper decision as to the time to operate, but a poorly performed operation will immediately negate the benefits of proper judgment. Of the preventable cases, 50.7 per cent showed an error in judgment on the part of the attendant evidenced by failure to make the diagnosis, undue delay in operating, or failure to fortify the patient properly for operation. In 49.3 per cent of the cases, there was fault in the technique of the operation as revealed by the development of either peritonitis or secondary hemorrhage.

In the deaths from hemorrhage, 62.6 per cent were found to be due to improper judgment, including a tendency to neglect warning hemorrhage and a failure to provide for prompt transfusion to combat the acute anaemia. The remaining 37.4 per cent were thought to show an error in technique, many in unsuccessful tamponade or failure to perform a version which would have controlled the bleeding.

When the group of deaths ascribed to septicaemia was examined, the opposite distribution was found. Only 34.5 per cent revealed the error to have been one of judgment, while 65.5 per cent showed errors of technique. In the cases where the error was one of judgment, it was most often the performance of an operation on a potentially infected patient, such as a classical type of caesarean section on a patient who had been long in labor with membranes ruptured for a prolonged period. The errors in technique were those in which the attendant or his assistant may justly be presumed to have been the source of an infection. Operative procedures followed by septicaemia were presumably not performed properly as to asepsis or the avoidance of trauma.

The deaths from albuminuria and eclampsia were due in all cases where the physician was thought responsible to errors in judgment. Clinic patients were often not properly advised or followed up to insure cooperation with the physician in charge of the case; there was a definitely discernible laxity in the intensive treatment of the early stages of the toxaemias, which allowed the impending disaster to occur. The same observations are true of the cases of pernicious vomiting, of which Table 6 shows the 2 who died without being aborted.

The 5 preventable deaths from emboli and similar accidents were divided into 2 due to error of judgment and 3 due to error in technique, but the figures are too small to be of any significance.

The accidents of labor for which the physician was held responsible show a preponderance of errors of technique. This is what prior judgments would lead one to expect. The large figure for errors of judgment (43.3 per cent) resulted from those cases where a faulty prognosis of delivery resulted in allowing the patient to exhaust herself, where the choice of operative procedure was wrong, and, in some instances, where the time for the performance of the operation was improper.

In the group of cases where death was due to causes other than puerperal, the preponderant errors were those of judgment. Many of the deaths were due to cardiac disease, and the series shows a definite failure to evaluate properly the relation of cardiac insufficiency to the strains of pregnancy and labor. This group also includes deaths directly due to the anaesthetic, which had been often incorrectly chosen for the type of procedure to be followed.

A similar analysis has been made of those cases in which the responsibility was ascribed to the patient. The results appear in Table 7. These cases were of two types: those in which there was a failure on the part of the patient to obtain any care, including failure to seek prenatal care or failure to call an attendant in the event of abnormal symptoms or disturbance of pregnancy; and failure to cooperate with the attendant who had been selected.

The whole series shows a predominance of the cases in which the patient did not seek care—59.2 per cent. This series

TABLE 7

ANALYSIS OF PREVENTABLE DEATHS FOR WHICH RESPONSIBILITY WAS ASCRIBED TO PATIENT

(Exclusive of deaths following abortion)

CAUSE OF DEATH	TOTAL		FAILURE TO OBTAIN SUITABLE CARE		LACK OF CO-OPERATION	
	Number	Per cent	Number	Per cent	Number	Per cent
Total	292	100	173	59.2	119	40.8
Ectopic gestation	16	100	12	75.0	4	25.0
Hemorrhage	27	100	18	66.7	9	33.3
Puerperal septicaemia	56	100	18	32.1	38	67.9
Albuminuria and eclampsia	116	100	81	69.8	35	30.2
Pernicious vomiting	6	100	4	66.7	2	33.3
Phlegmasia alba dolens and embolus	3	100	1	33.3	2	66.7
Accidents of labor	11	100	3	27.3	8	72.7
Extra-puerperal causes	57	100	36	63.2	21	36.8

of cases would indicate that there is still a great tendency to omit prenatal care. Careful, persistent education is required to produce in the less educated and less fortunate women of the city an attitude which will make prenatal care an accepted necessity. It seems that the large amount of propaganda and effort already put forth has failed to produce the desired results. Too often the woman goes to the clinic only to register for delivery and then fails to return regularly. The 40.8 per cent of the cases ascribed to lack of cooperation on the part of the patient include many cases of this type. One visit to the clinic, and then no further contact until labor sets in or there is some symptom so alarming that it cannot be disregarded is, far too often, the rule in these cases.

The 16 cases of death from ectopic gestation were divided into 12 which showed a failure to seek care and only 4 where the patient had refused to cooperate with the attendant. There is apparent a definite lack of knowledge of the symptoms of ectopic gestation—indeed very often the patient is unaware of her pregnancy. Some further instruction of women in the warnings which indicate a possible ectopic gestation is undoubtedly needed.

Of the cases of hemorrhage deaths in which the responsibility was ascribed to the patient, 66.7 per cent were due to the patient's failure to obtain care. In numerous instances the patient sought no attendant until an exsanguinating hemorrhage followed intermittent smaller hemorrhages. In only 33.3 per cent did she fail to follow the attendant's advice.

Most of the deaths from septicaemia, on the other hand, were laid to the patient's neglect. Here 67.9 per cent were ascribed to the neglect by the patient of the instructions of the physician or to her refusal to enter a hospital when the attendant felt that it was necessary. In the remaining 32.1 per cent, the patient failed to summon an attendant. Many of these were precipitate deliveries because the patient did not call the attendant or go to the hospital early in labor.

The toxaemias show a reversal of this distribution; 69.8 per cent of the patients neglected to seek any care at all, even in the face of unmistakable symptoms of dangerous disturbance. The large number of women who allowed total blindness or convulsive seizures to supervene before seeking medical care was astounding. The other 30.2 per cent refused to follow the regime established for them, failed to return as they were instructed to do, or refused to enter the hospital when advised to.

The pernicious vomiting deaths reveal the same state of affairs. The women were prone to regard the vomiting as a normal accompaniment of pregnancy and failed to obtain care in 4 of the 6 cases. The figures are small and are therefore unsafe as a basis for broad conclusions.

The 3 deaths from embolism or phlegmasia alba dolens, where the patient was judged responsible, are not significant.

The preponderance of responsibility rests upon the attendant in the deaths from accidents of labor. In 11 instances, however, the patient was judged responsible, 3 of these being due to her failure to obtain care and 8 to her lack of cooperation. Some of the patients refused to enter a hospital where difficult operative procedures could have been performed more expeditiously.

Among the deaths from extra-puerperal causes, 63.2 per cent of those ascribed to the patient were due to a failure to obtain care. Neglect of cardiac disease and other constitutional disturbances figure prominently in this group. The remaining 36.8 per cent refused to cooperate in the regime the attendant prescribed.

Table 8 shows the distribution of the cases in which the midwife was judged responsible, by errors of judgment and of technique.

Ten of the 14 cases of septicaemia were allocated to errors in technique. The decision in these cases was made on a different basis than in the cases attended by a physician. In cases

TABLE 8

ANALYSIS OF PREVENTABLE DEATHS FOR WHICH
RESPONSIBILITY WAS ASCRIBED TO MIDWIFE

CAUSE OF DEATH	TOTAL		ERROR OF JUDGMENT		ERROR IN TECHNIQUE	
	Number	Per cent	Number	Per cent	Number	Per cent
Total	30	*100*	19	*63.3*	11	*36.7*
Abortion	1	*100*	—	—	1	*100.0*
Hemorrhage	8	*100*	8	*100.0*	—	—
Puerperal septicaemia	14	*100*	4	*28.6*	10	*71.4*
Albuminuria and eclampsia	3	*100*	3	*100.0*	—	—
Accidents of labor	4	*100*	4	*100.0*	—	—

where the physician was held responsible, if the delivery was entirely spontaneous and if there was no trauma, the general rule was to consider the death not preventable. In the case of the midwives, the evaluation of each midwife entered into the formation of the judgment, and when there was doubt as to her competence, the case was classified as preventable.

The deaths from hemorrhage, albuminuria and eclampsia, and accidents of labor were due to the failure of the midwife to recognize the gravity of the situation with which she was confronted and to obtain the immediate assistance which might have averted the outcome.

The preventable deaths from abortions have been analyzed in the same manner, dividing them into two groups according to responsibility. We have divided them into the therapeutic abortions and all others. Table 9 gives the results of the analysis of the group of abortion deaths in which the physician was thought to be responsible, by error of judgment and error of technique. The figures are small and not to be used as a basis for valid conclusions. Most of the failures have seemed to be those of judgment, 71.4 per cent in the cases of

TABLE 9

ANALYSIS OF PREVENTABLE DEATHS FOLLOWING ABORTION, FOR WHICH RESPONSIBILITY WAS ASCRIBED TO PHYSICIAN

(*Exclusive of deaths following therapeutic abortion*)

CAUSE OF DEATH	TOTAL		ERROR OF JUDGMENT		ERROR IN TECHNIQUE	
	Num-ber	Per cent	Num-ber	Per cent	Num-ber	Per cent
Total	41	100	27	65.9	14	34.1
Hemorrhage	7	100	5	71.4	2	28.6
Puerperal septicaemia	32	100	20	62.5	12	37.5
Albuminuria and eclampsia	2	100	2	100.0	—	—

hemorrhage, 62.5 per cent in those of septicaemia, and 100 per cent in the toxaemia cases. The tendency to disregard hemorrhage until it becomes alarming, the performance of curettage on seriously infected patients, and the failure to use proper and intensive treatment for the toxaemias resulted in this large percentage.

The therapeutic abortions, as shown in Table 10, show a slight preponderance of those cases in which the technique was faulty, 53.6 per cent.

Three of the 4 deaths from hemorrhage were due to faulty judgment, while one arose out of failure in the technique of performing the measures directed toward the control of the hemorrhage.

Twelve of the 13 deaths from septicaemia following a therapeutic curettage were felt to be due to faulty technique. The operation was one of choice in which antecedent infection could not be shown to have existed and the presumption must be that there was infection introduced at the time of operation.

TABLE 10

ANALYSIS OF PREVENTABLE DEATHS FOLLOWING THERAPEUTIC ABORTION, FOR WHICH RESPONSIBILITY WAS ASCRIBED TO PHYSICIAN

CAUSE OF DEATH	TOTAL		ERROR OF JUDGMENT		ERROR IN TECHNIQUE	
	Num- ber	Per cent	Num- ber	Per cent	Num- ber	Per cent
Total	28	100	13	46.4	15	53.6
Hemorrhage	4	100	3	75.0	1	25.0
Puerperal septicaemia	13	100	1	7.7	12	92.3
Albuminuria and eclampsia	2	100	2	100.0	—	—
Pernicious vomiting	5	100	5	100.0	—	—
Accidents of labor	1	100	—	—	1	100.0
Extra-puerperal causes	3	100	2	66.7	1	33.3

Both deaths recorded in this group due to albuminuria and eclampsia as well as the 5 due to pernicious vomiting were judged to be the result of improper judgment. The operations were frequently postponed until the damage had become irreparable and the fatal outcome unavoidable.

The 3 deaths brought about by causes other than strictly puerperal ones included 2 due to faulty judgment and one due to improper technique. There was an inclination to delay operation too long and so pass that point in the progress of the disease when the patient could derive any benefit from emptying the uterus.

When we examine those preventable deaths from abortion which were judged to be the responsibility of the patient, we have divided them into two categories: the induced and the spontaneous. (See Table 11.) Many of those said to be spontaneous were, in the opinion of the investigators, indubitably induced, but the difficulty of getting accurate data about the entire group of abortions, except those which were therapeu-

TABLE 11

ANALYSIS OF PREVENTABLE DEATHS FOLLOWING
ABORTION, FOR WHICH RESPONSIBILITY WAS
ASCRIBED TO PATIENT

(*Exclusive of deaths following therapeutic abortion*)

CAUSE OF DEATH	TOTAL		SPONTANEOUS ABORTION				INDUCED ABORTION	
			LACK OF CARE		LACK OF CO-OPERATION			
	Number	Per cent	Number	Per cent	Number	Per cent	Number	Per cent
Total	197	100	81	41.1	9	4.6	107	54.3
Hemorrhage	9	100	7	77.8	—	—	2	22.2
Puerperal septicaemia	181	100	72	39.8	5	2.8	104	57.4
Albuminuria and eclampsia	1	100	1	100.0	—	—	—	—
Pernicious vomiting	2	100	1	50.0	1	50.0	—	—
Extra-puerperal causes	4	100	—	—	3	75.0	1	25.0

TABLE 12

ANALYSIS OF PREVENTABLE DEATHS FOLLOWING
THERAPEUTIC ABORTION, FOR WHICH RESPONSIBILITY
WAS ASCRIBED TO PATIENT

CAUSE OF DEATH	TOTAL		FAILURE TO OBTAIN SUITABLE CARE		LACK OF CO-OPERATION	
	Number	Per cent	Number	Per cent	Number	Per cent
Total	4	*100*	2	*50.0*	2	*50.0*
Hemorrhage	2	*100*	1	*50.0*	1	*50.0*
Puerperal septicaemia	1	*100*	—	—	1	*100.0*
Albuminuria and eclampsia	1	*100*	1	*100.0*	—	—

tic, is so great that we cannot feel that the findings based on the figures are reliable.

Among the deaths following abortions, 41.1 per cent were considered preventable because of failure of the patient to obtain care. In many of these cases the woman would entirely disregard an early miscarriage, presumably because she felt it was of minor importance. Many were incomplete and the patient only sought medical care because of the persistent vaginal bleeding or the beginning of septicaemia. Four and six-tenths per cent of these cases were due to a lack of cooperation on the part of the patient in following the advice of the attendant, and 54.3 per cent were known to be induced.

The most frequent cause of death in this group of cases was septicaemia (91.9 per cent). The patient failed to seek any care in 39.8 per cent and either induced the abortion herself or had it induced in 57.4 per cent of the cases.

The 4 cases in which the patient was held responsible for death following a therapeutic abortion are included merely to show the distribution and not with the idea that any justifiable conclusions arise out of them. (Table 12.)

The immediately striking element in the foregoing analysis is, of course, the enormously high proportion of the deaths which were thought to be avoidable. Any group of deaths in which two-thirds of the total could have been prevented becomes immediately a most pressing problem. The Advisory Committee always asked this question: If this patient had had the advantage of the best possible attention and care, would this death have occurred? Where the answer to the question was in the negative, they classified that death as preventable. It is realized that such a procedure is based on the assumption that there is a responsibility to see that every woman has such care and the Committee affirm their conviction that such a responsibility does exist. It lies with the medical profession as a whole, it lies with the individual members of that profession, it lies with society as it is represented in the numerous organizations for the improvement of the health conditions of that part of the social body which is forced into a greater or less degree of dependence on the public health facilities, and it lies finally with the woman herself. She will ultimately demand what she is trained or educated to recognize as the proper and minimum attendance and quality of care which is due. If she has no understanding of the situation, obviously she can only accept whatever type of attendance is available and within her capacity to pay for. She will be guided by one of two things—necessity to accept whatever is offered by the community to which she must look for care, or the habitudes and demands of her social group if she has the ability to make a choice. Under the first of these alternatives, society must assume the double responsibility of training the woman to avail herself to the full of the facilities which are provided, and of making those facilities measure up to the highest possible standards. Under the second, the responsibility is one of educating women to know what should be demanded and to refuse to accept less than that minimum. These two elements—education of the lay public to an understanding of what constitutes proper medical care and provision of that standard of medical attendance—are closely interdependent. It is futile to educate the public to recognize and demand certain minimum standards if the medical profession fails to make these standards available. Any such practice results in disregard of subsequent efforts at education and tends to undermine the confidence of the lay public in the medical profession. It is equally ineffective to provide care of the highest possible standards if the public does not understand the need to avail itself of such care. It is evident from the data in the previous paragraphs that there has been failure both in education and in provision of adequate professional service.

Sixty per cent of all the deaths which could have been avoided have been brought about by some incapacity in the attendant: lack of judgment, lack of skill, or careless inattention to the demands of the case. Some of these situations have arisen out of the fact that internes have been given too wide a field of independent activity. Most are plainly the results of incompetence. Prevention in this field will mean increasing the respect of the physician for the gravity of obstetrical operations and educating him to a greater caution in attacking problems which are properly the field only of the highly trained obstetrician.

More than a third of all preventable deaths were due to some failure on the part of the patient herself to take advantage of those facilities which are at hand for safeguarding her in the period of gestation and lying-in. This element in the situation is one of education entirely. For many women pregnancy is of such frequent occurrence that they cannot regard it as a condition meriting any special consideration. One uncomplicated delivery may lead a woman falsely to suppose that subsequent pregnancies are without hazards instead of being, perhaps, potentially more hazardous. She is unaware of the grave possibilities which arise with pregnancy, and the pressure of maintaining the home at its usual level is so great that her problems are prone to be disregarded. Education to instil the knowledge that with proper care during pregnancy and labor much of the discomfort and many, if not most, of the dangers of childbearing can be removed, has quite simply failed to reach these women. It must be constantly renewed and persistently maintained to have its full effect in altering the present situation. Furthermore, mere education to obtain care will not suffice. The lay public must know what constitutes proper care so that there may be discrimination in the choice of attendants. Those doctors who do not qualify will automatically be forced to meet the demands of an educated lay opinion.

This education is the field of the medical profession. From them has come the impetus leading to the prevention of all the conditions which, through prophylaxis, have been brought under control. Prevention of these deaths is possible, and the challenge of the situation must be accepted. In the detailed discussions which follow, we shall point out where, according to the data accumulated, the points of weakness lie and how there may be brought about the alterations which are imperative if the deaths of women which can be avoided are to be avoided.

IV

PUERPERAL AND EXTRA-PUERPERAL CAUSES OF DEATH

IN this chapter we shall discuss separately and in detail the data concerning each puerperal cause of death as well as those deaths from extra-puerperal causes. It will be seen that the entire series of 2,041 deaths has been divided into three groups. The first includes those following abortion; the second, those following extra-uterine pregnancy. The third group is composed as follows:

Deaths at 28 weeks of gestation or later, delivered

Deaths at 28 weeks of gestation or later, undelivered

Deaths at less than 28 weeks of gestation, undelivered.

Tables are based, for the most part, either on the total of 2,041 cases or on the third group, which numbers 1,564. Table 13 gives the distribution of the entire series by cause.

TABLE 13

DISTRIBUTION OF DEATHS BY CAUSE

CAUSE OF DEATH	NUMBER	PER CENT
Total	2,041	100.0
Septic abortion	262	12.8
Abortion	95	4.7
Ectopic gestation	120	5.9
Hemorrhage	197	9.7
Puerperal septicaemia	510	25.0
Albuminuria and eclampsia	231	11.3
Pernicious vomiting	14	.7
Phlegmasia alba dolens and embolus	89	4.4
Accidents of labor	171	8.4
Accidents of puerperium	8	.4
Extra-puerperal causes	344	16.9

ABORTION

ANY consideration of the subject of abortion is necessarily a most inaccurate and unsatisfactory one. To get information concerning any given death following an abortion is extraordinarily difficult and the value and truth of the information obtained are open to the most serious question. The difficulties surrounding the study and evaluation of abortion are, in many instances, those surrounding criminal activity. Deaths from abortion are frequently falsely reported. Many of the reports to the registrar's office, in failing to record the period of gestation, cause the death to be registered as of over 28 weeks' gestation, when further investigation has shown it to be of shorter duration. This error occurred in 33 out of the 357 cases of abortion which we studied.

Wilfully false reporting is the main source of error. The actual number of cases lies wholly in the realm of conjecture, but it is generally conceded to be of really significant proportions. Such cases, of course, do not appear in our figures, as they cannot be classified as puerperal deaths but are included in the general rates. Nor have proven criminal abortions been included in our figures. It must, however, be realized that cases where criminal intervention is evident to the degree required by law for such classification are comparatively rare; the legal requirements for such decisions are extremely stringent. If by error the death reports of cases which the registrar's office had classified as criminal abortions were sent to us, we excluded them. This decision to exclude abortions known to be illegal was based on two factors: first, this type of case is primarily a problem of social import and only secondarily a medical one; and second, the complexities surrounding these cases are of such magnitude that data concerning them would be almost entirely impossible to obtain and would be invalid if they were obtained.

But when all known illegal operations were excluded, the resulting collection of cases still remained a most confused one. There were undoubtedly among them many criminal cases, but where this had not been proved, we were forced to include them. There was no satisfactory way of determining which were induced and which were truly spontaneous. The patient almost invariably gave a history of spontaneous origin and the question resolved itself into a matter of suppositions which had no real validity in a scientific examination of the subject. A few patients gave a straightforward history of self-induction and then the problem was simplified. We based our decision on all the facts in the case. If the attendant had good reason to believe that the abortion was spontaneous, because of his knowledge of the patient and her attitudes, we have been content to regard it as such. Where there was doubt, and the indications pointed to the probability of induction, we have classed the case as an induced abortion. This was particularly true in the cases of septic abortions. It is the existing medical opinion that truly spontaneous abortions have no great hazard as far as the development of septicaemia is concerned. Therefore, those cases of septic abortion have been considered, in many instances, to be the result of induction, unless the investigation produced most convincing evidence to the contrary. As a result, the division of the cases has been arbitrary, based upon judgments, scraps of evidence of doubtful value, suppositions, and conjectures, and not upon demonstrable fact.

The material which was collected has been analyzed and studied for any possible valuable features. The therapeutic abortions, of course, were susceptible of the same investigation and analysis as the deaths from other causes. The data on these cases are entirely satisfactory.

We have divided all abortions into two groups: abortions,

TABLE 14

ABORTION DEATH RATES FOR THREE YEARS

	TOTAL DEATHS	DEATHS FOLLOW-ING ABORTION	PER CENT OF ALL DEATHS	RATE PER 1,000 LIVE BIRTHS
Total	2,041	357	*17.5*	1.0
1930	**675**	91	*13.5*	.7
1931	708	127	*17.9*	1.1
1932	658	139	*21.1*	1.3

and abortions with septicaemia. This is in accordance with the 1929 version of the *International List of Causes of Death*, where such a division is made for the first time.

During the three years of the investigation, abortions steadily increased as a cause of death, both actually and relatively, as is shown in Table 14. Abortions preceded 17.5 per cent of all puerperal deaths for the three years, but there was an increase in this percentage from 13.5 in 1930, a rate of .7 per 1,000 live births, to 21.1, a rate of 1.3, in 1932. This gives us no information regarding the actual death rate following abortions, as no figure which even remotely approaches accuracy is available for the total number of abortions occurring in the city.

The 357 deaths following abortion in the three years were classified as follows: abortion, 95, or 26.6 per cent; abortion with septicaemia, 262, or 73.4 per cent. A further analysis of the type of abortion is shown in Table 15. The large percentage of cases with septicaemia among the spontaneous group (69.8) casts considerable doubt upon the accuracy of this grouping. In the group of 95 who died of non-septic abortion only 3 cases were thought to be illegally induced, a fact which emphasizes the almost universal role of sepsis as the cause of death in the illegally produced abortion.

The causes of death among the 95 cases of non-septic abor-

TABLE 15

ABORTION DEATHS BY TYPE OF ABORTION

	TOTAL ABORTION DEATHS		WITHOUT SEPTICAEMIA		WITH SEPTICAEMIA	
	Number	Per cent	Number	Per cent	Number	Per cent
Total	357	100	95	26.6	262	73.4
Spontaneous	192	100	58	30.2	134	69.8
Induced	108	100	3	2.8	105	97.2
Therapeutic	47	100	32	68.1	15	31.9
Type not reported	10	100	2	20.0	8	80.0

tion were as follows: pernicious vomiting, 14; hemorrhage, 27; shock, 2; embolic processes, 3; pregnancy toxaemias, 9; extra-puerperal causes, 39. In one case the cause of death could not be determined. The bulk of the deaths resulted from hemorrhage and causes outside of the puerperal state. This is due largely to the tendency of abortion to occur in the course of constitutional disease. In this series, the occurrence of serious respiratory diseases in almost epidemic proportions several times during the period of study brought a concomitant increase in the number of early abortions.

The preventability of the deaths in the abortion group is high—271 out of the total 357 cases being judged preventable. (See Table 5A, page 32.) Eight of the 14 deaths from pernicious vomiting might have been avoided if the patient had realized the gravity of the symptoms and the attendant had undertaken a therapeutic interruption before serious damage had been done. Twenty-two of the 27 deaths from hemorrhage could have been prevented. The patients usually failed to seek a medical attendant until the condition was hopeless. Of 262 deaths from septicaemia, 226 were the result of factors which could have been controlled. This figure probably represents induced abortions. Only 9 of a total of 39 deaths from extra-puerperal causes were preventable. This relatively small ratio is due to the fact that in a large proportion of these cases the abortions were inevitable accompaniments of serious intercurrent illness, which in turn was the real cause of death.

Among the cases dying after the performance of a therapeutic abortion, the most important cause of death was, again, septicaemia. Fifteen of the 47 deaths were from this cause, and of the 15, 13 were considered preventable, the critical factor usually being the infection introduced at the time dilatation and curettage were performed. Hemorrhage caused 6 of the deaths, all of them being preventable. Of the 10 deaths from pernicious vomiting, 5 were preventable. In these instances, the operation was usually undertaken too late to be of value. Toxaemia of the albuminuric type caused 4 deaths, of which 2 were preventable. Extra-puerperal causes accounted for 8 out of the total of 47. Three of these were due to cardiac disease and one to tuberculosis. The causes of death were, in these cases, the indications for which the therapeutic abortion was undertaken, but the disease had progressed beyond the stage where the interruption of pregnancy could be of any benefit. In all, 32 out of the 47 deaths following therapeutic abortion were preventable. There was a tendency to postpone the operation until the patient's condition was beyond the hope of improvement.

The deaths following abortion represented 15.5 per cent of all the deaths among the women legitimately pregnant and 44.9 per cent of the deaths among those illegitimately pregnant. This is a reliable figure, since it is based not on the report on the death certificate but on information obtained by investigations. A figure derived from the death certificates would be smaller than the actual total, since the attendant frequently falsified this item under pressure from the family.

TABLE 16

ABORTION DEATHS BY AGE

	ALL DEATHS	ABORTION DEATHS	
		Number	Per cent of all deaths
Total	2,041	357	*17.5*
15 to 19 years	108	20	*18.5*
20 to 24 years	429	85	*19.8*
25 to 29 years	559	96	*17.2*
30 to 34 years	449	64	*14.3*
35 to 39 years	358	73	*20.4*
40 years and over	138	19	*13.8*

The truth, however, was easily brought out in personal conversations with him.

Deaths following abortion among Negroes were 23.1 per cent of the total puerperal deaths in that race, while among the white population they constituted 16.7 per cent. Only a slight difference appeared between native and foreign-born women, the deaths following abortions being 18.8 per cent and 15.7 per cent of the respective totals.

The distribution of these deaths according to age groups and gravidity offers some interesting features. It might be expected that the largest percentage of deaths following abortion would be among the primigravidae and in the lowest age groups, but this is not the case, as is shown in Tables 16 and 17. The age group having the highest proportion of deaths due to the effects of abortion was thirty-five to thirty-nine years, with 73 deaths, or 20.4 per cent of all deaths in this age group; the age group twenty to twenty-four years was next highest, with 85 deaths, or 19.8 per cent.

Table 17 shows the distribution by gravidity of deaths following abortion. The highest ratio of abortion deaths to all

TABLE 17

ABORTION DEATHS BY GRAVIDITY

	ALL DEATHS	ABORTION DEATHS	
		Number	Per cent of all deaths
Total	2,041	357	*17.5*
Primigravidae	867	134	*15.5*
Gravidae II	351	47	*13.4*
Gravidae III	236	33	*14.0*
Gravidae IV	176	37	*21.0*
Gravidae V	115	22	*19.1*
Gravidae VI	64	15	*23.4*
Gravidae VII	51	15	*29.4*
Gravidae VIII and over	127	20	*15.8*
Multigravidity not reported	16	8	*50.0*
Gravidity not reported	38	26	*68.4*

deaths was found in gravida six, 23.4 per cent, and gravida seven, 29.4 per cent; the lowest was found in gravida two, 13.4. Of all deaths among primigravidae, 15.5 per cent followed abortion, and among multigravidae, 17.3.

The problem of abortion is largely a social one. But since it is the cause of 17.5 per cent of all the deaths arising from the childbearing function, it has an important medical aspect. An extensive study of the entire problem from the social as well as the medical point of view would be desirable.

ECTOPIC GESTATION

AN analysis of the deaths from ectopic gestation cannot yield data of great significance because we do not have figures to show the death rate for this condition. The symptoms of ectopic gestation frequently lead to a diagnosis of a surgical abdomen, and the surgeon sees these cases more often than does the obstetrician or gynecologist. It is not a reportable disease, and our survey of the hospitals did not give us any figures on its incidence. Nevertheless the large number of deaths from this cause, 120, which was 5.9 per cent of the total deaths in the entire series, warrants a detailed examination of the cases. The Committee feels that in view of the large number of deaths from this cause, an exhaustive study of the whole subject would prove extremely valuable.

Of the total number of deaths from ectopic gestation, 29, or 24.1 per cent, died without operation. In many instances the true condition was not recognized; some of the patients were received in such critical condition that an operation was contra-indicated; and in some cases religious regulations prevented operation. A few of the cases were treated as threatened abortions, and in 11 cases a dilatation and curettage was performed for what was diagnosed as incomplete abortion. Fifteen of the cases had operative procedures performed because of faulty diagnosis.

Hemorrhage and shock were the chief actual causes of death, accounting for 63 of the 120 cases; in an additional 9 cases, secondary hemorrhage caused the death, bringing deaths from hemorrhage and shock up to 72, or 60 per cent of the total.

The causes of death in this group are as follows:

	Number	Per cent
Embolism	3	2.5
Hemorrhage and shock	63	52.5
Secondary hemorrhage	9	7.5
Septicaemia	35	29.2
Extra-puerperal causes: total	10	8.3
Pneumonia	4	3.3
Nephritis	1	.8
Ileus	3	2.5
Anaesthesia	1	.8
Accidental poisoning	1	.8

TABLE 18

DEATHS FOLLOWING ECTOPIC GESTATION, BY AGE

	ALL DEATHS	ECTOPIC GESTATION DEATHS		
		Number	Per cent of all deaths	Per cent distribution by age
Total	2,041	120	5.9	100.0
15 to 19 years	108	1	1.1	.8
20 to 24 years	429	20	6.2	16.7
25 to 29 years	559	31	7.2	25.8
30 to 34 years	449	34	9.7	28.3
35 to 39 years	358	26	10.0	21.7
40 years and over	138	8	7.2	6.7

The age distribution of the cases is shown in Table 18.

There was very little difference between multigravidae and primigravidae. The 51 deaths occurring in first pregnancies were 42.5 per cent of the deaths following ectopic gestation and 6.0 per cent of all the deaths among primigravidae. The 65 deaths of multigravidae were 54.2 per cent of the total for this cause and 5.7 per cent of all deaths of multigravidae.

One hundred and four of the 120 cases were legitimate pregnancies and 16 were illegitimate. Ninety-seven of the patients were white—5.4 per cent of all deaths among white women—and 23 were Negro—7.2 per cent of all deaths among Negro women. Seventy-four, 61.6 per cent of all deaths from ectopic gestation, occurred in native-born women, while 46, or 38.3 per cent, occurred in foreign-born. This represents 6.3 per cent of all deaths among native-born women and 5.3 per cent of all foreign-born.

Of the 120 women, 91 were operated upon. Of these 91, the greater proportion (79.1 per cent) had had symptoms of more than a week's duration before the operation was undertaken; 26 (28.5 per cent) for one to two weeks, 6 (6.5 per cent) from two to three weeks, and 30 (33.0 per cent) for over three weeks. The delay was due to faulty diagnosis on the part of the attendant, or to ignorance on the part of the patient. These elements in the picture seem most significant in accounting for the deaths.

The time of post-operative death is significant:

	Number	Per cent
Within 24 hours	36	39.5
2nd day	9	9.8
3rd day	7	7.7
4th day	10	10.9
5th day	2	2.2
Over 5 days	27	29.6

More than 70 per cent died within five days of operation, which indicates a very high percentage of women coming to operation in such critical condition that the shock incident to operation was too great for their reduced recuperative powers. Frequently there was failure to safeguard and fortify the patient by prior or simultaneous transfusion.

The group which survived operative procedure by more than five days died as a rule from peritonitis and septicaemia following operation. The supposition in these cases was always that the infection was introduced at operation and the patient's depleted condition was favorable to the development of an infection of such overwhelming proportions that she was unable to cope with it.

The initial symptom in 59 of the 120 cases was vaginal bleeding, but 53 had no vaginal hemorrhage at any time.

Eighty-nine of the deaths (74.2 per cent) were judged preventable, and 31 (25.8 per cent) not preventable. In 73 of the 89, or 82.0 per cent, the responsibility was ascribed to the attendant. The 16 deaths for which the patient was thought responsible were due to her failure to seek proper medical advice at the onset of abnormal symptoms and in a few instances her refusal to cooperate with the physician.

It is evident from these findings that a large number of patients are not receiving competent care. Better knowledge and accuracy in diagnosis, with increased appreciation of the necessity for transfusion as a vital accessory to the operative treatment of ectopic gestation, should serve to diminish appreciably the deaths from this cause. With this should go proper instruction of the woman in the possible gravity of symptoms which at first may seem mild in character.

HEMORRHAGE

THIS section is confined to the consideration of the deaths from hemorrhage and its immediate results, omitting those cases, already discussed, in which death was due to abortion or ectopic gestation.

In 125 cases which are also omitted from further discussion, hemorrhage was considered a contributory cause of death, distributed as follows: accidental or postpartum hemorrhage, 64 (51.2 per cent); abruptio placentae, 21 (16.8 per cent); placenta praevia, 40 (32.0 per cent). Cases in this group were classified under the following causes of death: operative shock, 51; septicaemia, 39; albuminuria and eclampsia, 14; embolism, 7; puerperal psychosis, 1; extrapuerperal causes, 13. The decision as to which factor was more important, the operation or the hemorrhage, was a most difficult one to make. While there was an effort to classify as deaths from hemorrhage all cases where the loss of blood was sufficient to cause death, it is quite possible that, in some instances, a different decision could have had an equal claim to validity.

Postpartum Hemorrhage

Postpartum hemorrhage was the direct cause of 117 of the deaths due to hemorrhage. These included bleeding associated with retention of the placenta and that due to the failure of the uterus properly to contract after the expulsion of the foetus and placenta.

TABLE 19

POSTPARTUM HEMORRHAGE DEATHS BY AGE

	TOTAL	15 TO 19 YEARS	20 TO 24 YEARS	25 TO 29 YEARS	30 TO 34 YEARS	35 TO 39 YEARS	40 YEARS AND OVER
Total deaths*	1,564	87	324	432	351	259	111
Postpartum hemorrhage deaths	117	5	21	28	27	29	7
Per cent of total	*7.5*	*5.7*	*6.5*	*6.5*	*7.7*	*11.2*	*6.3*

*Exclusive of deaths following abortion and ectopic gestation.

Table 19 shows the distribution of these cases according to age. These deaths show a marked tendency to increase with age—from 5 cases in the youngest group to 29 cases in the group from 35 to 39 years old, this representing 11.2 per cent of all the deaths in that group. The figures grouped for the two important decades show 49 cases (6.5 per cent of the deaths in this decade) in the third decade, and 56 cases (9.2 per cent) in the fourth to be due to postpartum hemorrhage. Gravidity, as shown in Table 20, is not so striking a factor. The 46 deaths of primigravidae are 6.7 per cent of all the fatalities occurring with the first pregnancy and the 71 of multigravidae represent 8.1 per cent for that group. While the increasing incidence with age is striking, that with gravidity is less so but still significant.

Among the 117 cases, 93 were preventable. In 79 of these the responsibility was ascribed to the attendant, the treatment in all of these being judged deficient. Only 11 in this group were given transfusions. In 16 tamponade of the uterus was

TABLE 20

POSTPARTUM HEMORRHAGE DEATHS BY GRAVIDITY

	TOTAL	PRIMI-GRAVIDAE	MULTI-GRAVIDAE	GRAVIDITY NOT REPORTED
Total deaths*	1,564	682	874	8
Postpartum hemorrhage deaths	117	46	71	—
Per cent of total	7.5	6.7	8.1	—

*Exclusive of deaths following abortion and ectopic gestation.

done but the blood loss was not replaced by transfusion. In 29, not even tamponade was resorted to, and in the remaining 23 cases details of treatment are not known. It is useless to arrest hemorrhage if the patient is so exsanguinated that she succumbs to acute anaemia. The omission of tamponade may be a most serious one in the treatment of this type of case. It appeared from some of the case histories that transfusion was not considered except as a final measure of desperation, and death frequently occurred before the arrival of a blood donor.

Placenta Praevia

There were 49 deaths from hemorrhage due to placenta praevia. In 40 additional cases, it was considered contributory.

Table 21 gives the distribution according to the gravidity of the patients in whom this was the principal cause of death. Eleven were primigravidae and 38 multigravidae. It was the cause of death of 1.6 per cent of the women dying during the first pregnancy, and of 4.3 per cent of those who died as the result of subsequent pregnancies.

The age distribution of this group is given in Table 22. In the later ages, there is a pronounced increase in the percentage of deaths associated with placenta praevia. In the three lower

TABLE 21

PLACENTA PRAEVIA DEATHS BY GRAVIDITY

	TOTAL	PRIMIGRAVIDAE	MULTIGRAVIDAE	GRAVIDITY NOT REPORTED
Total deaths*	1,564	682	874	8
Placenta praevia deaths	49	11	38	—
Per cent of total	*3.1*	*1.6*	*4.3*	—

*Exclusive of deaths following abortion and ectopic gestation.

TABLE 22

PLACENTA PRAEVIA DEATHS BY AGE

	TOTAL	15 TO 19 YEARS	20 TO 24 YEARS	25 TO 29 YEARS	30 TO 34 YEARS	35 TO 39 YEARS	40 YEARS AND OVER
Total deaths*	1,564	87	324	432	351	259	111
Placenta praevia deaths	49	—	6	11	19	6	7
Per cent of total	*3.1*	—	*1.9*	*2.5*	*5.4*	*2.3*	*6.3*

*Exclusive of deaths following abortion and ectopic gestation.

TABLE 23

PLACENTA PRAEVIA DEATHS BY PERIOD OF UTEROGESTATION

	TOTAL	UNDER 28 WEEKS	28 TO 31 WEEKS	32 TO 35 WEEKS	36 TO 39 WEEKS	40 WEEKS AND OVER
Total deaths*	1,564	79	118	82	219	1,066
Placenta praevia deaths	49	1	3	6	20	19
Per cent of total	*3.1*	*1.3*	*2.5*	*7.3*	*9.1*	*1.8*

*Exclusive of deaths following abortion and ectopic gestation.

age groups placenta praevia occurred in: no cases, 6 cases (1.9 per cent), and 11 cases (2.5 per cent), respectively. There is an abrupt increase to 19 cases (5.4 per cent) in the group from 30 to 34 years, a drop to 6 cases (2.3 per cent) from 35 to 39 years, and among those over 40 years old 6.3 per cent of the deaths (7 cases) were due to placenta praevia. The increase in the number of multigravidae in the later age groups is a possible factor in this variation.

There was very little difference between the native-born women, 25 of whom had placenta praevia, and the foreign-born, among whom 24 were affected.

Only 19 cases reached full term (see Table 23). Twenty were delivered or died undelivered in the last four weeks of pregnancy, 6 in the period from thirty-two to thirty-five weeks, 3 from twenty-eight to thirty-one weeks; one died before twenty-eight weeks' gestation. There was a noticeable tendency for the patient to develop serious symptoms prior to term.

Over one-half (28) of the babies were either stillborn or never delivered (see Table 24)—a greatly increased proportion over the rate of stillbirths in the general series.

Labor was spontaneous in 24 of the 49 cases. In 10 there was no labor, some of these being delivered by caesarean operation before labor set in. In 15 cases labor was induced; by

TABLE 24

LIVE BIRTHS AND STILLBIRTHS IN CASES OF PLACENTA PRAEVIA

	TOTAL	BORN ALIVE	STILLBORN	NOT DELIVERED
Total babies*	1,615	964	381	270
Placenta praevia	50	22	17	11
Per cent of total	*3.1*	*2.3*	*4.5*	*4.1*

*Exclusive of deaths following abortion and ectopic gestation.   Multiple births included.

bag insertion in 11 cases, vaginal tamponade in 1, manual dilatation in 2, and medication in 1 case.

Thirty-six of the 49 women gave a history of irregular vaginal bleeding at some time prior to death or labor, 9 had a definite history of no previous bleeding, and in 4 cases the record was not available on this point. In 23 of the total number, the condition was not diagnosed until the onset of labor or the fatal hemorrhage, 5 more went unrecognized until one week prior to the fatal hemorrhage or labor, while 19 of the remaining 21 were recognized more than one week before labor and 2 gave no history on this point. When it is realized that 36 of the women had symptoms which should have suggested the presence of placenta praevia, it is evident that the prenatal course of these women was improperly supervised, either through their own ignorance in disregarding what seemed to be trivial bleeding, or through the failure of the attendant to evaluate the symptoms and institute proper treatment. The frequency with which the patient was neglected, even after a really significant hemorrhage which pointed most emphatically to the existence of placenta praevia, is an indication that the gravity of the situation was only poorly grasped by the attendants.

Six of the patients were delivered spontaneously, 10 were undelivered, and 33 had operative deliveries. There were 34 operative procedures performed on these 33 women (one being a twin pregnancy) distributed as follows: 8 caesarean operations, 1 low forceps, 1 mid forceps, 2 version, 1 extraction, 20 versions and extractions, and 1 craniotomy.

Table 25 shows the relationship of preventability to the type of prenatal care. Eighteen women were properly cared for during pregnancy, and 13 of these cases were judged preventable and the responsibility ascribed to the physician. The tendency on the part of the physician to perform rapid ver-

TABLE 25

PLACENTA PRAEVIA DEATHS BY PREVENTABILITY
AND PRENATAL CARE

	TOTAL	NOT PRE-VENTABLE	PREVENTABLE			
			Total	Responsibility ascribed to		
				Physician	Patient	Mid-wife
Total placenta praevia deaths	49	9	40	31	8	1
Adequate prenatal care	18	5	13	13	—	—
Inadequate or no pre-natal care	31	4	27	18	8	1

sion and extraction in some cases and postpone urgently indicated operative procedures in other cases accounts for the apparent inconsistency here. In 31 cases prenatal care was
improper or lacking entirely, and 27 deaths were judged preventable; responsibility was ascribed to the physician in 18
cases, to the patient in 8, and to the midwife in 1.

This group of cases is significant for the light it throws
upon the handling of this condition. It is vital that the attendant inform the patient categorically that bleeding during
pregnancy is never trivial and may be and often is the warning of disaster. Furthermore, the treatment in these cases was
frequently improper. The choice of operation as well as the
time of its performance must be judicious. Rapid traumatizing delivery by the birth canal must be avoided as it increases
the hazard to the mother.

Premature Separation of the Placenta

This accident was the immediate cause of death in 31 cases.

Table 26 gives the distribution according to the gravidity
of the patients. Eleven were primigravidae and 18 multigravidae.

The variation according to the age of the patient, as shown

TABLE 26

DEATHS FOLLOWING PREMATURE SEPARATION OF THE PLACENTA, BY GRAVIDITY

	TOTAL	PRIMIGRAVIDAE	MULTIGRAVIDAE	GRAVIDITY NOT RECORDED
Total deaths*	1,564	682	874	8
Deaths following premature separation of the placenta	31	11	18	2

*Exclusive of deaths following abortion and ectopic gestation.

TABLE 27

DEATHS FOLLOWING PREMATURE SEPARATION OF THE PLACENTA, BY AGE

	TOTAL	15 TO 19 YEARS	20 TO 24 YEARS	25 TO 29 YEARS	30 TO 34 YEARS	35 TO 39 YEARS	40 YEARS AND OVER
Total deaths*	1,564	87	324	432	351	259	111
Deaths following premature separation of the placenta	31	—	4	8	8	8	3

*Exclusive of deaths following abortion and ectopic gestation.

TABLE 28

DEATHS FOLLOWING PREMATURE SEPARATION OF THE PLACENTA, BY PREVENTABILITY AND PRENATAL CARE

	TOTAL	NOT PREVENTABLE	PREVENTABLE			
			Total	Responsibility ascribed to		
				Physician	Patient	Midwife
Total deaths following premature separation of the placenta	31	13	18	6	11	1
Adequate prenatal care	10	8	2	2	—	—
Inadequate or no prenatal care	21	5	16	4	11	1

in Table 27, reflects the effect of gravidity, the later age groups showing the higher incidence. Only 4 patients of the 324 between 20 and 24 years died of this cause, and the ratio increased to 8 of the 259 women between the ages of 35 and 39 years. Ten patients had suitable care and 21 had either wholly inadequate care or none. One of the women was delivered spontaneously, 10 were not delivered, and 20 were delivered by operation, which included the following 21 procedures: caesarean section, 9; forceps of some type, 8; version, 1; and version and extraction, 3.

In Table 28, the quality of prenatal care is analyzed according to the preventability of the deaths. Eight of the 10 deaths which followed adequate prenatal care were not preventable, and the responsibility for the 2 which were preventable was ascribed to the physician, on the ground of his having conducted labor improperly. When we come to those cases without adequate prenatal care, only 5 of the 21 cases were not preventable. Four of the remaining 16 were thought to be the responsibility of the physician, 11 of the patient, and 1 of the midwife. The very frequent association of the prematurely separated placenta with pregnancy toxaemia accounts, in large measure, for this distribution. Frequently the presence of the toxaemia was not discovered, and among those women who had no care during pregnancy, the presence of the toxaemia was not known.

General Considerations

We cannot find in these data on deaths from hemorrhage any one particular defect which, if corrected, would serve to improve the situation. From the onset of pregnancy through the conduct of labor and delivery and the period immediately following the emptying of the uterus, there was repeated failure to achieve a consistently competent management. Where the hemorrhage arose without warning, following a normal pregnancy and spontaneous delivery, there was repeated failure to employ all the available procedures to control and combat it. Where the hemorrhage was quickly brought under control, there was laxity in replacing the blood loss by prompt transfusion. The number of cases in which transfusion was not undertaken until the situation was desperate in the extreme testifies to the negligence common in this regard. If transfusion had been used early its effectiveness would be increased. Among the cases where the hemorrhage resulted from a prematurely separated or abnormally situated placenta, there was, more often than not, warning of the impending danger. Neglect of these warnings on the part of the patient or her attendant repeatedly brought about a situation which could not be controlled. Hospitalization after the first hemorrhage would have allowed a proper study of the case and enabled the attendant to map out the correct line of treatment. Patients are prone to minimize a slight bleeding during pregnancy and the attendant must be vigilant to prevent such oversight. The conduct of delivery, as we have pointed out, was frequently improper. Rapid traumatizing operative delivery, such as version followed immediately by extraction—a procedure which increases the hazard to the patient—was frequently encountered in this series.

The remedy for this situation calls for improvement in all the elements of treatment. It must begin with the education of the woman regarding the seriousness of bleeding during pregnancy. Recognition and treatment of all pregnancy toxaemias should reduce the incidence of premature separation of the placenta. Delivery must be skilfully conducted, as to both the choice of type and the avoidance of trauma. There must be no delay in the use of all means for the control of the hemorrhage and for the treatment of the anaemia.

PUERPERAL SEPTICAEMIA

It has been a reproach to obstetrics that the high incidence of deaths from puerperal septicaemia has not materially lessened during the antiseptic and aseptic era, as it has in surgical practice. The reproach is only partly deserved, for the problem of preventing septic infection is a more difficult one in obstetrics than in surgery. This is due to the fact that the lower genital tract is always a potentially infected area and that the puerperal uterus always contains organisms and is a peculiarly suitable nidus for the growth of both non-pathogenic and pathogenic bacteria.

It is now a well-established fact that in the vagina and in the cervix of every pregnant woman there are organisms of various kinds. Most of these are non-pathogenic and some, such as the Doederlein bacillus, may be actually protective. In many women, however, the vagina contains organisms which, on culture, have all the characteristics of pathogens. Among the latter are non-hemolytic streptococci of different varieties, bacillus coli, and staphylococci. The hemolytic streptococcus, the organism causing one of the most virulent of puerperal infections, is seldom found in the vagina or cervix prior to labor. Most investigators have found it in not more than one per cent of patients. While all of these organisms in the vagina are identical in cultural characteristics with known pathogens, the consensus of opinion among those who have studied the subject is that, under ordinary circumstances, they are non-pathogenic for the individual. All are agreed, however, that if the resistance of the tissues is lowered by severe hemorrhage, shock, or tearing or bruising of the soft parts they may become virulent and cause severe and sometimes fatal infection.

At the end of pregnancy the uterine cavity is sterile, but in the course of labor, especially after rupture of the membranes, it begins to be invaded by organisms and by the third day of the puerperium the invasion is a heavy one. The organisms found at that time may be streptococci, hemolytic, non-hemolytic, and anaerobic; staphylococci, bacillus coli, and diphtheroids. Some of these organisms have ascended to the uterus from the vagina and cervix but some may be of extraneous origin. They cause no symptoms, are apparently non-pathogenic for the individual, but may acquire virulence under the circumstances previously mentioned.

Of late years, special attention has been directed to the anaerobic streptococci which are a frequent habitant of the vagina and cervix of the puerperal uterus, and which are usually harmless. They may, however, cause mild and sometimes severe or fatal infection if given the proper conditions, among which trauma, bruising, and devitalization of tissues seem to be the most important.

There are two ways in which the risk of infection by these various endogenous organisms can theoretically be minimized: (1) by disinfection of the vagina and cervix early in labor and throughout the course of labor as advocated by Mayes[3] who uses mercurochrome; and (2) by conducting labor in such a way that there is a minimum of hemorrhage, of shock, and of tearing and bruising of tissue. Mayes' figures show that he has diminished the morbidity incidence in those patients on whom he has used mercurochrome, but his method has not been generally accepted and it is doubtful if it would be efficacious if the second condition were not observed. Until some simple method can be devised it seems to the Committee that emphasis should be placed on the importance of the avoidance of unnecessary blood loss and trauma. Trauma, bruising, blood loss, and shock may result from a too-prolonged labor or they may be caused by inexpert or ill-advised attempts to shorten labor. The avoidance of this type of infection, therefore, depends on good obstetrical judgment and on the skilful performance of obstetrical operations when they are indicated. The Committee believes that in many of the deaths from sepsis under review these conditions have not been fulfilled.

All recent investigators and writers are agreed that in the majority of puerperal infections, especially in the fatal ones, the infecting organism has been introduced from without. In fatal cases the most frequently found organism is a hemolytic streptococcus. It is the opinion of a majority of those who have studied this organism that it is impossible to distinguish culturally or serologically between streptococci causing scarlet fever, pneumonia, mastoiditis, or puerperal sepsis. There is a seasonal incidence of hemolytic streptococcal puerperal sepsis corresponding to seasonal incidence of sore throat and other streptococcal diseases, all of them being most prevalent in the months from January to May. There is constantly increasing evidence that the streptococcus is disseminated by carriers who harbor the organism in the mouth, nose, or throat, and that they are responsible for many of the cases of puerperal infection. From the nasal and buccal cavity the organism is sprayed onto the hands of the attendants at the time of labor or in the early puerperium, and thence conveyed to the genital passage of the patient, or the transfer may be even more direct. It seems likely that this is the mode of epidemic spread in hospitals and communities. The hemolytic streptococcus does not long survive outside the body, so the transfer must be a fairly direct one from patient to attendant or from attendant to patient. In the winter months especially, many individuals are streptococcus carriers. In the Aberdeen inquiry,[1] Kinloch, Smith, and Stephen ascribed the higher incidence of hemolytic streptococcal infections among patients attended by doctors, as contrasted with those attended by midwives, to the fact that doctors are more likely to be streptococcal carriers than midwives.

The Committee believes that the deaths from streptococcal puerperal sepsis would be materially diminished if streptococcus carriers were excluded from attendance on the parturient and puerperal woman until they had become free of the organisms, and if everyone in attendance at labor and in the puerperium had, at all times, the mouth and nose efficiently masked.

The risk of infection from carriers is greater in instrumental than in spontaneous delivery and greater in hospital than in home delivery; the risk in hospital is again increased if the institution has no proper isolation unit or if the obstetrical division is not separated completely from other units.

There remain to be mentioned those cases of puerperal infection where the organism is conveyed to the patient directly from some septic lesion on the hands or person of the attendant, or in which unsterile instruments or dressings are used. These probably constitute a small proportion of all cases.

The foregoing is a brief résumé of an article by Watson on puerperal septicaemia.[4] He sums up thus the situation as he sees it today:

(1) Infection may be due to a variety of organisms;

(2) In a certain proportion of cases the organism may already be present in the vagina or cervix at the time of labor. The organism in this case is most likely to be one of the less virulent types, such as the anaerobic streptococcus, the non-hemolytic aerobic streptococcus, staphylococcus, or bacillus coli;

(3) Exhaustion, due to long labor, blood loss, and traumatization of tissue, favors this type of infection;

(4) In the majority of cases so infected, the infection is a mild one and the mortality rate is low;

(5) In exceptional cases, however, a severe general infection with prolonged illness and death may result;

(6) Exogenous infection by these organisms is probably more frequent than endogenous, the organism being introduced into the vagina in the course of obstetrical manipulations;

(7) Infection with the hemolytic streptococcus is practically always exogenous;

(8) Such infections constitute the majority of the severe and fatal cases of puerperal sepsis;

(9) The precise way in which the organism gets into the genital passages has not been proved;

(10) It may be air borne;

(11) But it is much more likely that it is by droplet infection of hands, gloves, instruments, and nursing appliances, from the noses and throats of doctors and nurses who are streptococcus carriers;

(12) When such an infection occurs in a patient in an institution the attendants on that patient are likely to become carriers and to pass the organism to others;

(13) Such patients and their attendants should, therefore, be strictly isolated;

(14) Thorough masking of the mouth and nose should be practiced by all those who come in contact with the parturient and postpartum woman;

(15) If an individual is proved to be a carrier he or she should be excluded from obstetrical practice until cultures from nose and throat are negative for hemolytic streptococcus.

The total number of puerperal deaths (exclusive of those following abortion and extra-uterine pregnancy) in New York City during the three years under review was 1,564 which gives a rate of 4.49 per 1,000 live births. The total number of deaths from sepsis was 510 which is 32.6 per cent of the total deaths and gives a septic death rate of 1.46 per 1,000 live births. When these are divided according to race

TABLE 29

PUERPERAL SEPTICAEMIA DEATHS BY RACE

(*Exclusive of deaths following abortion and ectopic gestation*)

	TOTAL LIVE BIRTHS	TOTAL DEATHS		TOTAL SEPTICAEMIA DEATHS		SEPTICAEMIA DEATHS EXCLUSIVE OF CAESAREAN SECTION		SEPTICAEMIA DEATHS FOLLOWING CAESAREAN SECTION	
		Number	Rate*	Number	Rate*	Number	Rate*	Number	Rate*
Total	348,310	1,564	4.49	510	1.46	362	1.03	148	.42
White	325,998	1,392	4.27	463	1.42	326	1.00	137	.42
Negro	21,863	170	7.77	47	2.14	36	1.64	11	.50
Yellow	449	2	4.45	—	—	—	—	—	—

*Per 1,000 live births.

(Table 29), the rate for the Negro is seen to be considerably in excess of that for the white race, 2.14 to 1.42. This difference is perceptible for all deaths from sepsis whether following caesarean section or other type of delivery.

The death rates by months from all causes during the period of the study appear to show some seasonal variation. The rates were somewhat higher during the winter months, December through March, than during the rest of the year.

In Chart A the death rates for all puerperal causes and for sepsis alone for 1930–1932 have been plotted, together with the mortality rates for pneumonia during the same period, the pneumonia rates being used as an index of the incidence of respiratory infections in the community. The rate for all puerperal causes follows in a general way the curve for pneumonia, but the sepsis rate shows a more marked variation of the same type except that there is no rise in November and December to correspond to the pneumonia rise.

In order to determine if the picture for 1930–1932 was characteristic of a general trend, similar data for the five-year period immediately preceding are also shown on the same

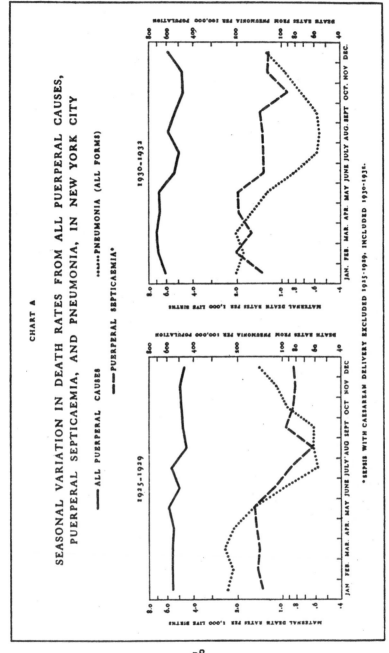

CHART A

SEASONAL VARIATION IN DEATH RATES FROM ALL PUERPERAL CAUSES,
PUERPERAL SEPTICAEMIA, AND PNEUMONIA, IN NEW YORK CITY

——ALL PUERPERAL CAUSES   ·····PNEUMONIA (ALL FORMS)

——PUERPERAL SEPTICAEMIA*

*SEPSIS WITH CAESAREAN DELIVERY EXCLUDED 1925-1929. INCLUDED 1930-1931.

78

TABLE 30

PUERPERAL SEPTICAEMIA DEATHS BY NATIVITY

(*Exclusive of deaths following abortion and ectopic gestation*)

	TOTAL LIVE BIRTHS	TOTAL DEATHS.		TOTAL SEPTICAEMIA DEATHS		SEPTICAEMIA DEATHS EXCLUSIVE OF CAESAREAN SECTION		SEPTICAEMIA DEATHS FOLLOWING CAESAREAN SECTION	
		Number	Rate*	Number	Rate*	Number	Rate*	Number	Rate*
Total	348,310	1,564	4.49	510	1.46	362	1.03	148	.42
Native	237,986	878	3.68	282	1.18	200	.84	82	.34
Foreign	109,619	686	6.25	228	2.07	162	1.47	66	.60
Unknown	705	—	—	—	—	—	—	—	—

*Per 1,000 live births.

chart. The mortality rate from all puerperal causes shows, if anything, less seasonal trend than during the period of the study and the sepsis rate shows more marked variation and a trend more nearly of the form of the pneumonia curve except for a still more decided tendency to remain low during the last two months of the year.

In Table 30 the rates are given according to nativity. Foreign-born women show a puerperal death rate from all causes in excess of that for the native-born, and this continues in the rates for puerperal septicaemia, where the rate for the foreign-born is 2.07 and for the native-born 1.18. Dividing the cases of septicaemia into those with caesarean operation and those without, the difference in rate remains: 1.47 and .84 for those not having had caesarean section and .60 and .34 in the cases following caesarean. The cause of this discrepancy is not clear and does not emerge from the figures alone. Other factors closely related to nativity, such as type of care and economic status, enter here to influence the result.

It is not at all unexpected to find a great disparity evident between the death rates from septicaemia following legitimate and illegitimate births—1.42 and 4.27 (Table 31).

TABLE 31

PUERPERAL SEPTICAEMIA DEATHS BY LEGITIMACY

(*Exclusive of deaths following abortion and ectopic gestation*)

	TOTAL LIVE BIRTHS	TOTAL DEATHS		TOTAL SEPTICAEMIA DEATHS		SEPTICAEMIA DEATHS EXCLUSIVE OF CAESAREAN SECTION		SEPTICAEMIA DEATHS FOLLOWING CAESAREAN SECTION	
		Number	Rate*	Number	Rate*	Number	Rate*	Number	Rate*
Total	348,310	1,564	4.49	510	1.46	362	1.03	148	.42
Legitimate	343,862	1,504	4.37	491	1.42	348	1.01	143	.41
Illegitimate	4,448	60	13.48	19	4.27	14	3.14	5	1.12

*Per 1,000 live births.

The difference is the same when the deaths from sepsis are divided with reference to caesarean operations. The frequency with which women who are illegitimately pregnant enter hospitals late in labor after a totally unsupervised pregnancy no doubt contributes to this result.

The proportion of septic deaths in women less than 30 years of age (64.6 per cent) was somewhat higher than the proportion of non-septic deaths in the same age group (51.1 per cent) (Tables 32 and 33).

In connection with operative deliveries, a larger percentage of septic than of non-septic deaths occurred in the age group 25 to 29 years. The greatest percentage of septic deaths among spontaneous deliveries was in the next younger age group (20 to 24 years).

Non-septic deaths had a fairly symmetrical age distribution even when operative and spontaneous cases were considered separately, with the peak at ages 25 to 29 years. Septic deaths had an asymmetrical distribution, when all cases were considered. The peak among operative deliveries was, however, the same as for non-septic cases (25 to 29 years), and the peak for spontaneous deliveries was well marked in the 20 to 24

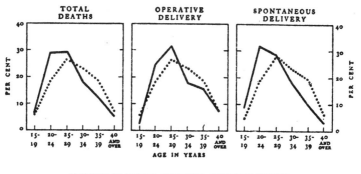

CHART B

PERCENTAGE DISTRIBUTION OF DEATHS FROM
SEPTICAEMIA AND OTHER PUERPERAL CAUSES
BY TYPE OF DELIVERY AND AGE

———SEPTICAEMIA   ······OTHER PUERPERAL CAUSES

EXCLUSIVE OF DEATHS FOLLOWING CAESAREAN SECTION

TABLE 32

SEPTIC DEATHS BY TYPE OF DELIVERY AND AGE

(*Exclusive of deaths following caesarean section*)

	TOTAL		OPERATIVE DELIVERY		SPONTANEOUS DELIVERY		NOT DELIVERED	
	Num-ber	Per cent	Num-ber	Per cent	Num-ber	Per cent	Num-ber	Per cent
Total	362	100.0	133	100.0	224	100.0	5	100.0
15 to 19 years	23	6.4	3	2.3	20	8.9	—	—
20 to 24 years	105	29.0	33	24.8	71	31.7	1	20.0
25 to 29 years	106	29.3	42	31.6	64	28.6	—	—
30 to 34 years	65	18.0	24	18.0	40	17.9	1	20.0
35 to 39 years	44	12.2	21	15.8	22	9.8	1	20.0
40 and over	19	5.2	10	7.5	7	3.1	2	40.0

TABLE 33

NON-SEPTIC DEATHS BY TYPE OF DELIVERY AND AGE

(*Exclusive of deaths following caesarean section*)

	TOTAL		OPERATIVE DELIVERY		SPONTANEOUS DELIVERY		NOT DELIVERED	
	Num-ber	Per cent	Num-ber	Per cent	Num-ber	Per cent	Num-ber	Per cent
Total	898	100.0	292	100.0	347	100.0	259	100.0
15 to 19 years	52	5.8	16	5.5	15	4.3	21	8.1
20 to 24 years	167	18.6	53	18.2	65	18.7	49	18.9
25 to 29 years	240	26.7	78	26.7	97	28.0	65	25.1
30 to 34 years	207	23.1	68	23.3	81	23.3	58	22.4
35 to 39 years	168	18.7	55	18.8	68	19.6	45	17.4
40 and over	64	7.1	22	7.5	21	6.1	21	8.1

age group. The asymmetrical age distribution of the septic deaths is, therefore, very largely determined by the spontaneous deliveries. This relationship is shown graphically in Chart B.

In Table 34, the percentage of septic and non-septic deaths according to the gravidity of the patients and type of delivery is exhibited. Of the non-septic deaths, 32.5 per cent were preceded by operative delivery and 38.6 per cent by spontaneous delivery, while 28.8 per cent of the cases were undelivered.

TABLE 34

SEPTIC AND NON-SEPTIC DEATHS BY TYPE OF DELIVERY AND GRAVIDITY

(Exclusive of deaths following caesarean section)

	TOTAL		OPERATIVE DELIVERY		SPONTANEOUS DELIVERY		NOT DELIVERED	
	Number	Per cent	Number	Per cent of total	Number	Per cent of total	Number	Per cent of total
Non-septic deaths: total	898	100	292	32.5	347	38.6	259	28.8
Primigravidae	364	100	147	40.4	106	29.1	111	30.5
Multigravidae	526	100	144	27.4	241	45.8	141	26.8
Gravidity not reported	8	100	1	12.5	—	—	7	87.5
Septic deaths: total	362	100	133	36.7	224	61.9	5	1.4
Primigravidae	157	100	79	50.3	77	49.0	1	.6
Multigravidae	205	100	54	26.3	147	71.7	4	2.0

In the same group, 40.4 per cent of primigravidous deaths followed operative delivery, while only 27.4 per cent of multigravidous deaths followed operative delivery. In the case of the septic deaths, 36.7 per cent were preceded by operative, and 61.9 per cent by spontaneous delivery. There was an almost even division between the two types of delivery in the case of the primigravidae while the percentage of spontaneous deliveries was greatly in excess of the operative in the case of multigravidae.

These figures are not to be considered as in any way indicative of the relative hazards from septicaemia in the two types, as the incidence of operative delivery is very much lower than that of spontaneous. Furthermore, a considerable number of the deaths following abnormal delivery take place immediately or very soon after delivery before the possibility of the development of septicaemia.

TABLE 35

PUERPERAL SEPTICAEMIA DEATH RATES BY
TYPE OF DELIVERY

(*Exclusive of cases not delivered*)

	TOTAL	OPERATIVE DELIVERY	SPONTANEOUS DELIVERY
Total live births	348,310	69,665	278,645
Total septicaemia deaths	505	281	224
Approximate rate per 1,000 live births	1.4	4.0	0.8

In Table 35 the rates per 1,000 live births following operative and spontaneous delivery give the true picture of the relative risks from septicaemia in the two types of delivery. The rate of deaths from septicaemia following operative delivery is seen to be five times that following spontaneous delivery. The causes and more detailed consideration of this

TABLE 36

PUERPERAL SEPTICAEMIA DEATHS BY PLACE OF DELIVERY

(Exclusive of cases not delivered)

	TOTAL LIVE BIRTHS	TOTAL DEATHS		TOTAL SEPTICAEMIA DEATHS		SEPTICAEMIA DEATHS EXCLUSIVE OF CAESAREAN SECTION	
		Number	Rate*	Number	Rate*	Number	Rate*
Total	348,310	1,300	3.73	505	1.47	357	1.04
Delivered in hospital	246,205	1,111	4.51	413	1.67	265	1.07
Delivered in home	102,105	189	1.85	92	.90	92	.90

*Per 1,000 live births.

variation will be considered under the discussion of operative and spontaneous deliveries in Chapter V (page 116).

In Table 36 are given the rates for all deaths, as well as for septic deaths, according to the place of delivery. The death rate from septicaemia following home delivery is 47 per cent below that following delivery in hospital. If caesarean sections are excluded, the excess of hospital over home is 18 per cent. This confirms the findings as to the relative safety of home and hospital deliveries which will be discussed in detail in Chapter V (page 139).

In Table 37, the deaths from septicaemia following operative delivery are classified according to the type of procedure. Thirty-eight and six-tenths per cent of all operative procedures were followed by septicaemia. In the case of caesarean sections, the percentage was in excess of the average—48.7 per cent. This was true also of destructive operations and extractions, among which the septicaemia percentage was 55.6 per cent and 41.2 per cent, respectively. The figures for "other operative procedures" are too small to be significant. They consisted of one laparotomy for abdominal pregnancy,

TABLE 37

PUERPERAL SEPTICAEMIA DEATHS BY OPERATIVE
PROCEDURE

	OPERATIVE PROCEDURES RESULTING IN DELIVERY			OPERATIVE ATTEMPTS ASSOCIATED WITH OPERATIVE DELIVERY		
	TOTAL	FOLLOWED BY SEPTICAEMIA		TOTAL	FOLLOWED BY SEPTICAEMIA	
		Number	Per cent		Number	Per cent
Total	747	288	38.6	46	19	41.3
Caesarean section	304	148	48.7	12	5	41.7
Version and extraction	113	31	27.4	22	9	40.9
Version	9	2	22.2	1	—	—
Extraction	29	12	41.2	—	—	—
High forceps	24	9	37.5	1	—	—
Mid forceps	91	27	29.7	—	—	—
Low forceps	145	41	28.3	—	—	—
Destructive operations	27	15	55.6	7	4	57.1
Other operative procedures	5	3	60.0	3	1	33.3

one vaginal caesarean section, 2 operative attempts followed
by spontaneous deliveries, and one in which the type of operation was not known.

In 46 instances, there had been operative attempts at delivery prior to the final operation. Among these the incidence
of septicaemia was 41.3 per cent. In instances where an operative attempt prior to delivery was followed by caesarean
section, the incidence was 41.7; in cases of this group where
delivery was by version and extraction, 40.9 per cent; and in
cases where delivery was by a destructive operation, 57.1 per
cent.

In considering the influence of operative delivery on the
incidence of sepsis, two other factors must be taken into account: (1) the length of time the membranes had been ruptured, and (2) the total duration of the labor. It would appear that these two factors have a greater influence than the
actual operative procedure. From Table 38 it is evident that
the ratio of septic deaths to total deaths increases as the time

TABLE 38

PUERPERAL SEPTICAEMIA DEATHS BY TIME OF RUPTURE OF MEMBRANES

(Exclusive of deaths following abortion and ectopic gestation)

	TOTAL DEATHS	SEPTICAEMIA DEATHS		EXCLUSIVE OF CAESAREAN SECTION			FOLLOWING CAESAREAN SECTION		
				TOTAL DEATHS	SEPTICAEMIA DEATHS		TOTAL DEATHS	SEPTICAEMIA DEATHS	
		Number	Per cent of total		Number	Per cent		Number	Per cent
Total	1,564	510	32.6	1,260	362	28.7	304	148	48.7
Membranes not ruptured prior to delivery	408	72	17.6	229	6	2.6	179	66	36.9
Membranes ruptured less than 6 hours	602	205	34.1	574	190	33.1	28	15	53.6
Membranes ruptured over 6 hours	427	187	43.8	336	123	36.6	91	64	70.3
Membranes ruptured—time not reported	127	46	36.2	121	43	35.5	6	3	50.0

elapsing between rupture of the membranes and delivery lengthens. There are approximately 10 per cent more septic deaths in patients with membranes ruptured for more than six hours than in those in which delivery occurred in less than six hours after rupture. This bears out what has been said regarding the ascent of organisms into the uterine cavity after the escape of the liquor amnii.

TABLE 39

PUERPERAL SEPTICAEMIA DEATHS BY DURATION
OF LABOR

(*Exclusive of deaths following abortion and ectopic gestation*)

	TOTAL DEATHS	TOTAL SEPTICAEMIA DEATHS		SEPTICAEMIA EXCLUSIVE OF CAESAREAN SECTION		SEPTICAEMIA FOLLOWING CAESAREAN SECTION	
		Number	Per cent	Number	Per cent	Number	Per cent
Total	1,564	510	32.6	362	23.1	148	9.5
Not in labor	316	33	10.4	5	1.6	28	8.9
Less than 1 hour	20	4	20.0	4	20.0	—	—
1 to 12 hours	556	186	33.5	158	28.4	28	5.0
12 to 24 hours	306	119	38.9	88	28.8	31	10.1
24 to 48 hours	190	89	46.8	53	27.9	36	18.9
48 hours and over	142	69	48.6	44	31.0	25	17.6
Duration not reported	34	10	29.4	10	29.4	—	—

In the same way there is a very definite relationship between the total duration of labor and the number of septic deaths (Table 39). Of the deaths following labor of forty-eight hours or more, 48.6 per cent were due to septicaemia; of those following labor of twelve hours or less, only 33.0 per cent were septic. It is in those cases of prolonged labor that frequent vaginal or rectal examinations are made, and these also increase the risk of sepsis, as is shown by Table 40.

Early rupture of the membranes, a slow first and second stage with inadequate uterine contractions, and a normal pelvis is a not infrequent combination. In the management of

TABLE 40

PUERPERAL SEPTICAEMIA DEATHS BY EXAMINATION BEFORE DELIVERY

(*Exclusive of deaths following abortion and ectopic gestation*)

	EXCLUSIVE OF CAESAREAN SECTION			FOLLOWING CAESAREAN SECTION		
	TOTAL DEATHS	SEPTICAEMIA DEATHS		TOTAL DEATHS	SEPTICAEMIA DEATHS	
		Number	Per cent		Number	Per cent
Total	1,260	362	28.7	304	148	48.7
No examination	406	82	20.2	79	23	29.1
Vaginal, rectal, or both	846	275	32.5	225	125	55.6
Not reported	8	5	—	—	—	—

such cases fine obstetric judgment is required to determine when assistance is best given and what the nature of that assistance should be. On the one hand, early interference, if it is determined upon, must be carried out without shock or laceration, and this calls for manipulative skill; on the other hand, delay in these procedures may render them easier but may also allow infection to occur with a risk of deeper inoculation of the organisms when they are carried out.

A realization by the practitioner of the danger of prolonged labor would make for more frequent and earlier consultation with the specialist, with a possible saving of human life.

ALBUMINURIA AND ECLAMPSIA

THE most frequent cause of death, with the exception of puerperal septicaemia, is the group of pregnancy toxaemias of various types included under the heading albuminuria and eclampsia. This classification includes only those kidney and liver disturbances which arise directly as the result of pregnancy and not true nephritis, chronic or acute. At times the differentiation was difficult as the symptom complex is very similar, but usually a careful history brought to light those cases in which true nephritis was present. A toxaemia can usually be detected during pregnancy by proper examination and can often be prevented from assuming dangerous proportions by proper attention to the regime. The cure lies in prevention, but prevention demands alertness in detecting the first sign of approaching breakdown and prompt and vigorous treatment to combat it. It requires the utmost in cooperation between physician and patient, and cooperation from the patient implies that she be properly instructed in the signs of danger. Once the toxic condition has been allowed to develop to the convulsive stage, the task of the attendant becomes infinitely more difficult and the results for the mother and foetus much more serious.

Of the 1,564 deaths from all conditions exclusive of abortions and extra-uterine gestations, 231, or 14.8 per cent of the total, were due to pregnancy toxaemia. An additional 95 women, 6.1 per cent, had toxic manifestations of sufficient proportions to make these a factor in the fatality. The causes of death among these 95 women were as follows: hemorrhage, 22; shock or accident of labor, 16; septicaemia, 34; phlegmasia alba dolens or embolism, 5; and extra-puerperal causes, 18.

Sixteen and five-tenths per cent of all the native-born women in the series died of this condition, but only 12.5 per cent of the foreign-born women. Among native women, albuminuria and eclampsia was the second greatest cause of death; it ranked fourth in importance among the foreign-born. However, the rate of death from this cause per 1,000 live births was .61 among native-born women against .78 for the foreign-born. While the mortality from this cause, then, was higher among foreign-born than among native-born, and thus was a partial cause of the higher general mortality rate, the importance of albuminuria and eclampsia as a factor in causing maternal deaths was considerably greater among native-born than among foreign-born. A more marked variation was evident in the distribution of deaths from this cause among Negro and white women. Among Negroes it comprised 19.4 per cent of all deaths, while among white women the corresponding ratio was 14.2 per cent.

It is not immediately evident why this should be so. One factor undoubtedly lies in the care received during the prenatal period. Prenatal care was strikingly deficient for both groups, but the foreign-born received less prenatal care than did the native women. Of the women of native origin who died of this condition, 30.0 per cent had sufficient care during pregnancy, but the corresponding figure for foreign-born women is only 24.0 per cent. A total of 377 native-born women in the entire series had adequate care, and of this number 45, or 11.9 per cent, died of albuminuria and eclampsia. Among the 223 foreign-born women who had sufficient prenatal care, 20 (9.0 per cent) died of toxaemia. Moreover, the general living level of the foreign-born is below that of the native-born, and this may have its effect upon the development of abnormalities. The precise relationship is not susceptible of evaluation, but it is to be considered as a possible factor. The foreign-born are, to a great extent, among the underprivileged group, and economic pressure prevents easy cooperation with the attendant in obtaining a suitable regime for the prevention of complications. Proper diet and adequate rest are frequently impossible. The demands of the family are paramount, and the woman, of necessity, neglects herself.

Table 41A gives the relation between this cause of death and the age and gravidity of the patient. The ratio of deaths

TABLE 41A

ALBUMINURIA AND ECLAMPSIA DEATHS BY AGE AND
GRAVIDITY

	TOTAL	15 TO 19 YEARS	20 TO 29 YEARS	30 TO 39 YEARS	40 YEARS AND OVER
Total deaths*	1,564	87	756	610	111
Albuminuria and eclampsia	231	21	114	85	11
Per cent of total deaths	*14.8*	*24.1*	*15.1*	*13.9*	*9.9*
Primigravidae: total†	682	78	428	157	19
Albuminuria and eclampsia‡	122	21	76	24	1
Per cent of total primigravidae	*17.9*	*26.9*	*17.6*	*15.3*	*5.3*
Multigravidae: total†	874	9	327	447	91
Albuminuria and eclampsia‡	106	—	38	58	10
Per cent of total multigravidae	*12.1*	—	*11.6*	*13.0*	*11.0*

*Exclusive of deaths following abortion and ectopic gestation.
†Excluding 8 cases of which the gravidity was unknown.
‡Excluding 3 cases of which the gravidity was unknown.

from albuminuria and eclampsia to all deaths was greatest in
the 15 to 19 year group (24.1 per cent) and declined with age
in each decade to a minimum of 9.9 per cent in the group 40
years and over. That this trend by age was largely determined by the group of primigravidae is shown by the separate age distributions for primigravidae and multigravidae.
Deaths from albuminuria and eclampsia formed 17.9 per cent
of all deaths among primigravidae, the highest proportion
falling in the youngest age group, 15 to 19 years, and the
lowest, following a steady decline by decades, in the group 40
years and over. Among multigravidae, on the other hand,
only 12.1 per cent of all deaths were due to albuminuria and
eclampsia, the maximum percentage being recorded in the 30
to 39 year group. A very definite relationship between age
and gravidity is evident in these figures. Primigravidae and
low age groups present a persistently higher proportion of
toxaemia deaths than do the older and multigravidae. The

disturbance of the usual trend in the figures for the multi-gravidae is not easily explicable, but is possibly affected by the constitutional changes brought about by repeated child-bearing. The variation here is not in the relation of multi-gravidae to primigravidae, but in that between multigravidae in the various age groups. Of all primigravidae between 15 and 19 years of age, 26.9 per cent died of toxaemia; 17.6 per cent of all primigravidae and only 11.6 per cent of all multigravidae between 20 and 29 died of this condition. The fourth decade shows the same relationship—primigravidae 15.3 per cent and multigravidae 13.0 per cent. In the group over 40 years of age the figures are so small that the reversed relationship, 5.3 per cent primigravidae and 11.0 per cent multigravidae, is not significant.

It is important to note that this condition was not precipitate except in a very few cases. The vast majority of the patients had warning symptoms which, if heeded, might have indicated the way toward prevention of the fatality. Among the 231 patients, only 9 gave a history of a fulminating onset; 217 had definite premonitory symptoms of albuminuria, elevated pressure, eye symptoms, or persistent headache; in 5 of the women, no definite history was obtainable. Among the 231 women who died, 176 had convulsions. In the neglect of these symptoms by both patient and attendant lies the key to the large number of these deaths.

Only 95 (41.0 per cent) of these women went to term before going into labor or developing symptoms of so serious a nature that death ensued without delivery or the attendant emptied the uterus artificially. Sixty-four of them died between the thirty-sixth and thirty-ninth weeks, 16 between the thirty-second and thirty-fifth, 38 between the twenty-eighth and thirty-first, and 18 prior to the twenty-eighth week of pregnancy.

For 24 women delivery was by caesarean operation, 15 before the onset of labor, and 9 after labor had set in. Ninety-five of the additional 207 went into labor spontaneously, 36 had it induced, 73 died before labor set in, 2 had *accouchement forcé*, and of one there is no history.

Delivery was effected before death in 140 cases. Sixty-six, less than one-half, were delivered spontaneously, the remaining 74 being subjected to operative procedures of one sort or another. Caesarean section was performed in 24 cases, version and extraction in 8, version alone in 1, extraction in 3, high forceps in 2, mid forceps in 15, low forceps in 22, and destruction of the foetus in 2 instances. There were five pairs of twins, two of which were delivered by section, one by version and extraction with a second extraction, one by version and extraction and low forceps, and one by mid forceps and extraction.

There were 146 babies delivered, of which 80, 54.8 per cent, were alive and 66, 45.2 per cent, were stillborn. When we add to this the 93 babies which were undelivered, the loss of foetal life associated with these fatalities becomes more startling, for out of 239 babies only 80, about one-third, were brought to term or near term and delivered alive.

In view of these facts, it is not surprising to find that, of the total number, the Advisory Committee found only 63 cases which could be considered unavoidable. The physician was held responsible in 49 of the 168 deaths which could have been prevented, the patient in 116, and the midwife in 3.

By consulting Table 41B, the relationship between preventability, prenatal care, and type of delivery may be seen. There were 74 operative deliveries. Thirty-two of these women had proper prenatal care, but 11 of the deaths were, none the less, preventable, 10 of them being ascribed to the physician. Forty-two had less than adequate care in the prenatal period, and of these the attendant was held responsible

TABLE 41B

ALBUMINURIA AND ECLAMPSIA DEATHS BY PREVENTABILITY AND PRENATAL CARE, ACCORDING TO TYPE OF DELIVERY

	TOTAL	NOT PRE-VENTABLE	PREVENTABLE			
			Total	Responsibility ascribed to		
				Physician	Patient	Midwife
Total albuminuria and eclampsia deaths	251	63	168	49	116	3
Operative delivery: total	74	26	48	23	25	—
Adequate prenatal care	32	21	11	10	1	—
Inadequate or no prenatal care	42	5	37	13	24	—
Spontaneous delivery: total	66	15	51	16	32	3
Adequate prenatal care	15	8	7	5	2	—
Inadequate or no prenatal care	51	7	44	11	30	3
Not delivered: total	91	22	69	10	59	—
Adequate prenatal care	18	14	4	3	1	—
Inadequate or no prenatal care	73	8	65	7	58	—

in 13 cases and the patient herself in 24. Of the 66 spontaneous deliveries, 51 deaths were preventable. Among the 15 with adequate care, 7 deaths were avoidable, 5 by the physician and 2 by the patient. In the remaining 51 without adequate care, death could have been avoided in 44 cases, 11 being the responsibility of the attendant, 30 of the patient, and 3 of the midwife. Sixty-nine of the 91 deaths occurring before the patient was delivered were avoidable. In 3 instances where the patient had had proper care, the physician was thought responsible for the outcome, and in one, the patient. Among those who had not had adequate care, the physician was held responsible in 7 cases and the patient in 58. The preventability in the series as a whole is due much more frequently to failure on the part of the patient than on the part of the physician. Prenatal care is strikingly deficient, only 65, 25.9 per cent, having received proper care.

This group of deaths, as a whole, reveals a serious defect in management in the large percentage of cases. The effort to induce patients to obtain suitable care during pregnancy has fallen far short of the mark. When we consider that only 9 of these cases had the fulminating type of eclampsia without previous symptoms, and that of those who received proper care only 35 per cent were preventable, while among those who failed to have proper care, 94 per cent were judged preventable, the possibilities of lowering the death rate from this cause become very significant. The tendency among these women was to postpone the first visit to a clinic or physician until the seventh or eighth month and to make following visits only rarely. Once the patient had registered in a hospital for delivery, there was a great tendency for her to neglect her visits. In such instances, it is of the greatest importance to have adequate social service personnel to see that all women who are registered in the prenatal clinics return at the time set by the clinic physician. There were numerous instances of the patient's refusal to enter the hospital when advised to do so at the time of onset of the mild symptoms. She returned at a later time in critical condition. The problem of the women who never come to the clinics is even more difficult. In numerous instances the woman was admitted to a hospital in convulsions with a history of prolonged symptoms for which she had made no attempt to seek medical advice. This again emphasizes the serious need of education that will be really effective. It is realized that recent years have greatly changed public attitude toward early and continuous observation during pregnancy, but the progress of such education is slow. The necessity for further effort along these lines is still present, if we are to expect that the large mass of women will be reached by it and brought to a realization of the great importance of this part of their care.

Among the deaths for which the attendant was held responsible, the largest proportion was among those patients having operative delivery. In view of the fact that non-intervention, with all treatment directed toward combating the toxaemia without regard for the onset of labor, is now accepted as the most effective method of handling a case of eclampsia, the number of caesarean sections and inductions of labor is significant of the quality of care these patients were receiving.

Further reduction of these deaths, a very large percentage of which can be prevented, will be brought about only by education of women to the vital necessity of putting themselves under supervision early in pregnancy and cooperating scrupulously with the physician throughout the prenatal period, and by assuring to every woman the services of highly trained specialists when those services are needed because of an abnormal development of pregnancy.

PERNICIOUS VOMITING OF PREGNANCY

WE have already considered the first two main divisions of the causes of death, abortions and ectopic gestations. In the group we are about to discuss, which is a subdivision of the third group, it is necessary to consider, besides the 14 deaths caused by pernicious vomiting, 14 cases which have already been discussed under abortions, because, while abortions did occur, the true cause of death was pernicious vomiting. It seems appropriate that all the cases in which this was the cause of death should be considered together.

Besides these 28 cases, there were 21 cases in which pernicious vomiting was a contributory factor in the death.

Pernicious vomiting primary cause of death
  With abortion   14
  Not delivered   14

Pernicious vomiting contributory cause of death
  With abortion   10
  Not delivered   11

The figures in these groups are too small to be statistically important, and we present the following analyses merely as a matter of interest.

Table 42 shows the age distribution in both groups.

TABLE 42

PERNICIOUS VOMITING DEATHS BY AGE

	TOTAL	15 TO 19 YEARS	20 TO 24 YEARS	25 TO 29 YEARS	30 TO 34 YEARS	35 TO 39 YEARS	40 YEARS AND OVER
All deaths	2,041	108	429	559	449	358	138
Pernicious vomiting deaths*	28	3	6	10	4	5	—
Pernicious vomiting contributory to death†	21	5	5	5	4	1	1

*Including 14 deaths following abortion.   †Including 10 deaths following abortion.

Eleven of the 28 women who died of pernicious vomiting and 10 of the 21 in whom it was only a contributory agent were primigravidae.

Of the primary cases, 8 of the women were Negroes, and 20 were white; 3 Negroes and 18 white women had vomiting which was a contributory factor.

In the first group, 15 of the women, 53.6 per cent, were native born, and 13, 46.4 per cent, were foreign born. In the group in which the condition was contributory, 19, or 90.5 per cent, were native and 2, or 9.5 per cent, foreign born.

The Advisory Committee considered that 15 of the 28 deaths could have been prevented. Seven of these 15 were laid to improper judgment or care on the part of the attendant and 8 to the patient's failure to seek medical care earlier.

Ten therapeutic abortions were performed in cases where pernicious vomiting was the cause of death, 3 abortions occurred spontaneously, and one was illegally induced. Among the 10 abortions in cases where pernicious vomiting was contributory, 6 were therapeutic and 4 spontaneous.

PHLEGMASIA ALBA DOLENS, EMBOLUS, AND SUDDEN DEATH

In ascribing the cases to this cause of death, the Advisory Committee has been at particular pains to discover whether or not a terminal embolism was associated with some underlying cause such as sepsis. Where this has been the case, the death has been ascribed to the underlying cause. In order to be as nearly certain as possible that the death was of embolic origin, the investigators have carefully examined the cases in which the death certificate has given embolism as the cause of death to determine in detail the symptoms present at the time of death. Furthermore, great care has been taken to discover whether or not there was a septicaemia which might give rise to fatal septic emboli. In these instances the true cause of death has been the septicaemia. We have recognized that even in some of the cases where there was no evidence to indicate its existence, a low-grade septicaemia may have, in fact, been present and was in reality the underlying cause of the embolism; but where it has been impossible to adduce any evidence whatever, we have been forced to ascribe the death to embolism.

After careful examination, 89 of the deaths were assigned to embolism; this is 5.7 per cent of all deaths, exclusive of abortion and ectopic gestation. Of these deaths, 48.3 per cent were in primigravidae and 51.7 per cent in multigravidae.

TABLE 43

DEATHS FROM PHLEGMASIA ALBA DOLENS AND
EMBOLUS BY AGE

	TOTAL	15 TO 19 YEARS	20 TO 24 YEARS	25 TO 29 YEARS	30 TO 34 YEARS	35 TO 39 YEARS	40 YEARS AND OVER
Total deaths*	1,564	87	324	432	351	259	111
Phlegmasia alba dolens and embolus deaths	89	3	13	27	27	12	7
Per cent of total	5.7	3.4	4.0	6.3	7.7	4.6	6.3

*Exclusive of deaths following abortion and ectopic gestation.

Table 43 gives the age distribution in this group. The age group in which embolism contributed most heavily to maternal deaths was 30 to 34 years. There is a gradual and consistent increase up to this age, after which the percentages are somewhat below the maximum. This would appear to be a phenomenon related strictly to age, since gravidity is not revealed as an important factor. Spontaneous deliveries greatly outnumber operative in this group, 54 to 29; 6 were not delivered. Twenty-two cases had other abnormalities of parturition and pregnancy as factors contributory to death. One had pernicious vomiting, 7 hemorrhage, 5 albuminuria and eclampsia, 9 extra-puerperal conditions.

This condition is fundamentally accidental and not to any extent preventable except by the prevention of those constitutional factors which may predispose to embolic processes. It probably represents a fixed and irreducible element in the inevitable deaths arising out of childbearing.

SHOCK AND ACCIDENTS OF LABOR

UNDER this caption are grouped all cases in which the death was ascribed to the effects of labor and the accidents occurring in its course, including the shock associated with operative delivery as well as that arising out of spontaneous delivery and of rupture and inversion of the uterus. These are the cases of greatly prolonged labor, with predominantly operative termination; the cases in which unsuccessful operative attempts preceded delivery; those with malposition which were mismanaged; and the neglected cases of obstructed labor.

In all, 171 women died as the direct result of labor and delivery, of which number 65 had a caesarean section done or attempted. These will be discussed under caesarean section (page 127). Fourteen women were delivered spontaneously, 144 by artificial methods, and 13 died undelivered.

The women who were delivered spontaneously had had no previous operative attempts at delivery made. Six had ruptured uteri, 3 inversion of the uterus, and 2 had postpartum hemorrhage; in 1 case, eclampsia was considered a contributory factor, and in 2 extra-puerperal conditions were so considered.

Labor was not unduly prolonged in most of the cases of spontaneous delivery. Eight women were delivered in less than twelve hours, 5 more in less than twenty-four hours, while in only 1 case was labor prolonged beyond twenty-four hours.

Nine of the 13 women who died without being delivered

TABLE 44A

DEATHS FOLLOWING ACCIDENTS OF LABOR, BY TYPE OF DELIVERY AND PREVENTABILITY

| | TOTAL* | | DEATHS FOLLOWING ACCIDENTS OF LABOR | | | | | | | |
| | | | TOTAL | | OPERATIVE DELIVERY | | SPONTANEOUS DELIVERY | | NOT DELIVERED | |
	Number	Per cent	Number	Per cent	Number	Per cent	Number	Per cent	Number	Per cent
Total deaths	1,564	100.0	171	100.0	144	100.0	14	100.0	13	100.0
Not preventable	581	37.1	22	12.9	16	11.1	5	35.7	1	7.7
Preventable: total	983	62.9	149	87.1	128	88.9	9	64.3	12	92.3
Responsibility ascribed to										
Physician	678	69.0	134	89.9	118	92.2	7	77.8	9	75.0
Patient	276	28.1	11	7.3	8	6.2	1	11.1	2	16.7
Midwife	29	2.9	4	2.7	2	1.6	1	11.1	1	8.3

*Exclusive of deaths following abortion and ectopic gestation.

had 14 attempts at operative delivery performed upon them, as follows: 2 caesarean sections, 2 destructive operations upon the foetus, 4 high forceps, 1 low forceps, 3 podalic version and extraction, and 2 podalic version alone.

Table 44A shows preventability according to the type of delivery. It is not surprising to find that in this group 87.1 per cent of the deaths were preventable, 24.2 per cent higher than for the series as a whole. The predominance of operative delivery in this group accounts, in large measure, for the percentage of cases in which the physician was held responsible. In the cases delivered by operative procedures, 88.9 per cent were considered preventable, the responsibility being ascribed to the physician in 92.2 per cent of the preventable deaths.

RUPTURED UTERUS

SEVENTY-ONE of the deaths studied followed rupture of the uterus. Slightly more than one-half of these cases were diagnosed at the time of or very soon after the rupture; others were not diagnosed until the autopsy was performed; still others were not reported as ruptured uterus, but were judged by the Obstetrical Advisory Committee, because of the significant symptoms, to be cases of rupture of the uterus and were accordingly classified as such. In a number of cases, the Committee felt that this was probably the true cause of death, but the data available were insufficient to permit a positive diagnosis. It should be emphasized that the number here presented as having had ruptured uteri prior to death represents, in the opinion of the Obstetrical Advisory Committee, a conservative figure.

Of these 71 deaths, 62 resulted directly from shock, 6 from puerperal septicaemia, 2 from hemorrhage, and 1 from an extra-puerperal cause.

TABLE 44B

DEATHS FOLLOWING RUPTURED UTERUS, BY AGE
AND GRAVIDITY

	TOTAL	PRIMIGRAVIDAE	MULTIGRAVIDAE
Total	71	16	55
15 to 19 years	1	—	1
20 to 24 years	10	5	5
25 to 29 years	14	—	14
30 to 34 years	15	4	11
35 to 39 years	21	7	14
40 years and over	10	—	10

In 40 of these patients, the pelvis was known to be normal, in 13 it was known to be abnormal, while in 18 the type of pelvis was not known.

Table 44B shows deaths according to age and gravidity. By far the larger number of these deaths were in multigravidae and women in the later age groups; of the 71 deaths, 55 were multigravidae and only 16 primigravidae. Among the multigravidae, only 6 were under twenty-five years of age; 14 were between twenty-five and twenty-nine, 11 between thirty and thirty-four, 14 between thirty-five and thirty-nine, and 10 over forty years of age.

In Table 44C these 71 deaths are analyzed according to gravidity. The 71 deaths represent 4.5 per cent of all the deaths occurring in women at or after the twenty-eighth week of gestation. Sixteen, or 2.3 per cent of all the primigravidae in this series, died following rupture of the uterus. Among the multigravidae, the highest percentage of deaths following rupture of the uterus was among the quartigravidae, 9.4 per cent of the cases. Gravidity thus appears to be a contributory factor in the production of rupture of the uterus.

Preventability is shown in Table 44D. Sixty-four, or 78.4 per cent of these deaths, were preventable—a percentage in

TABLE 44C

DEATHS FOLLOWING RUPTURED UTERUS, BY GRAVIDITY

	TOTAL DEATHS*	DEATHS FOLLOWING RUPTURED UTERUS	
		Number	Per cent of total
Total	1,564	71	4.5
Primigravidae	682	16	2.3
Gravidae II	277	14	5.1
Gravidae III	192	12	6.3
Gravidae IV	128	12	9.4
Gravidae V to VII	168	8	4.8
Gravidae VIII and over	105	9	8.6
Multigravidae, gravidity not reported	4	—	—
Gravidity not reported	8	—	—

*Exclusive of deaths following abortion and ectopic gestation.

TABLE 44D

PREVENTABILITY AND RESPONSIBILITY FOR DEATHS FOLLOWING RUPTURED UTERUS

	TOTAL DEATHS*	DEATHS FOLLOWING RUPTURED UTERUS	
		Number	Per cent of total
Total	1,564	71	4.5
Not preventable	581	7	1.2
Preventable: total	983	64	6.5
Responsibility ascribed to			
Physician	678	57	8.4
Patient	276	4	1.4
Midwife	29	3	10.3

*Exclusive of deaths following abortion and ectopic gestation.

excess of that for the series as a whole. Of the 64 preventable deaths, the responsibility was ascribed to the physician in 57 cases, to the patient in 4, and to the midwife in 3. It is apparent that the deaths following rupture of the uterus were due, in large measure, to the mismanagement of labor and delivery. Contracted pelvis was frequently overlooked; as often, improper operative procedures were undertaken and unskilfully performed by the attendant.

Any reduction in the deaths from this cause must be effected through an improvement in the skill and judgment of the accoucheur. He must have the training requisite to make accurate judgments as to prognosis for delivery; he must scrupulously avoid undertaking procedures for which his experience and training have not provided adequate preparation. More prompt procuring of competent consultation early in abnormal labor is also a requisite to a lessening of the number of deaths from ruptured uterus.

ACCIDENTS OF THE PUERPERIUM

THIS term is used to cover those conditions of the puerperal state not properly included in the previous classifications, such as the puerperal psychoses.

The 8 cases in this group were all puerperal psychoses in which the exhaustion attendant upon this condition was the actual cause of death. There were 6 additional deaths where the psychosis played a contributory part. Two of the women were between fifteen and nineteen years of age, 2 between twenty-five and twenty-nine, 2 between thirty and thirty-four, 1 between thirty-five and thirty-nine, and one over forty. They were equally divided between primigravidae and multigravidae. Five were delivered spontaneously, and 3 by operative procedure.

Only one of the cases gave a history of previous mental disease.

EXTRA-PUERPERAL CAUSES

WHEN all the deaths from strictly puerperal conditions had been considered, there remained a large group of deaths of which the actual cause was a condition not directly connected with the puerperal state, but one which was exacerbated by the pregnancy and delivery. Only those in which a definite causal relationship was thought to exist between the death and the pregnant or puerperal state were included in this category.

The group was a varied one, including many different diseases. The largest group was that of heart disease. We are discussing the 99 cases in which death was due to this condition in some detail, as a separate group.

Following cardiac disease in importance are the respiratory infections. Of 93 cases of this type, 52 were due to lobar pneumonia, 20 to the bronchial type, and 21 to influenza. During the winter months of 1931 and again in 1932, New York City experienced a mild but definite epidemic of influenza with the inevitable increase in deaths from all types of pneumonia. The great bulk of the deaths in our series occurred during these periods of greatly increased general morbidity and mortality from these diseases. Past experience has demonstrated that influenza is especially hazardous for the parturient, and a decided tendency to early miscarriage, in the course of an influenza, has a most serious effect in increasing the deaths from the respiratory infections. The inevitable question arises, in this connection, as to the validity of considering the pregnancy or postpartum condition a contributory factor in producing the fatality.

Chronic nephritis was the cause of death in 18 cases. There was, in these cases, an occasional history of toxaemia in previous pregnancy, but the story of a true nephritis was available in practically all of them, with the clinical course and laboratory findings as substantiating evidence. It was felt that the addition of the burden of pregnancy to already overstrained and failing kidneys contributed largely to the fatal outcome. Chronic nephritis should be regarded as a contra-indication to pregnancy, and the prevention of these deaths lies in the observance of this principle.

There were 16 deaths from pulmonary tuberculosis. Most of these women had no particular care. Many of them were unaware of the presence of tuberculosis, and some neglected serious symptoms. The group as a whole is too small to be of any significance and only serves to emphasize, again, the necessity for special treatment of the tuberculous woman.

The remaining 118 deaths were caused by various diseases. We have given the list with the itemized cause of death in the Appendix (page 233).

One hundred and fifteen of the 344 patients (33.4 per cent) died of the antecedent disease before delivery. The death of the mother followed the termination of pregnancy by less than twenty-four hours in 63 cases, by one to seven days in 83 cases, one to two weeks in 34 cases, two to three weeks in 20 cases, and more than three weeks in 29 cases. More than one-half (175) died prior to the fortieth week of pregnancy: 38 under twenty-eight weeks, 41 between twenty-eight and thirty-one weeks, 32 between thirty-two and thirty-five weeks, 64 between thirty-six and thirty-nine weeks. The remaining 169 died at or after forty weeks' gestation.

In a sense, these cases are not significant except for the group of cardiac cases which we discuss below. They are widely scattered and represent the accidents of morbidity to which the entire population, regardless of age or sex, is subject. They are of especial interest in so far as they show the increase in the risk assumed by women during pregnancy. Their prevention and control lie in the general field of disease prevention, but added precautions and safeguards should be provided for women at this time.

Cardiac Disease

It has long been recognized that any disease of the heart or its valves has a special significance in its relation to pregnancy. Serious heart damage is advanced as a contra-indication to pregnancy. The pregnant woman with an injured heart must have greatly increased rest in bed and very special treatment to minimize the strains incident to labor and delivery.

In considering the role of heart disease as a cause of death during pregnancy, a comparison between the death rate from heart disease among parturient women with that among the remaining female population of childbearing age is significant. These rates have been determined by subtracting from the sum of the estimated population of females from 15 to 46 years, for the three years, the number of live births during the same period. The resultant figure represents the sum of the non-pregnant female population of childbearing age. By subtracting the deaths occurring in pregnant women during this time from the total deaths from heart disease among the female population between ages of 15 and 46 years, the result is the number of deaths among non-pregnant women of the specified ages. The death rate for the group of pregnant women was .28 while that for the remainder was .58. The increased rate for the non-pregnant group may be accounted for by the facts that severe heart disease often prevents marriage, and among many married women is regarded as a contra-indication to pregnancy, and that the greatly improved type of care given to the woman who becomes pregnant helps to keep the rate low.

After a very careful study and examination of the cases, 99 women were judged to have died of heart disease, and an additional 74 had heart lesions which may have played a contributory part in causing death. Cases in which heart disease was contributory were distributed as follows: hemorrhage, 11; shock, 9; septicaemia, 26; embolism, 4; pneumonia, 8;

chronic nephritis, 5; anaesthesia, 5; and other extra-puerperal causes, 6. This does not include the large number of cases in which heart disease was reported on the death certificate as being the cause of death, but only those with an antecedent disease of the heart which was exacerbated by the pregnancy and delivery.

The white women were disproportionately affected, for while they included 90 per cent of the deaths from all causes (except abortion and ectopic gestation), they showed 97 per cent (96 out of 99 deaths) of the total deaths from cardiac disease. A similar preponderance of native-born over foreign-born is evident in the deaths from heart disease. Sixty-three (63.6 per cent) of all the deaths from this condition were among native-born women, and 36 (36.4 per cent) among the foreign-born, while the relation of native to foreign-born in the deaths from all causes was 56.1 per cent to 43.9 per cent.

There was a distinct percentage variation in the various age groups. In the earlier years, from fifteen to twenty-four, 4.6 per cent of all the deaths were caused by cardiac disease, while from twenty-five to twenty-nine, 7.2 per cent were due to this cause, and from thirty to thirty-four, 7.7 per cent. Following this age group there was a decrease to 6.2 per cent from thirty-five to thirty-nine and 5.4 per cent of the women over forty years of age. Gravidity plays a role in this variation, as 60 women, or 6.7 per cent of all fatal cases among multigravidae, died of this condition as compared with 39, or 5.7 per cent of the fatal cases among primigravidae.

Only 34 of the 99 gave a history of rheumatic fever, but the histories were, in many instances, so incomplete that this figure undoubtedly represents only a fraction of those from whom the story of some infection akin to rheumatic fever might have been elicited. However, 74 had a definite history of prior heart disease, some with attendant decompensation. In 70 of the patients the attendant discovered and diagnosed the heart damage during pregnancy. In the remaining 29, either it was overlooked in the course of a superficial examination, or the heart was not examined. In view of the very serious import of cardiac disease during pregnancy, it is significant to find that 29 per cent of these patients either did not consult a physician during pregnancy or, through the carelessness or incapacity of the physician consulted, were allowed to go through pregnancy and labor without any added care directed toward the support of the heart. Furthermore, whether or not the heart defect was discovered, only 41 women had what was considered proper care, such as rest in bed, whether at home or in hospital, and the use of supportive drugs, such as digitalis, where it was necessary. Among the 58 who failed to obtain this care, there were some who refused to cooperate with the attendant. Some refused therapeutic operations, and a greater number would not follow the strict regime which the attendant felt necessary to insure a satisfactory outcome.

The damage to the heart was so severe that in 70 instances compensation failed during pregnancy. Eleven of them decompensated in the course of labor and 15 following delivery, while in 3 the history was not available on this point.

Labor originated spontaneously in 48 cases, was induced in 5, and *accouchement forcé* was used in one instance. Forty-five of the patients were never in labor, 11 because a caesarean operation was done before labor set in. The duration of labor was short in the large majority of the 53 women who went into labor or in whom it was induced: 38 were delivered, or died without being delivered, in less than twelve hours, 9 died in less than twenty-four hours and 3 in less than forty-eight hours. The remaining 3 patients were in labor more than forty-eight hours.

Forty of the patients died without being delivered. Twenty-six were delivered spontaneously. Thirty-three were delivered by operation, 17 of these by caesarean operation; version and extraction were employed 3 times; high forceps, once; mid forceps, 4 times; and low forceps, 8 times.

In the opinion of the Advisory Committee, 53 of these deaths were unavoidable. Among the 46 cases which could have been prevented, the responsibility was ascribed to the attendant in 16, and to the patient in 30. The previously mentioned tendency of women with heart disease to ignore the situation, and, in the absence of decompensation, to refuse cooperation with the attendant or to fail to put themselves under competent care, is a decisive factor in preventability. The attendants, where the responsibility was ascribed to them, showed a failure to meet the situation with a sufficiently stringent regime to prevent the break in compensation, or did not properly safeguard the patient during labor.

The prevention of these deaths, as of all deaths from heart disease, will be best effected through a prevention of damage to the heart during the early years of life, since these diseases of the heart are primarily the acquired injuries to valves, and not the degenerative or later-age types. The prevention of repeated pregnancies together with a most careful supervision during pregnancy of every woman with a damaged heart, adequate provision for hospitalization during pregnancy where it is necessary, and finally a carefully conducted delivery, are all of the greatest importance in bringing about a decrease in the deaths associated with this condition.

V

VARIOUS FACTORS AFFECTING PUERPERAL MORTALITY

ANAESTHESIA

THE use of anaesthesia during labor and delivery has grown steadily in extent since its introduction in the last century, and is a problem of the most pressing importance, more so in the United States than in any other country. This has come about to a large extent through pressure from the lay public. The women of the large urban centers have become steadily more insistent in their demands for shorter and less painful parturition, and the accoucheur may disregard these demands only at great risk to his own practice. They reflect significant shifts in social attitudes, and as they have influenced the practice of obstetrics they are pertinent to this study. The wide effects of the increased use of anaesthesia can only be guessed at, but the direct effect of the administration of the anaesthetic in its tendency to lessen and enfeeble the expulsive powers of the uterine musculature must be reflected in an increased necessity for artificial assistance at delivery. The frequent use of instrumentation is based upon the easy accessibility of anaesthesia. It is the opinion of many observers that the increase in the use of anaesthesia is a factor in keeping the maternal mortality rate stationary.

The anaesthesia administered was considered the direct cause of death in 20 cases: 7 of these were spinal neocaine or novocaine; 7, ether; 3, gas oxygen and ether; 2, pernocton; and 1, avertin. There is a difference in the emphasis on these cases, for while the factor of maladministration did not arise in connection with the deaths caused by spinal neocaine, pernocton, and avertin, the deaths from the inhalation anaesthesiae were caused by poor technique on the part of the anaesthetist. There were a few additional deaths in which the anaesthetic was strongly suspected, but the evidence was not convincing enough to justify ascribing the death to the anaesthetic alone. The deaths from the use of spinal anaesthetic occurred in the first two years, 6 of them in 1930 and 1 in 1931. Furthermore, the number of deaths in which spinal anaesthetic was used, regardless of its role in causing death, were 53. Twenty-eight of these occurred in 1930, 17 in 1931 and 8 in 1932. There may be a presumption from this decrease in the general series that the use of this type of anaesthetic during labor is falling into disfavor.

Among all the deaths in the entire series, an anaesthetic was used in 1,017 and not used in 1,024 cases. However, there were 247 cases where delivery was not effected and no operative attempt was made at delivery so there would be that number in which the question of the administration of anaesthetic did not arise, and except for the therapeutic abortions, the question does not arise among the cases of abortion. Excluding the 247 cases in which no attempt was made at delivery and the 310 spontaneous and illegally induced abortions, there remain 1,017 cases in which anaesthesia was used, and 467 cases in which it was not used, giving a ratio of 69 per cent to 31 per cent.

Ether remains the most favored anaesthetic. It was used alone in 478 cases, with gas oxygen in 296 cases, with avertin in 6 cases, and with pernocton in 4 cases. Gas oxygen was used alone in 93 cases, chloroform in 38, spinal novocaine in 53, rectal instillation of ether in 10, local novocaine in 29, ethylene in 9, and pernocton in one. Of all the deaths in which ether, either alone or with gas oxygen, was used—a total of 774—10 (1.2 per cent) died of the effects of the anaesthetic, while with anaesthesia of the spinal type, 7 (13 per cent) died, and of the 5 cases in which pernocton was used, 2 died directly from the anaesthetic. Since the number of women who received ether during delivery is vastly greater than those having spinal anaesthesia, while the number of deaths from each is the same (7), the case fatality rate must be enormously higher for the latter.

Some type of anaesthetic was used with 87.7 per cent of all the patients dying of operative shock, 67.5 per cent of the deaths from septicaemia, 62.9 per cent of those from hemorrhage, 52.8 per cent of those from embolism, 38.5 per cent of those from albuminuria and eclampsia, and 34.9 per cent in those from extra-puerperal causes. The high figure for those who died of shock is quite to be expected and only re-emphasizes the association between anaesthesia and operative deliveries.

The figures are not significant inasmuch as the case rates are not available. If our assumptions are right, ether is still the safest anaesthetic, if one must be given. The undoubtedly high case fatality rate in the use of spinal anaesthetic confirms the Advisory Committee's conviction that this form is entirely unsuitable for use in the parturient. The same can be said of the use of the so-called basic anaesthesiae, pernocton and avertin. They are still in the experimental stage and until further evidence and work upon them can put them more safely into the control of the administrator, the weight of the evidence indicates their unsuitability for use except under the most experienced supervision and direction. Anaesthesia should not be undertaken casually, and should be used in the light of the known fact that an anaesthetic, of whatever type, is a dangerous and profoundly toxic drug. Before exposing the patient to the additional strain of its administration, satisfactory indication for its use must be present. Many multiparous labors are of such short duration that the use of an anaesthetic becomes unnecessary. The responsibility of the accoucheur is primarily to insure a living baby and mother and to accomplish these objectives with the least possible suffering compatible with proper management. The mere alleviation or the entire elimination of pain may be achieved at a cost to mother or infant which should be prohibitive.

OPERATIVE AND SPONTANEOUS DELIVERY

PERHAPS the most prominent feature of the development of modern obstetrical practice has been the steady increase in the proportion of operative deliveries. The termination and curtailment of labor by some intervention, either instrumental or manual, have come to be regarded quite casually and undertaken for indications which, at best, are dubious. This is particularly true in the large cities where the necessary hospital facilities are easily available.

This tendency is the subject of recurrent discussion and is regarded by most observers as one having dangerous potentialities for both mother and child. The rate of operative interference is variously estimated at 10 to 20 per cent, while the optimum is usually regarded as in the neighborhood of 5 per cent (Plass[5]). There are many factors entering into this high percentage: the greatly increased use of anaesthesia, the spread of the knowledge of surgical techniques, the pressure of time upon the attendant, particularly if he be a highly trained specialist, and the increasing demand on the part of the patient for shorter and less painful parturition. Plass regards the fact that the layman has come to consider an operative delivery as one which should command a higher price as a potent factor in increasing the incidence of intervention. The tendency is almost universally disparaged, and for a variety of reasons; the great danger of the misuse of operative procedures by the inexperienced and unskilled as well as the undoubted increase of morbidity and mortality associated with it are most frequently cited.

For the most part the estimate of the incidence of operation at delivery must be calculated from a variety of figures. As yet, except in isolated parts of the country, the birth certificate does not demand a statement of the type of delivery, and without this information no really accurate figures are available. For the three years during which this survey was under way, an effort was made to gain information on this subject by questionnaires issued to the various hospitals of the city. By this method we obtained detailed figures from 67 representative institutions, in which 74.7 per cent of all hospital deliveries occur. In these hospitals, 24.3 per cent of deliveries were operative. In attempting to arrive at an approximate figure for the operative deliveries in the city as a whole, we have considered the fact that the incidence of operative interference is far greater in the hospital than at home, and have estimated the proportion of operative deliveries as 20 per cent for the entire city. We believe this figure to be higher than the actual one, but the error will have the effect of lowering rather than raising the mortality rate following abnormal delivery. During the three years under survey, 348,310 live births occurred in the city. On the basis of the figure given above, 69,665 were operative deliveries and

TABLE 45

DEATHS BY TYPE OF DELIVERY

	TOTAL	OPERATIVE DELIVERIES	SPONTANEOUS DELIVERIES
Total live births	348,310	69,665†	278,645†
Total deaths*	1,300	729	571
Approximate rate per 1,000 live births	3.7	10.5	2.0

*Exclusive of 264 undelivered cases.
†Estimated.

the remaining 278,645 were estimated to be spontaneous deliveries. Table 45 gives the relative death rates based upon this approximation. A total of 1,300 deaths occurred in women who had been delivered at or after the twenty-eighth week of gestation. The 264 deaths which occurred prior to delivery are excluded. Of the 1,300 deaths, 729 followed operative delivery, a rate of 10.5 on the approximate figure of 69,665 operative deliveries, while the 571 deaths following spontaneous delivery represent a rate of 2.0 per 1,000 live births.

Table 46 gives the distribution of cause of death according to the type of delivery. Of all the deaths, 46.6 per cent followed operative delivery. Of the deaths from hemorrhage, 52.3 per cent followed operative delivery; from septicaemia, 55.1 per cent; and from accidents of labor, 84.2 per cent. In the remaining causes of death, the percentage which followed operative delivery was lower than that for the series as a whole. These figures are not at variance with prior assumptions. Hemorrhage not infrequently demands prompt operative interference, but if the operation were undertaken to increase the probability of a satisfactory outcome, and if the undertaking were judicious, one would expect a preponderance of deaths in cases in which such intervention was omitted. The

TABLE 46

CAUSE OF DEATH BY TYPE OF DELIVERY

	TOTAL		OPERATIVE DELIVERIES		SPONTANEOUS DELIVERIES		UNDELIVERED	
	Number	Per cent	Number	Per cent	Number	Per cent	Number	Per cent
Total	1,564	100	729	46.6	571	36.5	264	16.9
Hemorrhage	197	100	103	52.3	74	37.6	20	10.2
Puerperal septicaemia	510	100	281	55.1	224	43.9	5	.98
Albuminuria and eclampsia	231	100	74	32.0	66	28.6	91	39.3
Pernicious vomiting	14	100	—	—	—	—	14	100.0
Phlegmasia alba dolens and embolus	89	100	29	32.6	54	60.7	6	6.7
Accidents of labor	171	100	144	84.2	14	8.2	13	7.6
Accidents of puerperium	8	100	3	37.5	5	62.5	—	—
Extra-puerperal causes	344	100	95	27.6	134	39.0	115	33.4

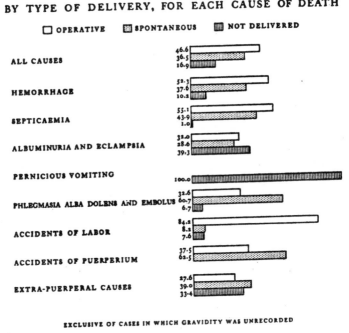

CHART C

PERCENTAGE DISTRIBUTION OF DEATHS
BY TYPE OF DELIVERY, FOR EACH CAUSE OF DEATH

☐ OPERATIVE   ▨ SPONTANEOUS   ▥ NOT DELIVERED

ALL CAUSES
46.6
36.5
16.9

HEMORRHAGE
52.3
37.6
10.2

SEPTICAEMIA
55.1
43.9
1.0

ALBUMINURIA AND ECLAMPSIA
32.0
28.6
39.3

PERNICIOUS VOMITING
100.0

PHLEGMASIA ALBA DOLENS AND EMBOLUS
32.6
60.7
6.7

ACCIDENTS OF LABOR
84.2
8.2
7.6

ACCIDENTS OF PUERPERIUM
37.5
62.5

EXTRA-PUERPERAL CAUSES
27.6
39.0
33.4

EXCLUSIVE OF CASES IN WHICH GRAVIDITY WAS UNRECORDED

results are unsatisfactory because, in numerous instances, the procedure was injudicious and unskilfully performed. In the case of accidents of labor, the vast majority of deaths inevitably followed operative interference, for, by definition, this cause of death includes the shock associated with delivery, and that associated with spontaneous delivery is very small. The difference between the percentages in the deaths from toxaemia was relatively small (32.0 per cent operative and 28.6 per cent spontaneous). The deaths from embolism are, to an overwhelming extent, purely accidental and the division between the normal and abnormal deliveries was probably fortuitous. Among the deaths from extra-puerperal causes, 27.6 per cent followed operative delivery and 39.0 per cent followed spontaneous. Many of these deaths were from cardiac disease, and the absence of any figure for the total incidence of constitutional disease associated with pregnancy makes it impossible to reach any conclusions concerning these cases. Chart C gives a graphic representation of the relations given numerically in Table 46.

There is a definite presupposition that operative procedures greatly increase the hazard from septicaemia. In Table 47 the death rates from septicaemia are divided according to opera-

TABLE 47

SEPTICAEMIA DEATHS BY TYPE OF DELIVERY

	TOTAL	OPERATIVE DELIVERIES	SPONTANEOUS DELIVERIES
Total live births	348,310	69,665†	278,645†
Total septicaemia deaths*	505	281	224
Approximate rate per 1,000 live births	1.4	4.0	0.8

*Exclusive of 5 undelivered cases.
†Estimated.

TABLE 48
AGE AT DEATH BY TYPE OF DELIVERY

	TOTAL		OPERATIVE DELIVERIES		SPONTANEOUS DELIVERIES		UNDELIVERED	
	Number	Per cent	Number	Per cent	Number	Per cent	Number	Per cent
Total	1,564	100.0	729	100.0	571	100.0	264	100.0
15 to 19 years	87	5.6	31	4.3	35	6.1	21	8.0
20 to 24 years	324	20.7	138	18.9	136	23.8	50	18.9
25 to 29 years	432	27.6	206	28.3	161	28.2	65	24.6
30 to 34 years	351	22.4	171	23.5	121	21.2	59	22.3
35 to 39 years	259	16.6	123	16.9	90	15.8	46	17.4
40 years and over	111	7.1	60	8.2	28	4.9	23	8.7

tive and spontaneous deliveries, the same figures being used as those in Table 45. From this, the approximate rate of fatal septicaemia following artificial delivery is seen to be five times that following spontaneous delivery (4.0 to .8).

Table 48 gives the distribution of spontaneous and operative deliveries according to the age of the patients, and in Chart D, the same relations are indicated diagrammatically. Age is apparently unconnected to any important extent with the incidence of operative interference. The increase of operative interference preceding death follows the increase in the percentage of total deaths in the various age groups and nothing significant is evident in the figures.

The distribution of types of operative procedure is given in Table 49, together with the operative attempts which were undertaken prior to the operation which resulted in delivery. Almost one-half of the operations, 304 out of 747, were cae-

TABLE 49

OPERATIVE PROCEDURES BY TYPE OF OPERATION

	OPERATIVE PROCEDURES RESULT-ING IN DELIVERY	OPERATIVE ATTEMPTS ASSOCIATED WITH OPERATIVE DELIVERY
Total	747	46
Caesarean section	304	12
Version and extraction	113	22
Version	9	1
Extraction	29	—
High forceps	24	1
Mid forceps	91	—
Low forceps	145	—
Destructive operations	27	7
Other operative procedures	5	3

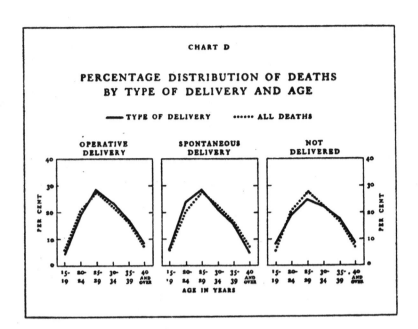

CHART D

PERCENTAGE DISTRIBUTION OF DEATHS
BY TYPE OF DELIVERY AND AGE

——— TYPE OF DELIVERY   ······ ALL DEATHS

124

sarean sections. The distribution of the remaining procedures is not unusual. The large number of high forceps as well as of destructive operations indicates a readiness to undertake operative measures whose usefulness is coming to be regarded with suspicion.

The decisions of the Committee as to the relative preventability of the deaths following normal and abnormal delivery reveal some striking variations. Of all the deaths in this series 64.2 per cent were judged avoidable, but of those following operative delivery, 76.8 per cent were so judged and of those associated with normal delivery, only 48.0 per cent were preventable.

When the preventable deaths are analyzed according to the allocation of responsibility, the physician was held responsible in 76.4 per cent of all cases, but among the cases of operative delivery, the responsibility was ascribed to the physician in 86.8 per cent, and in the spontaneous deliveries in only 55.1 per cent. In these cases incompetence on the part of the at-

TABLE 50

PREVENTABILITY AND RESPONSIBILITY BY TYPE
OF DELIVERY

	TOTAL*		OPERATIVE DELIVERIES		SPONTANEOUS DELIVERIES	
	Num-ber	Per cent	Num-ber	Per cent	Num-ber	Per cent
Total	1,300	100.0	729	100.0	571	100.0
Not preventable	466	35.8	169	23.2	297	52.0
Preventable	834	64.2	560	76.8	274	48.0
Responsibility ascribed to:						
Physician	637	76.4	486	86.8	151	55.1
Patient	170	20.4	67	12.0	103	37.6
Midwife	27	3.2	7	1.3	20	7.3

*Exclusive of 264 undelivered cases.

tendant was thought to be the decisive factor in producing the fatality, and it is of extraordinary significance to find so high a percentage in the deaths following operative delivery.

Out of the preceding tables and figures emerges a definite indication of the significant role played by high operative incidence in the production of a high mortality rate. That the increase in the use of instrumentation brings with it an increased hazard is evident if the relative rates for spontaneous and operative delivery are examined. We cannot disregard the enormous difference between them. The death rate for spontaneous deliveries is less than one-fifth that for the operative. Clearly this represents a serious defect in the management of these cases. It must indicate a broadening of the indications to a point where convenience is included. It is not contended that the rates can be made equal: the necessity for operative interference arises, at times, out of serious abnormalities or disturbances of the mechanism of labor, which, in themselves, greatly increase the hazards. But any such disparity as that shown in these figures is a certain indictment of those undertaking the interference. Frequently there was interference when such was contra-indicated; as often the operative procedure was injudiciously chosen and performed after an exhausting ineffective labor where the maternal resources had been vitiated. Caesarean operations of the classical type were repeatedly undertaken in the face of unmistakable contra-indications, such as prolonged labor with ruptured membranes, after repeated internal examinations, and in the face of existing infection as evidenced by an elevated temperature. The resultant extremely high rate for septicaemia following operative delivery is no more than should be expected. Little enough is known concerning the production of infections, but certainly injury and devitalization of tissue are contributory factors, and these are greatly increased by instrumentation and manual interference.

The Committee has felt that 76.8 per cent of all the deaths following abnormal delivery could have been prevented and, moreover, that the physician was responsible in 86.8 per cent of all the preventable cases in this group. Clearly a reduction of the mortality rate can be achieved through a reduction in operative interference. This may be brought about only through proper education of the lay public and even more of the medical profession. Greater emphasis on the fact that the prenatal period offers an opportunity for the attendant, if he is properly trained and capable, to inform himself with reasonable certainty of his patient's capacity to deliver herself without aid, will enable him to conduct the labor according to a previously determined plan and prevent recourse to artificial aids, which prove so disastrous. It is agreed that emergency measures are far more dangerous than those undertaken at a time and under circumstances which are elected. If all women who could do so were allowed to deliver themselves spontaneously and the indications for instrumentation were reduced to those having real validity, and, further, if the attendant were fully informed, before the onset of labor, as to each individual's capacity to deliver, there is every reason to believe that there would be a reduction in the deaths from childbearing.

CAESAREAN SECTION

WITH increasing use of all surgical maneuvers, the caesarean operation has grown in popularity and its incidence has greatly increased. Hawks[6] has shown that the incidence in the New York Nursery and Child's Hospital rose from 2 in 1,000 deliveries in 1910 to 25 in 1,000 in 1927. Moreover, during this period 3.8 per cent of all deliveries in the private pavilion were by caesarean section, while only 1.2 per cent of all ward deliveries were by caesarean section. Sacket[7] has reported similar distribution among private and ward patients in the New York Lying-In Hospital—4.98 per cent among private patients and 3.28 per cent among ward cases. Davidson[8] has compared the incidence in certain clinics here and abroad. For 1929–1930, he found the incidence at the Rotunda in Dublin to be 1 in 100 and in the Coombe 1 in 145, as compared to 1 in 12 at Boston Lying-In, 1 in 6 at Jefferson, and 1 in 48 at De Lee's clinic. Figures for the Boston City Hospital show an increase from 26 per 1,000 in 1920 to 33.7 per 1,000 in 1929; Chicago Lying-In reports an increase from 6 per 1,000 in 1915–1916 to 30 per 1,000 in 1928–1929. Various observers[6, 9, 10] agree that the incidence is greater among private patients than among those in the wards.

This increase in the relative frequency of the caesarean operation, in the opinion of many observers, is due to ill-advised widening of the indications. Smith[11] is of the opinion that too many caesarean sections are being done on women with borderline pelves where delivery from below would be possible. Miller[12] found a wide variety of indications listed, from "wrecked health" to "abdominal pains." Thompson[13] reviewed the caesarean sections in Los Angeles and found many questionable indications, request alone being sufficient in 4 cases. One hundred and ninety-seven out of his 1,225 operations were done because of previous caesarean sections, and of these women 119 had normal pelves.

Foetal indications have received increasing recognition, and Plass[5] believes the available statistics indicate that many operations done for foetal indications are responsible for infant deaths. When Max Hirsch,[14] in Germany, advocated an increase in the number of caesarean sections as a method of reducing maternal mortality, Winter[15] refuted his statistics by showing he had used only figures from selected clinics and that the general figures failed to indicate any advantage to be obtained from the wider use of this operation. Various observers give different figures for the case fatality rate in the caesarean operation. Martin and Spieckhoff[16] reported 4.4 per cent in 405 abdominal deliveries and 3.5 per cent in 1,114 vaginal operations. Krukenberg and Bodewig[17] found a 10.3 per cent mortality in 426 caesarean sections, while Schröder[18] had a 5 per cent mortality in 280 cases. In the University Gynecology Clinic in Berlin, Hornung[19] reported a caesarean mortality eight to ten times greater than that for vaginal procedures. Even when performed only for the strictest indications, he believes, its fatality rate is always 3 to 4 per cent higher than that of the major vaginal procedures.

The high case fatality rate, in Hawks'[6] opinion, is due to the poor selection of the type of operation. Most observers agree that the low type has great advantages over the classical.[12, 20, 21, 22] The figures indicate a pronounced difference in various hospitals and areas here and abroad. Chicago Lying-In reports 4.76 per cent fatality for the classical type and 1.26 per cent for the low type; in Evanston the comparable rates were 5.2 per cent and .80 per cent. Cleveland Registration Area had a classical section death rate of 7.6 per cent and a low cervical rate of 2.8 per cent. In Brooklyn, the classical section had a 5.9 per cent fatality and the low cervical 4.1 per cent. These figures, which could be repeated many times, indicate the general agreement as to the extra hazard associated with the classical type of section. In the presence of these data, Plass[5] reports a preponderance of the classical over the low cervical type of operation of 5 to 1 in general hospitals and 1.3 to 1 in special hospitals.

The chief argument against the use of the caesarean section

is the high mortality associated with it. In the hands of operators of sufficient judgment to use it only where the proper indications exist, and with surgical skill and experience commensurate with the technical demands of the operation itself, this mortality should be kept as low as that from any elective surgery. The danger lies in the fact that its use will not be confined to those qualified, but will be extended to those in whose inexperienced hands the hazard becomes greatly augmented. Moreover, Miller[12] believes that the proportion of living mothers and infants obtained by caesarean operation fails to justify its use and that average mortality figures show plainly that caesarean is a dangerous measure.

In view of these opinions from outstanding observers, the figures for caesarean operation in this series are significant.

Among all the deaths, 304 died following a caesarean section and 6 others died while a caesarean was being attempted —a total of 310 cases. This represents 19.8 per cent of all deaths in this group except those following the abortions and extra-uterine gestations. In the hospitals for which we have the detailed figures as to number and type of deliveries, 3,963 caesareans were performed, and this was 2.2 per cent of all deliveries. This is an average of wide variants, one of the largest hospitals averaging almost 1,000 deliveries a year, with an incidence of caesarean section of 5.3 per cent, while another having about the same number of deliveries had only .4 per cent caesarean section. Two hundred and forty of the 310 deaths occurred in these institutions, a case fatality of 6.1 per cent. The same variation was evident in this percentage: in 22 hospitals the case mortality was over 10 per cent and in 19 hospitals it was less than 4 per cent. There is, of course, a wide variation in the type of patient received, and this will affect both the number of sections performed and the results obtained, but the great differences in percentage of incidence and of mortality reflect more than a mere difference in the type of patient received. They are indicative also of the broad diversity in the indications accepted for the operation, and to some extent the quality of judgment and skill of the attendants.

One hundred and eighty-two, 20.7 per cent of the deaths among native-born women, and 128, 18.7 per cent of the deaths among the foreign-born, constitute this group. The operation is relatively of more frequent occurrence among the white women than among the Negro: it was performed for 285 (20.5 per cent) of the former and 25 (14.7 per cent) of the latter. Table 51 gives the distribution according to the age and gravidity of the patients. Throughout, it is seen that the ratio of deaths after caesarean section to all deaths increases with age. This is true for all cases as well as for primigravidae and multigravidae considered separately. Twenty-three and eight-tenths per cent of all deaths among primigravidae and

TABLE 51

CAESAREAN SECTION DEATHS BY AGE AND GRAVIDITY

	TOTAL	15 TO 19 YEARS	20 TO 29 YEARS	30 TO 39 YEARS	40 YEARS AND OVER
Total deaths*	1,564	87	756	610	111
Caesarean section†	310	12	141	129	28
Per cent of total deaths	*19.8*	*13.8*	*18.7*	*21.1*	*25.2*
Primigravidae: total‡	682	78	428	157	19
Caesarean section**	162	11	86	52	13
Per cent of total primigravidae	*23.8*	*14.1*	*20.1*	*33.1*	*68.4*
Multigravidae: total‡	874	9	327	447	91
Caesarean section**	147	1	55	76	15
Per cent of total multigravidae	*16.8*	*11.1*	*16.8*	*17.0*	*16.5*

*Exclusive of deaths following abortion and ectopic gestation.
†Including 6 attempted caesareans.
‡Excluding 8 cases of which the gravidity was unknown.
**Excluding one case of which the gravidity was unknown.

16.8 per cent of those among multigravidae followed caesarean section. In the age group 15 to 19 years, 14.1 per cent of the women dying in their first pregnancy and 11.1 per cent of those dying in later pregnancies had caesarean section prior to death. From 20 to 29 years, the percentages rose to 20.1 for the primigravidae and 16.8 for multigravidae. There is a still further increase to 33.1 per cent and 17.0 per cent for primigravidae and multigravidae, respectively, between the ages of 30 and 39 years, while over 40 years, 68.4 per cent of all primigravidous deaths were preceded by caesarean section and the figure for multigravidae dropped to 16.5 per cent. In general, and in all age groups, a larger proportion of the deaths among primigravidae than among the multigravidae followed caesarean operation. The naturally longer and somewhat more difficult first labor, as compared to subsequent labors, no doubt accounts for the increased proportion. The tendency to regard late primigravidity as an indication for the performance of a caesarean section is reflected in the later age groups.

The principal cause of death was some form of infection, which occurred in 148 cases (47.7 per cent of all deaths following caesarean); 65 died as the direct result of the shock of the operation; 24 from albuminuria and eclampsia, 23 from hemorrhage, 9 from embolism, 1 from puerperal psychosis, and 40 from various extra-puerperal causes.

The indications given for the operation were as follows: abnormal pelvis, 114; cephalo-pelvic disproportion, 19; inertia and prolonged labor, 22; dystocia including Bandl's ring, 17; fibroids, 12; previous section, 7; malpresentation, 5; previous operation on the soft parts, 3; placenta praevia, 26; premature separation of the placenta, 16; albuminuria and eclampsia, 33; ruptured uterus, 5; cardiac disease, 33; and extra-puerperal conditions, other than cardiac, 8. In some instances, the indication for which the operation was undertaken was, in turn, the ultimate cause of death. Thus 42 cases were operated upon because of antepartum hemorrhage from a prematurely separated or abnormally situated placenta; 23 of these subsequently died of hemorrhage. Twenty-four of the 33 cases of albuminuria and eclampsia which had caesarean sections died of the toxaemia and to this extent the operation must be considered as having failed of its objective. Further consideration of the indications reveals others which are of doubtful validity. Posterior or other abnormal presentation or position are not generally regarded as sufficient indication for so radical a procedure, nor is the caesarean operation regarded as the treatment of choice in the case of pregnancy toxaemia, for which it was undertaken in 33 cases. In cases of prolonged or obstructed labor, every effort should be directed toward delivery by the normal route, since the incidence of infection following caesarean sections under such circumstances is extremely high. In many instances, careful prenatal examination might have brought to light the condition which was the underlying cause of the prolonged or obstructed labor. A proper prognosis having been made, then the necessary operation could have been performed at the proper time. The same might apply to the dystocias. One would derive the impression that among these operations there were a large number which could have been avoided had there been proper care during pregnancy with correct prognosis of labor and delivery and the avoidance of those developments of labor which make the caesarean operation especially hazardous.

The classical type of operation was greatly preponderant, occurring in 61.9 per cent of the deaths following caesarean. There were 68 low flap operations, 13 Porro type, 4 Latzko, and 1 De Lee, and in 32 cases the type was not recorded.

There were 100 operations performed before the onset of labor, in 120 labor had been in progress less than 24 hours, in 89 more than 24 hours, and in one case the duration of labor was not known. In 182 cases the operation was undertaken as an emergency measure, and in the remaining 128 the attendant had chosen the operation in advance or had allowed a trial labor to make certain that caesarean would be required. In 129 cases the membranes had been ruptured prior to operation.

While a previous caesarean section was given as the principal indication in only 7 cases, it had been performed in previous pregnancies on 37 of the patients. Twenty-six had had only one caesarean section, 8 had had 2, and 3 had had 3 prior to the fatal one.

Ether, following a nitrous oxide and oxygen induction, was the most common anaesthetic, being used in 215 of the cases; spinal neocaine or novocaine was used in 37 cases, in many of which the operation was undertaken because of eclampsia; nitrous oxide and oxygen were used alone in 29; local infiltration in 15; ethylene in 7; avertin in 4; pernocton in 2, and chloroform in 1 case.

The operations resulted in 257 live babies, 80.1 per cent of the total babies delivered or on whom delivery was attempted by this method. This is a larger percentage of live babies than that in the series as a whole, where only 59.7 per cent were born alive, 23.6 per cent were stillborn, and 16.7 per cent were never delivered. This preponderance of live babies may be due to the tendency to accept foetal indications as valid for the performance of a caesarean section and to hold the outcome for the foetus of greater importance than that for the mother.

Peritonitis and septicaemia as the predominant cause of death following caesarean section require special mention, and have been considered in detail in the discussion of puerperal septicaemia, but it will not be out of place to re-state some of the facts here. There were 148 deaths from peritonitis or septicaemia out of the 304 caesarean sections in the series. This is 48.6 per cent of all deaths following this operation.

We have mentioned previously the frequent performance of the classical section on potentially infected patients. Other deaths from septicaemia have undoubtedly taken place because of faulty technique at operation on the part of the physician. The use of the caesarean section as a measure of desperation has been a factor in the high rate of infection, and the Committee feels that its performance at an inauspicious time is, in large measure, responsible for the very unsatisfactory results. In Table 52, the type of operation performed in the cases which subsequently died of infection is shown according to the length of labor: 22.7 per cent of the intra-peritoneal type were performed before the onset of labor, 42.3 per cent when labor had been in progress less than twenty-four hours, and 35.0 per cent on women who had been in labor more than twenty-four hours. Half of the women who

TABLE 52

SEPTICAEMIA DEATHS FOLLOWING CAESAREAN
SECTION, BY TYPE OF OPERATION AND
DURATION OF ANTECEDENT LABOR

	TOTAL		INTRA-PERITONEAL*		EXTRA-PERITONEAL		TYPE UNKNOWN	
	Number	Per cent	Number	Per cent	Number	Per cent	Number	Per cent
Total	148	*100.0*	97	*100.0*	39	*100.0*	12	*100.0*
Not in labor	28	*18.9*	22	*22.7*	5	*12.8*	1	*8.3*
Less than 24 hours	59	*39.9*	41	*42.3*	11	*28.2*	7	*58.3*
24 to 48 hours	36	*24.3*	20	*20.6*	14	*35.9*	2	*16.7*
48 hours and over	25	*16.9*	14	*14.4*	9	*23.1*	2	*16.7*

*Includes 5 Porros.

had caesarean sections after more than twenty-four hours of labor were subjected to the greatly augmented risk of infection attendant upon the classical type of operation.

Table 53 shows the same relationship according to the rupture of the membranes. Twenty and six-tenths per cent of the women who died of infection following an intra-peritoneal section had had membranes ruptured for more than twenty-four hours at the time of operation.

TABLE 53

SEPTICAEMIA DEATHS FOLLOWING CAESAREAN
SECTION, BY TYPE OF OPERATION AND
TIME OF RUPTURE OF MEMBRANES

	TOTAL		INTRA-PERITONEAL*		EXTRA-PERITONEAL		TYPE UNKNOWN	
	Number	Per cent	Number	Per cent	Number	Per cent	Number	Per cent
Total	148	100.0	97	100.0	39	100.0	12	100.0
Membranes not ruptured prior to operation	66	44.6	51	52.6	10	25.6	5	41.7
Membranes ruptured less than 24 hours	45	30.4	25	25.8	14	35.9	6	50.3
Membranes ruptured 24 to 48 hours	16	10.8	10	10.3	6	15.4	—	—
Membranes ruptured over 48 hours	18	12.2	10	10.3	7	17.9	1	8.3
Membranes ruptured—time not reported	3	2.0	1	1.0	2	5.1	—	—

*Includes 5 Porros.

Table 54 shows the type of operation in relation to the question whether it was undertaken as an elective or emergency measure. It is significant to note that 62.9 per cent of the intra-peritoneal operations which were followed by a fatal infection were undertaken as emergency measures. Case No. 1143 is illustrative of this type of case: a primigravida of 32 who had insufficient prenatal care went into labor spontaneously. Presentation was breech, and in the course of attempt-

TABLE 54

SEPTICAEMIA DEATHS FOLLOWING CAESAREAN
SECTION, DISTRIBUTED BETWEEN ELECTIVE
AND EMERGENCY OPERATIONS

	TOTAL		INTRA-PERITONEAL*		EXTRA-PERITONEAL		TYPE UNKNOWN	
	Num-ber	Per cent	Num-ber	Per cent	Num-ber	Per cent	Num-ber	Per cent
Total	148	100.0	97	100.0	39	100.0	12	100.0
Elective	53	35.8	36	37.1	9	23.1	8	66.7
Emergency	95	64.2	61	62.9	30	76.9	4	33.3

*Includes 5 Porros.

ing to deliver from below, the foetal body was accidentally severed and the contents of its abdominal cavity then presented. At this time the head was found to be too large to deliver and the attendant performed a classical caesarean section. Death from peritonitis followed four days later.

The preponderance of responsible opinion and the weight of evidence point to the fact that the classical type of caesarean operation carries with it an increased danger of infection and the risk is still further increased when the patient, by reason of antecedent labor with ruptured membranes, is already potentially infected. All the data obtained concerning the women who died of infection following caesarean section confirm this assumption.

In summary, the incidence of caesarean section in the hospitals of the city is seen to be high—2.2 per cent of all deliveries, while it preceded almost a fifth of all deaths (19.8 per cent). This extremely high incidence in the series is a matter of concern. The indications as given on the records include some, such as toxaemia, which some authorities no longer regard as valid. Slight degrees of pelvic contraction, in many instances, do not preclude delivery by the normal route, while malpresentation should rarely make a caesarean section necessary. Dystocia, prolonged labor, and similar terms are not definite ones, and doubt must be expressed as to the propriety of many of the operations undertaken for these reasons.

More serious and closely related to the indications is the question of the choice of operation and the time of its performance. There is little doubt that in these two elements the greatest danger lies. We have indicated the great preponderance of the classical type. There were only 128 elective operations, but the classical type was used in 192 cases. Furthermore, the use of the low flap operation was common among the elective operations, so that the discrepancy between these two figures is greater than it appears. Many of the operations were performed after twenty-four hours of labor, as extreme emergency measures, and in these cases the use of the classical type was not uncommon, although entirely contra-indicated. The repeated failure to make an accurate prognosis of labor and delivery contributed to the high proportion of emergency operations. The performance of a caesarean section is technically less demanding than the more difficult vaginal procedures. Consequently, it is subjected to misuse and pressed into service when better judgment and greater skill would permit delivery by the less hazardous normal route.

It seems to the Advisory Committee that the foregoing data reveal an excessive use of the caesarean section, and, as a result, a great increase in the mortality. Only 54 of these deaths could be considered not preventable. The great majority of the remainder were the result of faulty judgment and lack of skill on the part of the attendants. This immoderate use of so dangerous a procedure is traceable to a variety of influences. The lack of appreciation of the surgical demands of the procedure itself, the unwarrantable widening of the indications, the possible use of the operation merely because of the desire on the part of some physicians to increase their surgical experience, are all contributory.

The indications for the caesarean operation need re-statement and further limitation to really valid causes, such as severe degrees of contraction of the pelvis. More careful observation during the prenatal period should provide the opportunity for making a proper prognosis of labor and delivery, and so eliminate the use of the caesarean section as a last resort. The use of the classical type should be limited to the elective operation. The provision of the most highly trained specialist for every woman whose labor shows any abnormality will prevent the use of the caesarean section when less dangerous methods of delivery could be used by those having the requisite training and skill. Sharp reduction in the number of caesarean sections performed is to be strongly recommended. Where the operation is required, only those whose training in abdominal surgery is adequate to insure proper performance of the operation should be considered suitable operators. Only by this definite narrowing of its use to the legitimate occasion demanding it, as well as the provision of capable operators, can a decrease in these deaths be achieved.

HOSPITAL AND HOME DELIVERY

In discussing these cases, we will base our figures on the cases in which delivery was effected at or after the twenty-eighth week of gestation, excluding all abortions, ectopic gestations, and deaths which took place prior to delivery.

For the three-year period under examination, 102,105 deliveries, 29.3 per cent of the 348,310 live births, occurred in the home. During the same period, 189 deaths, 14.5 per cent of the 1,300 deaths under consideration, followed delivery in the home. The relative death rates per 1,000 live births for

TABLE 55

DEATHS BY PLACE OF DELIVERY

	TOTAL	HOSPITAL DELIVERIES	HOME DELIVERIES
Total live births	348,310	246,205	102,105
Total deaths*	1,300	1,111	189
Rate per 1,000 live births	3.7	4.5	1.9

*Exclusive of 264 undelivered cases.

hospital and home deliveries are given in Table 55. The rate
for deliveries at home is 1.9, and for hospital deliveries, 4.5.
This very great difference may be partly accounted for by the
equally great difference between types of delivery done in
the two places. Only those deliveries which are unassociated
with serious abnormalities or require the less hazardous and
difficult operative terminations will be undertaken at home.
Where the labor becomes unduly prolonged or serious accidents occur in its course or the prognosis is unfavorable for a
spontaneous termination, the attendant will attempt to place
the case in a hospital. There are always a certain number of
patients who refuse hospitalization under any circumstances
and for whom the accoucheur must undertake delivery at
home regardless of the operative requirements.

Table 56 shows the relation between cause of death and
place of delivery. Since the greatest percentage of all deliveries occurred in hospitals, it is inevitable that this proportion
will be maintained throughout the various causes of death.
The ratio of hospital to home deliveries in the total series was
85.5 per cent to 14.5 per cent. Among the deaths from hemorrhage, the percentage of home deliveries (15.3) exceeded
the general average; this was true of puerperal septicaemia
also where the percentage rose to 18.2, and in the group of
phlegmasia alba dolens and embolism, where it was 15.7. In

TABLE 56
CAUSE OF DEATH BY PLACE OF DELIVERY

	TOTAL*		HOSPITAL DELIVERIES		HOME DELIVERIES	
	Number	Per cent	Number	Per cent	Number	Per cent
Total	1,300	100	1,111	85.5	189	14.5
Hemorrhage	177	100	150	84.7	27	15.3
Puerperal septicaemia	505	100	413	81.8	92	18.2
Albuminuria and eclampsia	140	100	128	91.4	12	8.6
Phlegmasia alba dolens and embolus	83	100	70	84.3	13	15.7
Accidents of labor	158	100	146	92.4	12	7.6
Accidents of puerperium	8	100	8	100.0	—	—
Extra-puerperal causes	229	100	196	85.6	33	14.4

*Exclusive of 264 undelivered cases.

TABLE 57
OPERATIVE AND SPONTANEOUS DELIVERIES BY PLACE OF DELIVERY

	TOTAL		HOSPITAL DELIVERIES		HOME DELIVERIES	
	Number	Per cent	Number	Per cent	Number	Per cent
Total deaths*	1,300	100	1,111	85.5	189	14.5
Operative delivery	729	100	690	94.7	39	5.3
Spontaneous delivery	571	100	421	73.7	150	26.3

*Exclusive of 264 undelivered cases.

TABLE 58
DEATHS BY NATIVITY AND PLACE OF DELIVERY

	TOTAL		HOSPITAL DELIVERIES		HOME DELIVERIES	
	Number	Per cent	Number	Per cent	Number	Per cent
Total deaths*	1,300	100	1,111	85.5	189	14.5
Native-born	723	100	629	87.0	94	13.0
Foreign-born	577	100	482	83.5	95	16.5

*Exclusive of 264 undelivered cases (155 native-born and 109 foreign-born).

the remainder, the percentage of home deliveries was lower than the average. The relations here are those to be expected. The serious eclampsias and the difficult, obstructed, and prolonged labors are the cases that most surely require and receive hospital treatment, and the proportions of deaths reflect this relationship between the two.

Of all the operative deliveries in this series, 94.7 per cent were performed in hospital (Table 57); 73.7 per cent of the spontaneous deliveries were also in hospital. The 39 operative deliveries performed at home, which represent 5.3 per cent of the total operative deliveries, were divided as follows: 12 versions and extractions, 5 extractions, 3 high forceps, 10 mid forceps, 9 low forceps, and 1 operation of which the type was unknown. The extra operative procedure is accounted for by the fact that one pair of twins required two operative procedures—a version and extraction with an additional extraction.

Table 58 gives the distribution of hospital and home deliveries according to the nativity of the patient. Of the fatal confinements among native-born women, 87.0 per cent occurred in hospital and 13.0 per cent at home, while among foreign-born women, 83.5 per cent occurred in hospitals and 16.5 per cent in the home. The figures are significant only in so far as they reflect the probable attitudes of foreign and native-born women to home confinement.

It is to be regretted that the figures which are available do not make possible any estimate of true relative death rates for home and hospital deliveries. Without accurate figures as to the type of delivery done in the home, no true evaluation would be possible. There are factors operating in each place which indubitably affect the rates, but the extent to which they do so is not susceptible of measurement. One outstanding difference between the two sets of cases is the great disparity between the number of operative deliveries done in

hospitals and at home. To a great extent this difference is in-
herent in the types of cases, but there can be little doubt that
the ready facilities of a hospital tend to casual operative interference, while conditions at home preclude operation unless
there are urgent indications. The busy specialist in a well-
equipped hospital may readily apply forceps to terminate a
labor which would, in a slightly longer time, come to a spontaneous termination, while the practitioner at home must
avoid undertaking maneuvers which demand equipment and
assistance not easily obtainable there. In the discussion on
midwife practice in Chapter VIII, attention is called to a factor which is pertinent to the present question, namely, that
the patient who is delivered at home is subjected to fewer potential sources of danger. There are fewer attendants in home
deliveries, and the possibility of infection from other patients
is eliminated entirely.

The hospital is and will remain the only proper environment for the care and management of the abnormalities of
pregnancy, labor, and delivery. The great increase in the hospitalization of the normal parturient has failed to bring the
hoped-for reduction in puerperal morbidity and mortality,
and this in spite of great advances in our knowledge of the
processes involved and the proper way of treating them. It
would seem that the present attitude toward home confinement requires re-examination, and a program looking toward
an increase in the practice of domiciliary obstetrics deserves
careful investigation.

PRENATAL CARE

As we noted in Chapter III, in passing judgment on the total
care received in any given case the quality of the prenatal
care was taken into account and a decision as to preventability
was frequently based upon this factor. It is very difficult to
offer any conclusions in regard to the influence of prenatal

care upon the outcome of the case. The improper conduct of delivery will vitiate adequate care during pregnancy, and the two elements become confused and inseparable. We cannot, therefore, do more than offer the data without attempting to draw conclusions from them, and this section will be devoted chiefly to an explanation of the basis on which we have judged the adequacy of prenatal care. The criteria given here do not, of necessity, represent an ultimate decision as to the requirements for proper and satisfactory prenatal care; recommendations arising out of the study will be submitted in Chapter IX.

The requirements of the "Fifteen States Study"[1] were set out with the definiteness and inflexibility that was necessary to assure uniformity in reporting, where the investigators were widely separated and not in association with those handling, studying, and correlating the accumulated material. There was no necessity for such rigidity in this inquiry, because the field investigators were in constant close association with the material and if the information on any given case proved an insufficient basis for the Advisory Committee's judgment, further and more extensive data were requested and obtained. As a basis for comparison, however, we were guided in our analysis and recording of prenatal care by the recommendations and forms of the Children's Bureau of the Department of Labor, as follows:

First visit to clinic or physician to be made at or before the fifth calendar month of gestation. A general physical examination [see sample of form used, reproduced on page 261] including an examination of the heart and lungs, at this time. Pelvic measurements at or before the seventh month. Urinalysis and systolic and diastolic blood pressure readings at the time of the first visit and at all subsequent visits. Visits to the clinic or physician monthly up to the ninth month and weekly thereafter.

We accepted these requisites established by the Children's Bureau of the Department of Labor. We did not require a Wassermann examination, but we added certain requirements, as follows:

A careful personal history including infectious diseases and past pregnancies. A history of the present pregnancy to elicit any symptoms bearing on possible abnormalities or a toxaemia. Social service for clinic patients adequate to insure the patient's cooperation with the clinic.

Because of the detailed information which was made available on almost every case investigated, it was possible to vary from the inflexible standards outlined above and, it is hoped, to arrive at a truer judgment of the quality of the prenatal care obtained. If a patient actually received care by which her health was safeguarded, if deviations from normal were promptly observed and correctly treated and accurate prognosis of labor was arrived at in advance, such care was regarded as adequate whether or not it fitted exactly into the schedule. The emphasis was not on how much care the patient received, but rather on its quality. Where there was negligence or incompetence on the part of the attendant, care could not be classified as adequate. The patient who visited her physician at regular, frequent intervals and received examination at each visit, but after more than forty-eight hours of active labor required a caesarean section because of a generally contracted pelvis, cannot be thought to have had adequate prenatal care, and to this mismanagement the circumstances terminating in her death are attributable.

Throughout the foregoing pages we have indicated the probable relation of prenatal care to particular causes of death or other factors in mortality. In Table 59 the adequacy of prenatal care is indicated for each group of deaths by cause.

TABLE 59

PRENATAL CARE, BY CAUSE OF DEATH

(Exclusive of deaths following abortion and ectopic gestation)

	TOTAL		ADEQUATE PRENATAL CARE		INADEQUATE OR NO PRENATAL CARE	
	Number	Per cent	Number	Per cent	Number	Per cent
Total	1,564	*100*	600	*38.3*	964	*61.6*
Hemorrhage	197	*100*	72	*36.6*	125	*63.5*
Puerperal septicaemia	510	*100*	199	*39.0*	311	*61.0*
Albuminuria and eclampsia	231	*100*	65	*28.1*	166	*71.9*
Pernicious vomiting	14	*100*	2	*14.3*	12	*85.7*
Phlegmasia alba dolens and embolus	89	*100*	52	*58.4*	37	*41.6*
Accidents of labor	171	*100*	79	*46.2*	92	*53.8*
Accidents of puerperium	8	*100*	4	*50.0*	4	*50.0*
Extra-puerperal causes	344	*100*	127	*36.9*	217	*63.1*

Cases with inadequate care and those with none have been placed together; very often those with inadequate care had, in reality, so little that it amounted to none at all. The percentage of cases which had proper prenatal care is extremely low—38.3 for all deaths; considerably less for toxaemia and pernicious vomiting, as would be expected; slightly less for hemorrhage and extra-puerperal causes; and more for septicaemia, emboli, accidents of labor, and accidents of the puerperium.

LIVE BIRTHS AND STILLBIRTHS

THERE were 381 stillbirths in this series, giving a percentage of 28.3. Table 60 shows their distribution according to cause of the mother's death. As was to be expected, hemorrhage, albuminuria and eclampsia, and accidents of labor showed the highest percentages of stillbirths, 34.8, 45.2, and 46.0 per cent, respectively.

TABLE 60

LIVE BIRTHS AND STILLBIRTHS BY CAUSE OF DEATH

(*Exclusive of 270 not delivered, or delivered postmortem*)

	TOTAL BABIES		BORN ALIVE		STILLBORN	
	Num-ber	Per cent	Num-ber	Per cent	Num-ber	Per cent
Total	1,345	100	964	71.7	381	28.3
Hemorrhage	184	100	120	65.2	64	34.8
Puerperal septicaemia	520	100	409	78.7	111	21.3
Albuminuria and eclampsia	146	100	80	54.8	66	45.2
Phlegmasia alba dolens and em-bolus	86	100	74	86.0	12	14.0
Accidents of labor	161	100	87	54.0	74	46.0
Accidents of puerperium	8	100	6	75.0	2	25.0
Extra-puerperal causes	240	100	188	78.3	52	21.7

Table 61 shows the relationship of stillbirths to adequate prenatal care. To mothers who had adequate care, 21.2 per cent of the babies were stillborn; to those who had inadequate or no care 33.3 per cent were stillborn. Prenatal care is of significance in the causes of death associated with the higher foetal mortality, and the figures probably reflect this relationship.

TABLE 61

LIVE BIRTHS AND STILLBIRTHS BY PRENATAL CARE

(*Exclusive of 270 not delivered, or delivered postmortem*)

	TOTAL BABIES		BORN ALIVE		STILLBORN	
	Num-ber	Per cent	Num-ber	Per cent	Num-ber	Per cent
Total	1,345	100	964	71.7	381	28.3
Adequate prenatal care	556	100	438	78.8	118	21.2
Inadequate or no prenatal care	789	100	526	66.7	263	33.3

ECONOMIC STATUS

THE subject of maternity care is one of wide social and economic as well as medical concern. Any and all of the elements of the woman's life that bear on her procreative function are a part of that subject, and it is difficult to find any element in her life that does not impinge upon that function. Her racial and national origin will influence her physical development and endowments for childbearing; her social status will condition her attitudes toward her problem, which attitudes are of the utmost importance in determining the type of care she will seek for herself; her economic position with its effect on her diet and living conditions will not only alter, to some extent, the operation of the previous factors, but will fix the type of care to which she will have access. The structure of the medical service of a community is keyed to these social and economic variants. To the economically fortunate, there is offered the service of the private practitioner graded in cost to meet the resources of each group. To the underprivileged there is supplied free medical service through the agencies of the community, both public and private. In supplying this service, the complexity and wide ramifications of the problem are recognized. The establishment of a social service department in every hospital testifies to the fact that the community has accepted the responsibility for more than the purely medical aspect of health care. It is one function to determine the condition and needs of each woman during her pregnancy, delivery, and puerperium. It is another, perhaps more difficult and certainly more important, so to adjust the woman that she can and will take full advantage of the services offered for her welfare. The mother of small children, in a very poor home entirely cared for by herself, needs more than the advice given her by the clinic physician. If she requires special treatment, perhaps added rest and special diets, some way must be provided to make it possible for her to avail herself of them. Household cares must be adjusted or relieved, and all the multifarious details of the program be made practically possible. An efficient, properly functioning service must be measured by the extent to which there is success in removing the economic barriers to the individual woman's enjoyment of satisfactory maternity care.

In Chapter VI the available hospital facilities in the city are analyzed. From that chapter it is evident that, in theory at least, the organization of the medical services of the city and coordinated private agencies provides adequate medical care of high quality to those who are unable to purchase it. It is the aim of these agencies to assure to all members of the community as good a quality of medical care as is available to any. Such service is based on the principle that the economic status of the individual shall never operate to deprive her of what is held to be a necessity.

In any examination of maternity care the point at issue is to determine to what extent such services measure up to their theoretical commitments. Do they, in fact, provide the sufficient and proper care for which they were designed? Does the economic status of the individual affect the hazards of childbearing? Are those who are able to pay for their care being provided with as high a quality of professional service as they believe themselves to be?

In order to judge this element of the situation properly, an elaborate study of the social and economic factors operating in every case would be required. This has not been possible, but we have attempted to make an approximation. To do this, we have used material very generously made accessible by the research department of the Welfare Council of New York City—a complete survey of the homes of the city according to costs and rentals, by health areas.[23] Since our figures for individual health areas are too small to be of significance, it was necessary to combine the data to make a few larger areas. This was done by making four groupings according to the approximate average rentals of the homes in every area. In this way all the health areas in which the average rentals were from $10.00 to $20.00 per month were placed in one group; those in which the rentals were $20.00 to $50.00 in a second group; those with an average rental between $50.00 and $100.00 per month in a third group, and those few areas in which the average monthly rental was over $100.00 in the fourth group. The health areas of the city were thus gathered into four large economic groups. We have designated these groups by the letters, A, B, C and D, running from the lowest to the highest economic stratum, and will use those designations throughout the succeeding paragraphs.

Some factors are accepted as being definite and certain concomitants of economic status. Group A represents slum population: extreme poverty with intense overcrowding, filth, and widespread ignorance. The population of this group is, to a large extent, foreign born or of foreign extraction, and represents predominately the day-laborer class. It is from these areas that the bulk of those requiring free medical care is drawn.

Group B also represents a depressed economic group, the artisan class, but here the living conditions are of a slightly improved quality; congestion is less pronounced and the general standard of living is superior to that in the slum areas. This population, to a large extent, must also rely on municipal and voluntary hospitals to supply medical care for which it cannot pay.

Group C represents a distinct improvement in standards of living, as well as in general education. The residents of these areas are largely the so-called white-collar group. They are able, as a group, to pay for their medical care, and represent the clientele of the general practitioner and less highly trained specialists.

Group D is composed of those most favorably situated economically. The highest grade of living standards with the most widespread education prevails in this group, in which women are able to avail themselves of the services of the ablest physicians and the best equipped hospitals.

In Table 62 the puerperal death rates for the four groups are given. The general rate is 4.4 per thousand live births. In Group A, the rate of 4.9 is above the average; in Group B, it drops to 4.2, slightly below; in Group C, it rises to 4.6, and in Group D, drops well below the average to 3.9. The highest death rate is among the slum population, and the lowest rate among the members of the most fortunate group. This might be expected, although it is at variance with a study made in Aberdeen on the relation between slum conditions and the incidence of puerperal septicaemia.[1] However, it is in accord with the assumption based on the conditions which prevail in these groups. When we examine the rates for the other two groups, there is a reversal of the expected order. For in Group B the rate is lower than in Group C, where the standard of living is appreciably higher. The reason for this variation is not apparent in the form of conclusive data. Consideration of the groups themselves offers some possible clues.

TABLE 62
DEATHS BY ECONOMIC GROUP

	TOTAL	GROUP A	GROUP B	GROUP C	GROUP D
Live births	341,879	56,019	155,457	125,241	5,162
Deaths* Rate per 1,000 live births	1,520 4.4	275 4.9	653 4.2	572 4.6	20 3.9

*Exclusive of deaths following abortion and ectopic gestation and of non-residents.

Groups A and B include the bulk of the patients seeking admission to the free wards in the city and other hospitals offering medical care without cost. In Group C a smaller percentage of the population seeks free medical care. They are able to pay a physician, but they are not in a position to avail themselves of the services of the most highly trained and skilful specialists. They are, consequently, cared for by the general practitioner or the younger and less experienced specialist, and the difference in the results may be related to the difference in the ability of the two groups of physicians.

In Table 63, we have classified the deaths according to the place of delivery, and in the case of hospital deliveries, according to the type of hospital: whether municipal, obstetrical, voluntary, or proprietary. (The classification of hospitals is considered in detail in Chapter VI.)

Twenty-nine per cent of the deaths occurring in Group A were preceded by delivery in a municipal hospital. This is the highest percentage of any group, the percentage of patients delivered in municipal hospitals declining rapidly to 5.0 for Group D. Sixteen and three-tenths per cent of the deaths in Group A followed delivery in obstetrical hospitals, 22.6 per cent in voluntary hospitals, 11.3 per cent in proprietary hospitals, and 20.8 per cent in the home. The bulk of these deliveries, even those performed outside municipal hospitals, were on the ward services, except for the 25 deliveries performed in proprietary hospitals.

In Group B, 21.8 per cent of the deliveries in the series were in municipal hospitals, 7.3 per cent in obstetrical, 36.6 per cent in voluntary, and 18.7 per cent in proprietary institutions, while 15.7 per cent were performed at home. This distribution shows a decrease in the percentage seeking care in municipal and obstetrical hospitals and a marked increase in those going to the voluntary and proprietary types.

TABLE 63

DEATHS BY ECONOMIC GROUP AND PLACE OF DELIVERY

(Exclusive of deaths following abortion and ectopic gestation and of undelivered cases)

	TOTAL		GROUP A		GROUP B		GROUP C		GROUP D		NON-RESIDENT	
	Number	Per cent	Number	Per cent	Number	Per cent	Number	Per cent	Number	Per cent	Number	Per cent
Total	1,300	100.0	221	100.0	536	100.0	487	100.0	20	100.0	36	100.0
Deliveries in hospitals:												
Municipal hospitals	272	20.9	64	29.0	117	21.8	89	18.3	1	5.0	1	2.8
Obstetrical hospitals	148	11.4	36	16.3	39	7.3	59	12.1	7	35.0	7	19.4
Voluntary hospitals	425	32.7	50	22.6	196	36.6	160	32.9	5	25.0	14	38.9
Proprietary hospitals	266	20.5	25	11.3	100	18.7	126	25.9	6	30.0	9	25.0
Home deliveries	189	14.5	46	20.8	84	15.7	53	10.9	1	5.0	5	13.9

Group C shows a decrease in the use of the municipal and voluntary hospitals, and an increase in the percentage delivered in the obstetrical and proprietary hospitals.

In Group D the use of the municipal hospital is negligible, and the same is true of home confinements, the remaining deliveries in the series being divided between the three types, 35.0 per cent occurring in obstetrical hospitals, 25.0 per cent in voluntary, and 30.0 per cent in proprietary.

It is significant to note especially the distribution in the obstetrical hospitals and in the proprietary, since the municipal hospitals receive only those whose economic position excludes any choice, and the voluntary receive a variety of patients depending on whether the admission is to the ward or private service. The highest percentages delivered in obstetrical hospitals occur in Groups A and D, 16.3 per cent and 35.0 per cent, respectively. The percentage of cases in the series delivered in proprietary hospitals increases in each area from 11.3 per cent in Group A to 30.0 per cent in Group D.

In Table 64, the classification according to medical attendants is shown. In the series as a whole, physicians were in attendance in 92.2 per cent of the cases, midwives in 3.1 per cent, and in 4.7 per cent there was no attendant. Of all the cases 8.7 per cent were delivered by a physician at home. Among the cases in Group A physicians attended 85.5 per cent, midwives 7.6 per cent, and there was no attendant in 6.9 per cent. Of the deaths preceded by home delivery, physicians attended 9.5 per cent. In Group B there is an increase to 91.9 per cent in the cases attended by physicians, and a corresponding drop in the percentage delivered by midwives to 2.6 per cent, while 5.5 per cent of the cases had no attendant. Very little change is seen in the percentage of cases attended by physicians in the home (10.0 per cent). Group C shows still further alteration, but in the same trend. More

TABLE 64

DEATHS BY ECONOMIC GROUP AND ATTENDANT AT DELIVERY

(Exclusive of deaths following abortion and ectopic gestation)

	TOTAL		GROUP A		GROUP B		GROUP C		GROUP D		NON-RESIDENT	
	Number	Per cent	Number	Per cent	Number	Per cent	Number	Per cent	Number	Per cent	Number	Per cent
Total: Number	1,564	100.0	275	100.0	653	100.0	572	100.0	20	100.0	44	100.0
Per cent	100		17.6		41.8		36.6		1.3		2.8	
Physician: Number	1,442	92.2	235	85.5	600	91.9	547	95.6	20	100.0	40	90.9
Per cent	100		16.3		41.6		37.9		1.4		2.8	
Physician (home delivery):* Number	136	8.7	26	9.5	65	10.0	41	7.2	1	5.0	3	6.8
Per cent	100		19.1		47.8		30.1		.7		6.8	
Midwife: Number	48	3.1	21	7.6	17	2.6	10	1.7	—	—	—	—
Per cent	100		43.8		35.4		20.8					
None or other: Number	74	4.7	19	6.9	36	5.5	15	2.6	—	—	4	9.1
Per cent	100		25.7		48.6		20.3				5.4	

*Included under "Physician."

patients are delivered by physicians and fewer allow themselves to go unattended or choose a midwife attendant. The percentage of home deliveries attended by a physician drops to 7.2. Finally, in Group D all cases in the series are attended by physicians, none are unattended, and only 5 per cent are cared for at home.

Table 65 gives the distribution of the various causes of death by economic group. Hemorrhage, causing 14.2 per cent of the deaths in Group A, decreased steadily to 10.0 per cent in Group D. Septicaemia was the cause of death in 30.5 per cent of the cases in Group A, 33.2 per cent in Group B, 32.9 per cent in Group C, and 25.0 per cent in Group D. Albuminuria and eclampsia was most important in Group A, where 19.6 per cent of all deaths were from this cause. It accounted for 13.2 per cent of the deaths in Group B, 14.2 per cent in Group C, and 15.0 per cent in Group D. Accidents of labor were the cause of death in 12.4 per cent of the cases in Group A, decreasing in the other groups to the very low figure of 5.0 per cent in Group D. The figures for extra-puerperal causes varied from 20.0 per cent in Group A to 25.0 per cent in Group D.

The deaths in the slum areas are indicative of the faulty elements in the care of these patients. The high percentage of deaths from toxaemia bespeaks the very low percentage who had adequate prenatal care. The high percentages of deaths from hemorrhage and accidents of labor also point to this lack, as well as to the tendency of these women to enter the hospitals only after labor has been in progress for some time.

Septicaemia as the most important cause of death is analyzed in Table 66. The 519 deaths, including 9 cases which had septicaemia but died of other causes, represent 33.2 per cent of the entire series. In Group A, 30.9 per cent of the deaths were from septicaemia, 10.2 per cent being associated

TABLE 65

DISTRIBUTION OF CAUSE OF DEATH ACCORDING TO ECONOMIC GROUP

(Exclusive of deaths following abortion and ectopic gestation)

	TOTAL		GROUP A		GROUP B		GROUP C		GROUP D		NON-RESIDENT	
	Number	Per cent	Number	Per cent	Number	Per cent	Number	Per cent	Number	Per cent	Number	Per cent
Total	1,564	100.0	275	100.0	653	100.0	572	100.0	20	100.0	44	100.0
Hemorrhage	197	12.6	39	14.2	86	13.2	67	11.7	2	10.0	3	6.8
Puerperal septicaemia	510	32.6	84	30.5	217	33.2	188	32.9	5	25.0	16	36.4
Albuminuria and eclampsia	231	14.8	54	19.6	86	13.2	81	14.2	3	15.0	7	15.9
Pernicious vomiting	14	.9	1	.4	3	.5	9	1.6	—	—	1	2.3
Phlegmasia alba dolens and embolus	89	5.7	6	2.2	38	5.8	40	7.0	4	20.0	1	2.3
Accidents of labor	171	10.9	34	12.4	73	11.2	59	10.3	1	5.0	4	9.1
Accidents of puerperium	8	.5	2	.7	5	.8	—	—	—	—	1	2.3
Extra-puerperal causes	344	22.0	55	20.0	145	22.2	128	22.4	5	25.0	11	25.0

157

TABLE 66

SEPTICAEMIA DEATHS BY ECONOMIC GROUP

	TOTAL		GROUP A		GROUP B		GROUP C		GROUP D		NON-RESIDENT	
	Number	Per cent of total	Number	Per cent of total	Number	Per cent of total	Number	Per cent of total	Number	Per cent of total	Number	Per cent of total
Total deaths*	1,564	100.0	275	100.0	653	100.0	572	100.0	20	100.0	44	100.0
Total septicaemia deaths†	519	33.2	85	30.9	222	34.0	191	33.4	5	25.0	16	36.4
Without caesarean	369	23.6	57	20.7	170	26.0	131	22.9	1	5.0	10	22.7
With caesarean	150	9.6	28	10.2	52	8.0	60	10.5	4	20.0	6	13.6

*Exclusive of deaths following abortion and ectopic gestation.
†Inclusive of 9 cases who had septicaemia but died of other conditions.

158

TABLE 67

TYPE OF PRENATAL CARE, BY ECONOMIC GROUP

(Exclusive of deaths following abortion and ectopic gestation)

	TOTAL		GROUP A		GROUP B		GROUP C		GROUP D		NON-RESIDENT	
	Num-ber	Per cent	Num-ber	Per cent	Num-ber	Per cent	Num-ber	Per cent	Num-ber	Per cent	Num-ber	Per cent
Total	1,564	100.0	275	100.0	653	100.0	572	100.0	20	100.0	44	100.0
Adequate prenatal care	600	38.4	73	26.5	223	34.1	265	46.3	13	65.0	26	59.1
Inadequate or no prenatal care	964	61.6	202	73.5	430	65.9	307	53.7	7	35.0	18	40.9

159

with caesarean section. There is an increase in the percentage of the deaths in Groups B and C to 34.0 and 33.4 per cent, respectively, with 8.0 per cent in Group B, and 10.5 per cent in Group C following caesarean. In Group D, however, there were only 5 septicaemia deaths, amounting to 25.0 per cent of total deaths in this group, and in all but one of the 5 cases the septicaemia followed caesarean section.

Prenatal care varies greatly in the different areas, as shown in Table 67. Only 26.5 per cent of the cases in Group A had adequate care during pregnancy. This percentage increases steadily to 65.0 in Group D. These figures point to the fact that a great deal of the propaganda directed toward educating the lay public in the value of care during pregnancy has failed. It has reached the upper economic strata to a far greater extent than the lower. Patients in the latter groups are to a large degree being cared for by municipal or private hospitals which give free medical care, but which have not succeeded in inducing their clientele to avail itself of their facilities for prenatal care. More thorough social service follow-up to insure the return of those patients who do register in the clinics, as well as active teaching in the communities they serve, will be required to increase the number of women who receive adequate prenatal care.

In relation to care during pregnancy, the relative preventability as shown in Table 68 is interesting. The general series showed 62.9 per cent preventable deaths. Percentage of preventability decreased as the percentage of those having had proper prenatal care increased. In Group A, 70.2 per cent of the deaths were preventable, and from this peak there was a steady decrease to 50.0 per cent in Group D. More significant is the division of the responsibility in the cases which were preventable. In Group A, where the percentage of adequate prenatal care was the lowest, the percentage of cases where

TABLE 68

PREVENTABILITY AND RESPONSIBILITY, BY ECONOMIC GROUP

(*Exclusive of deaths following abortion and ectopic gestation*)

	TOTAL		GROUP A		GROUP B		GROUP C		GROUP D		NON-RESIDENT	
	Number	Per cent	Number	Per cent	Number	Per cent	Number	Per cent	Number	Per cent	Number	Per cent
Total	1,564	100.0	275	100.0	653	100.0	572	100.0	20	100.0	44	100.0
Not preventable	581	37.1	82	29.8	246	37.7	227	39.7	10	50.0	16	36.4
Preventable: total	983	62.9	193	70.2	407	62.3	345	60.3	10	50.0	28	63.6
Responsibility ascribed to												
Physician	678	69.0	115	59.6	278	68.3	254	73.6	9	90.0	22	78.6
Patient	276	28.1	67	34.7	114	28.0	88	25.5	1	10.0	6	21.4
Midwife	29	3.0	11	5.7	15	3.7	3	.9	—		—	

the physician was held responsible was also the lowest (59.6 per cent). As the percentage of cases having had adequate prenatal care increases, so does the percentage of deaths in which the physician was held responsible: 68.3 per cent in Group B, 73.6 per cent in Group C, and 90.0 per cent in Group D.

It is evident there is a difference in the risk assumed during pregnancy which depends upon the economic situation of the woman. This difference is most marked between the most depressed economic group and the most privileged. We have previously pointed out that, in theory, the quality of medical service does not vary with the economic situation. In practice, it does.

Much of the difference lies with the women in their failure to take advantage of the facilities provided. The reason for this failure, however, reverts to the quality of the service. The failure properly to educate the women of these groups to an understanding of the necessity for using the facilities put at their disposal is in itself a failure to realize the whole function of the service. Greater responsibility for the proper education of the lay public must be assumed by the medical profession in order to obtain the results that are being sought. Furthermore, we have seen that the difference between the death rate in Group A and that in Group C is very slight (4.9 and 4.6). (See Table 62.) Group C is able to purchase its own medical care and in general does not rely on municipal or other free care; the general standard of living and education is much higher than in Group A; and these women are seeking prenatal care to a far greater extent than those in Group A (26.5 per cent in Group A and 46.3 per cent in Group C). (See Table 67.) It is apparent that these patients are not receiving the highest type of medical attention, nor are they able to avail themselves of the services of the most highly trained specialists where those are needed. Further education of this group to an understanding of proper standards for obstetrical care, as well as education of the medical profession in the obligation to supply the services of the best obstetricians wherever these are needed, regardless of the economic status of the patient, are prerequisites to the removal of these economic hazards.

RACE

THE death rate from puerperal causes for the Negro population throughout the country greatly exceeds that for the white population. This is quite as true in New York City. The 251 deaths among Negroes in the series represent a puerperal death rate of 11.5 per 1,000 live births, more than twice as large as that among the white women (5.5).

Table 69 gives the distribution according to cause of death.

TABLE 69

CLASSIFICATION OF DEATHS BY RACE

	TOTAL		WHITE		NEGRO	
	Num-ber	Per cent	Num-ber	Per cent	Num-ber	Per cent
Total	2,041*	*100.0*	1,788	*100.0*	251	*100.0*
Septic abortion	262	*12.8*	217	*12.1*	45	*17.9*
Abortion	95	*4.7*	82	*4.6*	13	*5.2*
Ectopic gestation	120	*5.9*	97	*5.4*	23	*9.2*
Hemorrhage	197	*9.7*	171	*9.5*	26	*10.4*
Puerperal septicaemia	510	*25.0*	463	*25.9*	47	*18.7*
Albuminuria and eclampsia	231	*11.3*	198	*11.1*	33	*13.1*
Pernicious vomiting	14	*.7*	12	*.7*	2	*.8*
Phlegmasia alba dolens and embolus	89	*4.4*	84	*4.7*	5	*2.0*
Accidents of labor	171	*8.4*	155	*8.7*	16	*6.4*
Accidents of puerperium	8	*.4*	7	*.4*	1	*.4*
Extra-puerperal causes	344*	*16.9*	302	*16.9*	40	*15.9*

*Includes 2 Orientals who died of extra-puerperal conditions.

CHART E

PERCENTAGE DISTRIBUTION OF DEATHS
BY RACE, FOR EACH CAUSE OF DEATH

☐ WHITE   ▓ COLORED

ALL CAUSES*	89.0 10.9	
HEMORRHAGE	86.8 13.2	
SEPTICAEMIA	90.8 9.2	
ALBUMINURIA AND ECLAMPSIA	85.7 14.3	
PERNICIOUS VOMITING	85.7 14.3	
PHLEGMASIA ALBA DOLENS AND EMBOLUS	94.4 5.6	
ACCIDENTS OF LABOR	90.6 9.4	
ACCIDENTS OF PUERPERIUM*	87.5 12.5	
EXTRA-PUERPERAL CAUSES	87.8 11.6	

* TWO ORIENTALS WERE ALSO INCLUDED IN THIS GROUP

EXCLUSIVE OF CASES IN WHICH GRAVIDITY WAS UNRECORDED

The percentage of those dying following abortion was much larger for Negroes than for white women (23.1 and 16.7, respectively). The percentage of the deaths caused by septicaemia (except that following abortion) was lower among the Negroes than among the whites (18.7 and 25.9). Albuminuria and eclampsia caused a larger percentage of the deaths among the Negroes (13.1) than among the white women (11.1).

Prenatal care was adequate in only 15 per cent of the deaths among Negro women, while among the white women 43 per cent had adequate care.

Eighteen and two-tenths per cent of the Negro women and 14.1 per cent of the white women were delivered at home.

Preventability of death in the two groups varied only slightly, 67.7 per cent of the deaths among Negroes and 65.5 per cent of those among the white women being classed as preventable.

NATIVITY

THERE were 878 native-born women and 686 foreign-born in the series. This distribution leads to a death rate for native women of 3.69 and for foreign women of 6.26 per 1,000 live births. Table 70 shows the death rates for both native and foreign-born women by cause of death. In the last column is the percentage by which the rate for the foreign-born exceeds that for the native-born for each cause. Except for accidents of the puerperium, for which the figures are insignificant, the rate for the foreign women exceeds that for the native in all the causes of death. It is especially striking for hemorrhage where the excess is 109.5 per cent, for septicaemia (76.3 per cent), and for accidents of labor (138.0 per cent).

TABLE 70

CLASSIFICATION OF DEATHS BY NATIVITY

(Exclusive of deaths following abortion and ectopic gestation)

	TOTAL		NATIVE-BORN		FOREIGN-BORN		PERCENTAGE DIFFERENTIAL‡
	Number	Rate per 1,000 live births	Number	Rate*	Number	Rate†	
Total	1,564	4.5	878	3.69	686	6.26	69.6
Hemorrhage	197	.57	101	.42	96	.88	109.5
Puerperal septicaemia	510	1.5	282	1.18	228	2.08	76.3
Albuminuria and eclampsia	231	.66	145	.61	86	.78	27.9
Pernicious vomiting	14	.04	8	.03	6	.05	66.7
Phlegmasia alba dolens and embolus	89	.26	52	.22	37	.34	54.5
Accidents of labor	171	.49	82	.34	89	.81	138.0
Accidents of puerperium	8	.02	6	.03	2	.02	—33.3
Extra-puerperal causes	344	.99	202	.85	142	1.29	51.8

*Death rate per 1,000 live births to native-born mothers.
†Death rate per 1,000 live births to foreign-born mothers.
‡Percentage by which rate for foreign-born exceeds that for native-born.

TABLE 71

PRENATAL CARE, BY NATIVITY

(Exclusive of deaths following abortion and ectopic gestation)

	TOTAL		NATIVE-BORN		FOREIGN-BORN	
	Number	Per cent	Number	Per cent	Number	Per cent
Total deaths	1,564	100.0	878	100.0	686	100.0
Adequate prenatal care	600	38.4	377	42.9	223	32.5
Inadequate or no prenatal care	964	61.6	501	57.1	463	67.5

Prenatal care, as Table 71 exhibits, was more satisfactory for the native-born group than for the foreign, 42.9 per cent of the former and 32.5 per cent of the latter having had adequate care.

Type of pelvis did not show any marked variation for the two groups, being normal in 60.5 per cent of the foreign-born cases and in 66.6 per cent of the native-born.

We do not feel that the data offer any reliable evidence as to the cause of the extremely high rate among the foreign-born women. It may be presumed to lie in factors which we could not determine. These women are among the depressed

TABLE 72

TYPE OF PELVIS, BY NATIVITY

(Exclusive of deaths following abortion and ectopic gestation)

	TOTAL		NATIVE-BORN		FOREIGN-BORN	
	Number	Per cent	Number	Per cent	Number	Per cent
Total deaths	1,564	100.0	878	100.0	686	100.0
Normal pelvis	1,000	63.9	585	66.6	415	60.5
Abnormal pelvis	179	11.4	94	10.7	85	12.4
Pelvis not recorded	385	24.6	199	22.7	186	27.1

CHART F

PERCENTAGE DISTRIBUTION OF DEATHS
BY NATIVITY, FOR EACH CAUSE OF DEATH

☐ NATIVE-BORN   ▓ FOREIGN-BORN

	Native-Born	Foreign-Born
ALL CAUSES	56.1	43.9
HEMORRHAGE	51.3	48.7
SEPTICAEMIA	55.3	44.7
ALBUMINURIA AND ECLAMPSIA	62.8	37.2
PERNICIOUS VOMITING	57.1	42.9
PHLEGMASIA ALBA DOLENS AND EMBOLUS	58.4	41.6
ACCIDENTS OF LABOR	48.0	52.0
ACCIDENTS OF PUERPERIUM	75.0	25.0
EXTRA-PUERPERAL CAUSES	58.7	41.3

EXCLUSIVE OF CASES IN WHICH GRAVIDITY WAS UNRECORDED

economic groups, with the most unsatisfactory living conditions, and have in general the poorest type of attendance during both pregnancy and confinement.

BOROUGHS

In Chapter I we indicated the variability in size and population as well as in types of population, degree of congestion, and quality of housing in the five boroughs of New York City. The economic distribution of the population of the various boroughs is also significant. It is only in Manhattan and Brooklyn that there are any slum areas. Richmond falls entirely into Group B, as described on page 150 of this chapter. The Bronx and Queens are divided almost equally between Groups B and C. Manhattan, Brooklyn, and the Bronx contain all the institutions for medical teaching as well as the hospitals whose facilities are used for teaching purposes. This factor in the medical alignment of the city may have its effect upon the standards of the various hospitals.

The following tables are based on the place of death and not the residence of the mother, since the object was to determine any wide variations in the quality of the professional services in the five boroughs.

Table 73 shows cause of death according to the borough in which it occurred. Very few striking differences are revealed. Hemorrhage was the cause of death in approximately 9 to 10 per cent of the cases in Manhattan, Brooklyn, and the Bronx, and only 7.8 per cent in Queens, while it rose to 17.4 per cent in Richmond. As the figures for Richmond are extremely small, they cannot be regarded as significant. The percentage of deaths from septicaemia did not vary greatly, except in the Bronx, where it rose to 33.3 per cent. Albuminuria and eclampsia was a more frequent cause of death in Queens, where

TABLE 73
CAUSE OF DEATH, BY BOROUGH

	TOTAL		MANHATTAN		BROOKLYN		BRONX		QUEENS		RICHMOND	
	Number	Per cent	Number	Per cent	Number	Per cent	Number	Per cent	Number	Per cent	Number	Per cent
Total	2,041	100.0	748	100.0	826	100.0	252	100.0	192	100.0	23	100.0
Septic abortion	262	12.8	99	13.2	106	12.8	28	11.1	26	13.5	3	13.0
Abortion	95	4.7	36	4.8	44	5.3	8	3.2	7	3.6	—	—
Ectopic gestation	120	5.9	49	6.6	54	6.5	8	3.2	8	4.2	1	14.3
Hemorrhage	197	9.7	74	9.9	81	9.7	23	9.1	15	7.8	4	17.4
Puerperal septicaemia	510	25.0	162	21.7	213	25.8	84	33.3	44	22.9	7	30.4
Albuminuria and eclampsia	231	11.3	80	10.7	95	11.5	25	9.9	27	14.1	4	17.4
Pernicious vomiting	14	.7	2	.3	4	.5	6	2.4	2	1.0	—	—
Phlegmasia alba dolens and embolus	89	4.4	27	3.6	37	4.5	16	6.3	8	4.2	1	4.3
Accidents of labor	171	8.4	74	9.9	54	6.5	26	10.3	15	7.8	2	8.7
Accidents of puerperium	8	.4	4	.5	4	.5	—	—	—	—	—	—
Extra-puerperal causes	344	16.9	141	18.9	134	16.2	28	11.1	40	20.8	1	4.3

TABLE 74

NATIVITY, BY BOROUGH

(Exclusive of deaths following abortion and ectopic gestation)

	TOTAL		MANHATTAN		BROOKLYN		BRONX		QUEENS		RICHMOND	
	Number	Per cent	Number	Per cent	Number	Per cent	Number	Per cent	Number	Per cent	Number	Per cent
Total	1,564	100.0	564	100.0	622	100.0	208	100.0	151	100.0	19	100.0
Native-born	878	56.1	277	49.1	378	60.8	105	50.5	107	70.9	11	57.9
Foreign-born	686	43.9	287	50.9	244	39.2	103	49.5	44	29.1	8	42.1

TABLE 75

TYPE OF PRENATAL CARE, BY BOROUGH

(Exclusive of deaths following abortion and ectopic gestation)

	TOTAL		MANHATTAN		BROOKLYN		BRONX		QUEENS		RICHMOND	
	Number	Per cent	Number	Per cent	Number	Per cent	Number	Per cent	Number	Per cent	Number	Per cent
Total	1,564	100.0	564	100.0	622	100.0	208	100.0	151	100.0	19	100.0
Adequate prenatal care	600	38.4	218	38.7	226	36.3	87	41.8	64	42.4	5	26.3
Inadequate or no prenatal care	964	61.6	346	61.3	396	63.7	121	58.2	87	57.6	14	73.7

it accounted for 14.1 per cent of the cases. In general, these variations, with the possible exception of the rather high percentage of septicaemia deaths in the Bronx, do not indicate any significant differences.

Table 74 shows that the deaths in Manhattan and the Bronx were almost equally divided between native and foreign-born women.

In Table 75 prenatal care is reported by boroughs. The highest percentage showing adequate prenatal care was found in Queens—42.4 per cent of the cases. Forty-one and eight-tenths per cent in the Bronx, 38.7 per cent in Manhattan, 36.3 per cent in Brooklyn, and 26.3 per cent in Richmond had adequate care during pregnancy.

In Table 76 the figures on preventability are given. The lowest was that for Richmond, where 60.9 per cent of the deaths were classified as preventable, but the figures for this borough are small and justify no conclusions. The variation in the other boroughs was not great—from 67.3 per cent in Brooklyn to 63.5 per cent in Queens—and the figures do not reveal any wide variation in the quality of the professional service in the five boroughs.

A further analysis in this table shows where the responsibility for the preventable deaths was placed by the Advisory Committee. Here the percentages vary much more widely. In the Bronx 73.7 per cent of the preventable cases were considered to be the responsibility of the physician, while in Queens only 55.7 per cent were so classified. Manhattan and Brooklyn showed a responsibility on the part of the physician of 58.1 per cent and 61.0 per cent, respectively—a difference which is not significant. For Richmond, the figures are again too small to be valuable.

In Table 77 prenatal care is analyzed to show its relationship to preventability and the responsibility for the prevent-

TABLE 76

PREVENTABILITY AND RESPONSIBILITY FOR DEATH, BY BOROUGH

	TOTAL		MANHATTAN		BROOKLYN		BRONX		QUEENS		RICHMOND	
	Num-ber	Per cent	Num-ber	Per cent	Num-ber	Per cent	Num-ber	Per cent	Num-ber	Per cent	Num-ber	Per cent
Total	2,041	100.0	748	100.0	826	100.0	252	100.0	192	100.0	23	100.0
Not preventable	698	34.2	264	35.3	270	32.7	85	33.7	70	36.5	9	39.1
Preventable: total	1,343	65.8	484	64.7	556	67.3	167	66.3	122	63.5	14	60.9
Responsibility ascribed to												
Physician	820	61.1	281	58.1	339	61.0	123	73.7	68	55.7	9	64.3
Patient	493	36.7	197	40.7	197	35.4	42	25.1	52	42.6	5	35.7
Midwife	30	2.2	6	1.2	20	3.6	2	1.2	2	1.6	—	—

173

TABLE 77

PREVENTABLE DEATHS FOR WHICH RESPONSIBILITY
WAS ASCRIBED TO PHYSICIAN, PATIENT HAVING HAD
ADEQUATE PRENATAL CARE, BY BOROUGH

	TOTAL	MAN-HATTAN	BROOKLYN	BRONX	QUEENS	RICH-MOND
Deaths following adequate prenatal care: total	600	218	226	87	64	5
Preventable (physician responsible)	305	113	114	49	27	2
Per cent preventable (physician responsible)	50.8	51.8	50.4	56.3	42.2	40.0

able cases. The percentage of preventable cases in which the responsibility was ascribed to the doctor increased as the percentage of those having had adequate prenatal care increased. This was, however, not true in Queens, where the percentage of adequate care was highest (42.4), and the percentage of preventable cases in which the doctor was responsible was lowest (42.2).

In general, the figures do not reveal any important differences in the five boroughs, with the exception of the fact that in the borough of the Bronx the proportion of preventable cases ascribable to the incompetence of the physician was very much higher than in any of the other boroughs.

VI

HOSPITAL PRACTICE

SEVENTY and seven-tenths per cent of all the births in New York City occur in hospitals. To give a complete picture of the maternity care situation, it is necessary to examine all available data concerning hospitals, both as to the amount of work done and the quality of the results, but it is first necessary to set out, in some detail, the varied character of the hospital facilities available in New York City.

The hospitals of the city fall into four groups: municipal, voluntary, obstetrical, and proprietary.

The municipal hospitals are, of course, those maintained by the city out of municipal funds. They are all directly under the supervision of the Department of Hospitals and have a uniform organization and method of administration. Except for the special institutions for the care of communicable diseases, tuberculosis, orthopedic conditions, and cancer, they are all large general hospitals, with affiliated out-patient departments, housing all the branches of medicine as different departments of one unit. Their primary function is the care of the indigent sick, but they are all prepared to receive emergencies of whatever type, regardless of the economic status of the patient. They have no provision for the care of those able to pay for hospital facilities. The attending medical staffs of the city hospitals are all organized according to the requirements of the American College of Surgeons. They all have interne staffs and, with four exceptions, have also resident staffs composed of the more advanced grades of house physicians. The nursing staff is composed either entirely of registered nurses or, in those which conduct nurses' training schools, of student nurses under the supervision of registered nurses. Their records are comprehensive and uniformly kept. The municipal hospitals are distributed through three of the city boroughs, Manhattan having five, Brooklyn four, and the Bronx three. The boroughs of Richmond and Queens are unprovided with general municipal hospitals.

The voluntary hospitals are privately maintained institutions, organized generally after the manner of the city hospitals, with separate services for the different medical specialties, each service in charge of a responsible graded staff of specially qualified visiting physicians. These hospitals are variously owned and maintained—by the medical schools, both graduate and undergraduate, for the provision of the necessary teaching materials; by different church institutions; or by private corporations. None of them is operated for the purpose of making money. Their charges are designed to meet their expenses as far as possible, but never to yield a profit. These hospitals are all organized similarly in that they receive both paying patients and those unable to pay. All have interne staffs and many have resident staffs as well. Certain of them act also as adjunct municipal hospitals by maintaining an ambulance service for emergency work and by receiving indigent patients for whose care the city reimburses the hospitals at a fixed rate. This arrangement is made necessary by three factors: the total lack of municipal hospitals in two boroughs of the city, the inaccessibility of the city hospitals to certain areas of the other boroughs, and the inadequate bed capacity of the municipal hospitals. These hospitals, then, are receiving all types of emergent cases, frequently including obstetrical emergencies, whether advanced labor, hemorrhage, or eclampsia. In this connection, it is necessary to call attention to a ruling of the Department of Hospitals which states that no hospital may receive reimbursement for the care of an obstetrical case if that case has received prenatal care in the same hospital. It is not difficult to imagine the serious effects of such a ruling. These voluntary hospitals are unable, through lack of funds, to accept for prenatal care any woman who would be entitled to free care in a municipal hospital. They must advise her to seek her prenatal care at the nearest city hospital or public health prenatal station. Where such facilities are distant, the woman with pressing home duties will frequently abandon the effort to obtain care during her pregnancy. If she does persist in this effort and presents herself to the city clinic for care, she is received into the clinic of any municipal hospital without regard to the number of beds to be available at the time of her expected delivery. The woman thus receives no assurance that facilities will be available for her at the time of confinement.

Since a large part of the value of prenatal care lies in the information made available as to the prognosis for delivery, it is difficult to understand just what the value of such uncorrelated care may be. Such a regulation forces these general hospitals to receive patients about whose physical condition they are ignorant, of whose prenatal course they know nothing, and for whom they have been able to make no prognosis for delivery. They are consequently put at a grave disadvantage. There is no possible justification for or advantage in such a regulation, but rather every possible disadvantage to both patient and hospital.

The third classification—the obstetrical hospitals—includes those restricted to the care of obstetrical and gynecological cases. These are all prepared to receive both private and ward cases. They are staffed exclusively by highly trained specialists and have both interne and resident staffs. They are recognized as centers for the teaching of their speciality and some are affiliated with teaching institutions. The proprietary hospital devoted to obstetrics is not included in this classification but is discussed under the fourth group.

This fourth group, the proprietary hospitals, is a diverse one, ranging from the large, well-equipped private hospital to the small five or six-bed sanatorium with almost no equipment. They are under no public control, the licensure by the Department of Hospitals being concerned only with the enforcement of certain minor sanitary laws and not at all with the type of medical care provided. They have one characteristic in common: they are operated for the purpose of making money. They receive no non-paying patients. They have no organized staff which is responsible for the conduct of the major procedures or is charged with the duty of establishing certain minimum standards and certain principles of practice. The standards, therefore, vary with each physician. These hospitals are not affiliated with any teaching institutions. There are no interne or resident staffs, but in a few instances there is a paid resident physician to assist the doctors and to take care of sudden emergencies. The nursing staff is more often than not composed of a few registered nurses acting as supervisors while attendants give the actual nursing care. They are frequently operated by private individuals who solicit the patronage of the physician without regard to his ability or ethical standards.

This lax organization necessarily leads to uncertainty as to the quality of work of which such a hospital is capable. Its standard is the standard of the physicians who work in it. Where there is no responsible direction, no uniformity of ability can be demanded of the individual physicians.

Physicians who do not measure up to the standards necessary to obtain appointments to the organized staffs of the general hospitals, either municipal or voluntary, are free to organize sanatoria for themselves. Such physicians practice without the advantage of having highly trained and capable superiors. At their best, these institutions may, and some do, maintain a standard which is entirely satisfactory. In some, radical obstetrical procedures, caesarean operations for no better reason than that the attendant, because of his incapacity, was unable to deliver the patient by a less hazardous but more difficult procedure, so-called trial labors lasting upwards of forty-eight hours, ruptured uteri from unskilled vaginal maneuvers, successive cases of septicaemia, are all too common.

Perhaps the most dangerous element in the situation is that these hospitals are accepted by the lay public as of the same quality as the organized, well-staffed hospitals. To the laity the word "hospital" has but one meaning—an institution where one receives scientific, skilful, and scrupulous care. Obviously, if the community allows both types to operate under one designation, the layman cannot be expected to discriminate. The city establishes certain minimum standards for the institutions charged with the care of the sick who cannot afford to pay for their care. By so doing, it has tacitly put the stamp of approval on the type of hospital where skill and scrupulousness are demanded of the medical attendant. It should do no less for those who can pay for their own care.

In justice to these institutions, we must call attention to a recent development: the organization of certain of these private hospitals into a group which calls itself the Association of Private Hospitals, Inc., with the announced purpose of standardizing medical service and raising it to the highest level of efficiency, and of correcting certain abuses now ascribed to them. Such a move, honestly undertaken, should do much to ameliorate the conditions to which allusion has been made. It is now in its inception, and only its history will answer the question as to its value.

In this study an attempt was made to obtain, by questionnaire (reproduced in Appendix, page 257), detailed figures
as to number and type of delivery in all the hospitals of the
city. Data were obtained from 67, in which approximately 75
per cent of the total hospital deliveries occur. In the Appendix, the figures in detail are given grouped according to number of deliveries; Table 78 is a summary of this information,
by type of hospital. These figures do not include any of the
proprietary hospitals.

The corrected death rate was based on cases delivered in

TABLE 78

SUMMARY OF DATA FOR 1930, 1931, AND 1932 FROM SIXTY-SEVEN HOSPITALS ANSWERING QUESTIONNAIRE

	TOTAL	MUNICIPAL HOSPITALS	OBSTETRICAL HOSPITALS	VOLUNTARY HOSPITALS
Deliveries: total*	181,097	45,859	35,661	99,577
Maternal deaths: total	1,482	606	178	698
Death rate per 1,000 deliveries	8.2	13.2	5.0	7.0
Maternal deaths: corrected total†	1,209	450	173	586
Corrected death rate†	6.7	9.8	4.9	5.9
Septicaemia deaths, cases delivered in hospital only	380	138	57	185
Preventable septicaemia deaths:				
Number	221	64	35	122
Per cent	*58.6*	*46.4*	*61.4*	*65.9*
Operative deliveries:				
Number	44,022	4,729	10,747	28,546
Per cent of all deliveries	*24.3*	*10.3*	*30.1*	*28.7*
Caesarean sections:				
Number	3,963	571	1,152	2,240
Per cent of all deliveries	*2.2*	*1.2*	*3.2*	*2.2*
Caesarean section deaths:				
Number	240	58	50	132
Per cent of caesarean sections	*6.1*	*10.1*	*4.3*	*5.9*
Preventable deaths:				
Number	531	154	89	288
Per cent of corrected total deaths	*43.9*	*34.2*	*51.4*	*49.1*

*This represents approximately 75 per cent of total deliveries in all hospitals in New York City.

†Cases delivered in hospital regardless of place of death, and cases dying in hospital without being delivered.

the hospital regardless of the place of death, and those who died in the hospital without being delivered. This was necessary to give a more equitable view of hospital results than the gross total of deaths would yield. For example, the municipal hospitals receive any and all patients; often patients already delivered in other hospitals or at home who become septic are transferred to them. Even this correction does not result in a fair estimate because the hospital may receive cases on whom delivery has been attempted outside or who have been long in labor under the care of an outside physician or midwife. The tabulated figures for septicaemia deaths include only those who were delivered in the hospital and developed sepsis there.

The death rate for the municipal hospitals is 13.2 per 1,000 live births; that for the obstetrical hospitals, 5.0; and for voluntary hospitals, 7.0. When these rates are corrected, as explained above, they are 9.8, 4.9, and 5.9, respectively. The percentage of preventable septicaemia deaths is much lower in the municipal hospitals (46.4) than in either the obstetrical (61.4) or the voluntary (65.9). The same is true of the percentage of operative deliveries: in the municipal hospitals, it is 10.3, in the obstetrical 30.1, and in the voluntary 28.7. The percentage of caesarean sections is 1.2 in the municipal hospitals, 3.2 in the obstetrical, and 2.2 in the voluntary. However, the case fatality rate is higher in the municipal hospitals (10.1) than in the obstetrical (4.3) or voluntary (5.9). The percentage of preventable deaths is 34.2 in the municipal hospitals, 51.4 in the obstetrical, and 49.1 in the voluntary hospitals. While the death rate in the municipal hospitals is extremely high, the percentage of preventable deaths is lower than in the other two types. The key to this may be found in the fact that the percentage of caesarean sections in the municipal hospitals is less than one-half that in the obstetrical hospitals, and only little more than one-half that in the voluntary hospitals. In the case of operative deliveries, the obstetrical and voluntary hospitals show a percentage about three times that of the municipal hospitals.

It is to be regretted that accurate data from the proprietary hospitals could not be obtained. Consequently it is not possible to present any rates or percentages which could be used for comparison.

The real index of the results obtained by any hospital or group of hospitals lies in the percentage of preventability. The wide variety of the cases admitted to the various types of hospital makes a mere comparison of death rates valueless. The municipal hospitals must receive any emergency case; the obstetrical hospitals do receive emergencies, but exercise some selection of their cases and send those which are properly city cases to the hospitals obligated to receive them. In the case of the voluntary hospitals, there is a variation. If they provide an ambulance and are empowered to receive cases which are properly the responsibility of the city, they accept some emergencies but will attempt to exercise some selection in the matter. Comparisons between one type of hospital and another must take these facts into consideration.

VII

ATTENDANT AT DELIVERY

IT is of the greatest importance, in evaluating maternity care, to consider the type of medical attendant. This was regularly done in the present study: a record was kept of every physician associated at any time with one of the deaths in this series. The facts concerning each physician were obtained from the *Medical Directory of New York, New Jersey and Connecticut,* published annually by the Medical Society of the State of New York. Details of the individual physician's training and present appointments to hospital staffs as well as the specialty to which he was devoting himself were included in the record. In classifying the physician according to his specialty, we were guided by the record of his appointment to special staffs in the recognized hospitals, as given in the directory. We made four classifications as follows: obstetrician and gynecologist, general practitioner, surgeon, and all other specialties.

It is realized that in a great many instances a physician obtains a hospital staff appointment in order to qualify himself to undertake specialized work and not because he is so qualified. In the staff, the attendant physician is graded according to his experience and training, and there can be no intention on the part of the chief of the staff to regard his junior colleagues as qualified specialists. There is, however, no method of preventing the individual physician from so regarding himself and offering his services to his clientele on the basis of such an appointment. In a carefully supervised staff, due recognition is taken of the qualifications of the members and the work is so allotted as to prevent the less experienced members from undertaking the more exacting and difficult tasks. The individual, however, may not exercise any such objective attitude toward his own capabilities and may be ready to undertake all the activities of the fully trained and experienced specialist; indeed he may be eager to undertake, in his private practice, exactly those things which his position on the staff of the hospital precludes his undertaking there except under supervision. The lay public must take the individual physician at his own evaluation. At most, the patient will know that his physician is a member of a certain staff in a given hospital. We have, therefore, classified the physician according to the specialty he is following as indicated by the appointments he holds, regardless of the grade of those appointments.

In Table 79 we group all deaths (except those following abortions or extra-uterine gestations) according to attendant at delivery or, if undelivered, the attendant during the fatal illness. It is not surprising to find that 68.4 per cent of the cases were attended by obstetricians, as defined in the preceding paragraphs. The group "Other specialists" was sub-

TABLE 79
DEATH RATES ACCORDING TO ATTENDANT AT DELIVERY

	LIVE BIRTHS		PUERPERAL DEATHS*		PUERPERAL DEATH RATE PER 1,000 LIVE BIRTHS
	Number	Per cent	Number	Per cent	
Total	346,863	*100.0*	1,564	*100.0*	4.5
Obstetrician	196,287	*56.6*	1,070	*68.4*	5.4
General practitioner	98,247	*28.3*	247	*15.8*	2.5
Surgeon	10,686	*3.1*	106	*6.8*	9.9
Other specialists	8,628	*2.5*	47	*3.0*	5.4
Midwife	32,076	*9.5*	48	*3.1*	1.4
None or unknown	939	*.3*	46	*2.9*	48.9

*Exclusive of deaths following abortion and ectopic gestation.

divided, according to specialty as given in the Medical Directory, as follows, with the number of cases attended by each:

Pediatrician	20
Oto-laryngologist	11
Orthopedist	5
Urologist	3
Ophthalmologist	3
Radiologist	3
Anaesthetist	1
Dermatologist	1
	47

No accurate information concerning the relative quality of
the services given by the various groups can be obtained unless the number of live births attended by each group is
known. To obtain these numbers, we examined all the birth
certificates for 1931 and counted the live births attended by
each specialty group. The figures are as follows:

Obstetrician	65,429
General practitioner	32,749
Midwife	10,692
Surgeon	3,562
Pediatrician	1,189
Oto-laryngologist	302
Dermatologist	240
Ophthalmologist	239
Urologist	203
Neurologist	188
Radiologist	174
Orthopedist	136
Anaesthetist	62
Pathologist	55
Gastro-enterologist	51
Proctologist	30
Psychiatrist	7
None or other	12
Doctor not listed	301
	115,621

To secure estimated three-year totals we tripled these figures. Since the total number of live births in 1931 (115,621) lies about midway between that in 1930 (122,811) and that in 1932 (109,878), and since the total obtained by tripling the figure for 1931 (346,863) differs by only 1,447 from the actual total for the three years (348,310), we considered this method of calculation sufficiently accurate to provide bases for the determination of differential rates, as shown in Table 79.

The general death rate on the calculated total of live births for the three years is 4.5. The rate in the case of obstetricians is 5.4; that for the group of general practitioners is 2.5, well below the general rate, while that for surgeons is 9.9, greatly in excess of any of the rates for the other groups as well as of the general rate. The group of other specialists has a rate of 5.4, and the midwives a rate of 1.4, the lowest of all.

These rates, of course, cannot be accepted as entirely satisfactory criteria of the abilities of the respective groups. There are many factors which create special situations for one group or another. The obstetricians are repeatedly called upon to deliver patients when the previous attendant has found the situation too difficult. The obstetrical staffs of the large municipal and voluntary hospitals cannot select their cases, but must receive any case which requires treatment. A great many neglected and complicated cases are thus thrust upon the obstetricians after other physicians have failed. Moreover, many of the cases which are seen in pregnancy and found to have abnormalities which will complicate labor are quite properly referred to an obstetrician. Most abnormal, complicated, neglected, and mismanaged cases thus fall to the share of the obstetrician and contribute to the high death rate of this group. However, it is unlikely that one-half of all the cases delivered by obstetricians fall into this category, as would be necessary if the rate were to be lowered to that of the general practitioners. There are undoubtedly other factors. We have previously mentioned one which we believe to be important: the probable inclusion in the group of obstetricians of many physicians who are entirely unqualified, by either training or experience, to be considered specialists in this field, but who, nevertheless, are assuming the prerogatives of the highly trained specialist in making exacting judgments and performing operative procedures for which they cannot be considered adequately trained.

The extremely high death rate for the surgeons may be due in part to the higher percentage of caesarean sections among their cases. Of the total fatal cases attended by surgeons, 30.0 per cent had caesarean operations, while only 23.6 per cent of the fatal cases attended by obstetricians had caesarean section. The rate, even with this factor considered, remains extremely high and must reflect, to some extent, the quality of the professional services of surgeons in this field. It is not unlikely that their training and attitude incline them to an excessive use of instrumentation.

The low rates for the general practitioners and the midwives are due, in part at least, to the selection of cases. The midwives attend only uncomplicated and spontaneous deliveries. The general practitioners attend many of the deliveries performed at home, and undoubtedly do fewer operative deliveries.

In Table 80 cases are classified according to the responsibility of each group of attendants for preventable deaths. All cases for which the attendant was considered responsible are grouped together; the remaining deaths are those for which the attendant was not held responsible, including those for which the patient was considered responsible as well as those considered not preventable. In the group as a whole, 45.1 per

TABLE 80

DEATHS CLASSIFIED ACCORDING TO RESPONSIBILITY OF THE ATTENDANT AT DELIVERY

(Exclusive of deaths following abortion and ectopic gestation)

| | TOTAL DEATHS | | | | | | SEPTICAEMIA DEATHS | | | | | |
| | TOTAL | | ATTENDANT RESPONSIBLE | | ATTENDANT NOT RESPONSIBLE | | TOTAL | | ATTENDANT RESPONSIBLE | | ATTENDANT NOT RESPONSIBLE | |
	Number	Per cent	Number	Per cent	Number	Per cent	Number	Per cent	Number	Per cent	Number	Per cent
Total	1,564	100	706	45.1	858	54.9	510	100	325	63.7	185	36.3
Obstetrician	1,070	100	475	44.4	595	55.6	347	100	231	66.6	116	33.4
General practitioner	247	100	118	47.7	129	52.2	85	100	52	61.2	33	38.8
Surgeon	106	100	52	49.1	54	50.9	29	100	18	62.1	11	37.9
All other specialists	47	100	20	42.6	27	57.4	7	100	3	42.9	4	57.1
Midwife	48	100	21	43.8	27	56.2	23	100	15	65.2	8	34.8
None or unknown	46	100	20	43.5	26	56.5	19	100	6	31.6	13	68.4

TABLE 81

DEATHS FOLLOWING CAESAREAN SECTION CLASSIFIED
ACCORDING TO OPERATOR

	TOTAL CAESAREAN SECTIONS		ATTENDANT RESPONSIBLE		ATTENDANT NOT RESPONSIBLE	
	Num-ber	Per cent	Num-ber	Per cent	Num-ber	Per cent
Total	304	100	233	76.6	71	23.4
Obstetrician	253	100	193	76.3	60	23.7
General practitioner	17	100	12	70.6	5	29.4
Surgeon	32	100	26	81.3	6	18.8
All other specialists	2	100	2	100.0	—	—

cent of the deaths could have been prevented by the attendant:
among the cases attended by obstetricians, 44.4 per cent; by
general practitioners, 47.7 per cent; by surgeons, 49.1 per
cent; by all other specialists, 42.6 per cent; and by midwives,
43.8 per cent.

Responsibility for preventable deaths from septicaemia was
attributed to the attendant in 63.7 per cent of all the cases: in
66.6 per cent of those attended by obstetricians; in 61.2 per
cent by general practitioners; in 62.1 per cent by surgeons;
in 42.9 per cent by all other specialists; and in 65.2 per cent
by midwives.

In Table 81 a similar classification is made of the deaths
following caesarean section. Of those following operation by
obstetricians, 76.3 per cent were preventable; of those following operation by general practitioners, 70.6 per cent were preventable, by surgeons, 81.3 per cent; in each case with responsibility ascribed to the attendant. The obstetricians performed
the great bulk of these operations; the figures for the other
groups are too small to admit of any true conclusions.

VIII

MIDWIFE PRACTICE

IN the United States the midwife has been regarded until recently as a necessary evil to be done away with as soon as possible and in the interval to be disregarded on the general principle, one supposes, that if she is not noticed she will cease to exist. Provisions for the proper education, registration, and supervision of midwives, who attend approximately 10 to 12 per cent of the births in the country, are exceedingly inadequate in most states of the Union.

These conditions are the result of various factors. In the early history of the country and throughout the expansion westward, attention to social and medical problems was subservient to the immediate necessities of food and shelter. Since there was neither time nor money to set up schools for midwives, every woman was a potential midwife as she is today in many rural areas of the country. But in this country the midwife had no such status as in Europe, where by long custom a male attendant at delivery was unthinkable, and the population was trained to regard the midwife as the normal and most suitable attendant for all but the difficult and complicated confinements.

By the time training for specialized types of professional service became a possibility in the new country that the United States still was, the principle of male midwives was gaining wide acceptance in Europe. Thus it came about that the only training in midwifery provided in this country was designed to prepare the physician to act as accoucheur as well as general medical practitioner. This did not mean that the midwife was not practicing widely; she was, but without training or supervision of any kind. The woman who lived at long distance from a doctor, as the frontier women did, had to accept the hazard of attendance by a midwife. Those to whom a doctor was available and who could afford his services sought him out. The midwife was accepted by those who could do no better. This resulted in a social barrier to the use of midwives which still exists today. With the beginning of large-scale immigration, foreign-born groups settled in various communities, bringing Old-World attitudes toward midwives and the midwives themselves, who had been trained in the countries of their origin. This factor also strengthened the feeling which exists today that only the foreign-born or the very poor should be attended by midwives, and then only because they can afford no better.

A large number of the practicing midwives in New York City are foreign-born women who were trained in the country of their birth and came to this country and began the practice of midwifery before the present laws regarding licensure were put into effect. There is no provision in the law for examination or required "refresher" courses. It is a little hard to believe that a woman of sixty, wholly illiterate, trained forty years ago and having had no further study since that time, can be a safe attendant for a woman during her pregnancy and delivery. Yet just such women are practicing midwifery in New York City.

Laws designed to regulate midwife practice came long before any attempt to provide proper and sufficient training. The result can be imagined. Training, purely by practice or apprenticeship, could not long keep pace with the advances in the theory and practice of obstetrics. There were large numbers of women who practiced casually as midwives without training and without sufficient clientele to gain that training or increase it by experience. Such a condition of affairs, while not officially accepted, is tacitly condoned in those states where there is no provision for training.

The practice of the midwife in New York City, as elsewhere in this country, is of course confined to the home, and that factor alone tends to determine the type of patient who comes to the midwife. Domiciliary obstetrical practice is largely confined to the foreign-born and the economically less fortunate portions of the population. The average American woman living in a city has come to believe, rightly or wrongly, that a hospital is the only safe and proper place in which to be delivered. But this is not so true of the foreign-born woman nor, in many cases, of the woman of foreign extraction. She prefers being delivered at home and her training and attitudes lead her to seek a midwife. Her assimilation in this country is altering those attitudes, but it is questionable whether that alteration is working to her advantage.

It was not until 1911 that the first school for midwives was established at Bellevue Hospital. That school is still in operation and while there have been others at different times in recent years, there is, at present, only one other school in New York City. This was recently established for the training of nurses in midwifery. There are now only three or four schools for midwives in the entire United States, although this does not give a fair estimate of the attempts at training. Many private physicians train midwives informally by giving them practical instruction as assistants in their regular obstetrical practice. This is a casual, unregulated, and variable type of training which should not be looked upon as any solution of a pressing problem.

In New York City the problem of the midwife is a special one as it relates to her integration into a densely peopled urban community where she cannot be regarded merely as a stop-gap.

The regulation and licensure of midwives in New York City is a function of the Board of Health. At present there are 863 licensed midwives who attend approximately 10 per cent of the births annually. The law requires the midwife, in order to qualify for a license, to be a graduate of a school of midwives which is accepted by the Board of Health, but there are still many midwives in practice who obtained their licenses before this ruling went into effect. No annual re-registration is required, as is the case with physicians licensed to practice in the state. Supervision of the midwife includes a monthly visit by a nurse appointed by the Board of Health who examines her bag and her home conditions. The midwife must make quarterly reports to the Board of Health of all cases delivered by her during the period. She must report births within ten days. She is subject to an investigation in the case of a maternal death. This is the extent of the meager supervision exercised over her. No properly trained supervisor ever sees the patients delivered, and the quarterly reports may or may not be an indication of the quality of her work. There is no rule which requires the midwife to call a physician after a stipulated number of hours of labor. In many instances the midwife would be very grateful for such a rule to uphold her in her demand for help when the family refuses to accept her advice. So long as she does not get into trouble through the misfortune of having a maternal death, she is allowed to go along practically unsupervised.

In addition to this lack of official supervision and help, the midwife is constantly suffering from difficulty in the attitude of the agencies and individuals to which she ought to look for help, guidance, and cooperation. She is taught to make an attempt to have her patients get adequate prenatal care, but when she tries to do this she may meet with obstruction or entire refusal to cooperate. Clinics to which she sends her patients for care will attempt to dissuade the patient from entrusting herself to the midwife and to induce her to come to the hospital instead. Doctors will, more often than not, refuse any cooperation in the matter of prenatal care. Even when the midwife seeks assistance during delivery, she may meet with a lack of cooperation that cannot be too emphatically censured.

In marked contrast to this state of affairs is the European attitude. There the midwife is accepted by all elements of the population, official and social. She is properly trained and adequately supervised and always integrated into the general community plan of maternity service and care. The leaders of the medical profession regard her generally with respect, not disdain. She is a member of a skilled profession with a professional dignity and professional standards.

In only a few parts of this country is she so regarded. In the Kentucky mountain regions, where doctors are few, there has arisen a frontier nursing service for the care of the mountain women during pregnancy and delivery as well as for general medical care of the population. This service is performed by nurse-midwives under the most difficult and hazardous circumstances in a population where poverty, ignorance, inadequate feeding, and uncleanliness are the rules of life. A doctor is available for consultation and assistance in difficulties and for performing obstetrical operations.

In this study we visited and interviewed every midwife who was in any way associated with one of the deaths under examination. We attempted to discover from the midwife her complete professional history: her training and length of time in practice, her technique and routine methods, her results as she viewed them, as well as the details of the case under consideration. From all the data and from the general impression arising out of the interview, we have attempted an evaluation of the midwife's competence. The usual procedures have been followed in recording the case and determining the cause of death and preventability.

We were able to locate and interview 59 midwives who had either delivered or been in contact with a patient preceding her death.

Thirty-one were either Italian-born or of Italian extraction; 22 had been practicing without additional training for twenty years or more; 17 were graduates of the Bellevue School of Midwifery; 17 had been trained in European schools; 10 had been trained by private physicians; 1 had been trained forty years ago by a sister who was a midwife in Italy.

Nineteen we judged to be competent, 20 were thought to be only fairly competent, and 20 were incompetent. In judging competence, some effort was made to determine what knowledge the midwife had of the possible complications of pregnancy and how she was prepared to meet them: her ability to judge presentation, her technique as to sepsis, the use or non-use of gloves, method of making examinations, preparation for delivery as regards antiseptics, sterile goods, etc. In addition, an effort was made to evaluate her personal qualifications for her work. There were all gradations—from the seventy-six-year-old Italian who had never heard of prenatal care and had no idea of even ordinary cleanliness and was in every way inadequate to her task, to the intelligent young graduate of the Bellevue School of Midwifery who usually saw her patients early in their pregnancies, gave prenatal care under the supervision of a doctor, was thoroughly clean, understood asepsis, and was in every way equipped for the work she was doing.

Among all the deaths, exclusive of those following extrauterine gestation or abortion, 48 followed delivery by a midwife. In 2 other cases death occurred before delivery could be effected; in 30 cases the midwife had been in attendance on the patient for a more or less protracted period during labor; in 5 cases, the midwife's contact with the patient had been brief—merely seeing the patient and immediately calling a doctor or sending her to a hospital. The midwife thus had contacts with 85 of the patients, or 5.4 per cent of the total number.

Tables 82 and 83 give the puerperal death rate per 1,000 live births classified according to attendant. These rates are

TABLE 82

DEATHS CLASSIFIED BY ATTENDANT AT DELIVERY

(Exclusive of deaths following abortion and ectopic gestation)

	TOTAL	PHYSICIAN		MIDWIFE, DELIVERY ONLY	NONE OR OTHER
		TOTAL	HOME DELIVERY*		
Total live births	348,310	318,701	72,496	29,519	90
Total deaths	1,564	1,442	136	48	74
Death rate per 1,000 live births	4.5	4.5	1.9	1.6	—

*Included under "Physician, total."

TABLE 83

DEATHS CLASSIFIED BY ATTENDANT AT DELIVERY, WITH CORRECTION FOR MIDWIFE CONTACTS

(Exclusive of deaths following abortion and ectopic gestation)

	TOTAL	PHYSICIAN		MIDWIFE, DELIVERY AND CONTACT	NONE OR OTHER
		TOTAL	HOME DELIVERY*		
Total live births	348,310	318,701	72,496	29,519	90
Total deaths	1,564	1,406	130	85	73
Death rate per 1,000 live births	4.5	4.4	1.8	2.9	—

*Included under "Physician, total."

presented only for those cases dying at or after the twenty-eighth week of gestation and those cases of less than twenty-eight weeks' gestation who died undelivered. The midwife does not deal with abortions or ectopic gestations and for that reason it was thought just to exclude those figures entirely when the data are shown in reference to the midwife. To insure still further accuracy in attempting to compare the results obtained by midwives with those obtained by physicians, the cases attended by physicians were considered in two ways: all cases attended by physicians, and cases attended by physicians at home. This last group offers the fairer ground for comparison.

The general maternal death rate for all cases, exclusive of abortions and ectopic gestations, is 4.5 per thousand live births, while that for cases delivered by the physician at home is 1.9 and for cases delivered by the midwife, 1.6. This last figure is 64 per cent below the general rate and slightly lower than the rate for cases delivered by physicians at home. It is proper to note that not all deliveries attended by physicians at home terminate spontaneously, as do those attended by the midwife, and the comparability of the two series is thus somewhat vitiated. It must, however, be accepted that there is no great disparity in the results obtained under circumstances almost exactly similar. We shall analyze still further the other variable factors.

Table 83 presents the figures and rates in the same way with the figures reclassified to include in the group ascribed to the midwife all those cases in which the midwife had any contact with the patient during her pregnancy or labor as well as those actually delivered by midwives. Out of the total of 1,564 deaths, the midwife attended 48 cases at delivery, which represents a rate of 1.6 per 1,000 live births. The midwife attended at some time, but without delivering, 37 additional cases—a total of 85 cases in which the midwife either delivered or had some contact with the patient. This figure gives a rate of 2.9, which is still lower than the rate of 4.4, the corrected figure for physicians, and 1.1 higher than the resulting rate for physicians delivering at home.

In drawing any conclusions from these figures, two factors must be considered. First, the nature of the contact varied from the cases in which the midwife saw the patient only once and immediately called a physician or sent her to the hospital, to the cases in which she remained with the patient while in labor and only called assistance when some disquieting symptom became evident. It did not appear that in any large percentage of these cases the midwife could properly be held accountable for the outcome of the case. Further, it must be remembered that there were cases delivered in hospitals which had been previously treated by physicians at home, and in order properly to compare the two groups, it would be necessary to add this number to those delivered by physicians at home. Where this is done we find an additional 33 patients who had care at home during labor by a physician before being removed to a hospital where the delivery was completed by another physician. Thus the physician delivered at home, or had home contact with, 163 patients, which is a rate of 2.2 per 1,000 births, while the midwife had contact with, or delivered, 85 patients with a resultant rate of 2.9.

The conclusions arising from these figures must be that there is no great disparity between the results of the work done by the two groups.

In Table 84 the distribution of all the deaths is given according to the cause of death and the attendant. Though the total figure is too small to make percentages significant, it is convenient to present the data in the form already established. Septicaemia is seen to be the cause of death in the

TABLE 84

DEATHS BY CAUSE AND ATTENDANT AT DELIVERY

(Exclusive of deaths following abortion and ectopic gestation)

| | TOTAL | | PHYSICIAN | | | | MIDWIFE | | NONE OR OTHER | |
| | | | TOTAL | | HOME DELIVERY* | | | | | |
	Number	Per cent	Number	Per cent	Number	Per cent	Number	Per cent	Number	Per cent
Total	1,564	100.0	1,442	100.0	136	100.0	48	100.0	74	100.0
Hemorrhage	197	12.6	174	12.1	7	5.1	9	18.8	14	18.9
Puerperal septicaemia	510	32.6	473	32.8	58	42.6	24	50.0	13	17.6
Albuminuria and eclampsia	231	14.8	208	14.4	15	11.0	5	10.4	18	24.3
Pernicious vomiting	14	.9	10	.7	3	2.2	—	—	4	5.4
Phlegmasia alba dolens and embolus	89	5.7	85	5.9	12	8.8	2	4.2	2	2.7
Accidents of labor	171	10.9	168	11.7	10	7.4	2	4.2	1	1.4
Accidents of puerperium	8	.5	8	.6	—	—	—	—	—	—
Extra-puerperal causes	344	22.0	316	22.1	31	22.8	6	12.5	22	29.7

*Included under "Physician, total."

largest proportion of cases for all attendants. The second most important cause of death among those cases which were attended by a midwife was found to be hemorrhage, while extra-puerperal causes occupied this position in the series as a whole. These results are to be expected in view of the fact that the midwife is not attending those cases requiring operative interference or having grave pregnancy toxaemias or serious illness of any sort.

Table 85 shows the distribution of deaths according to gravidity and attendant. The table lacks rates per 1,000 births, since figures for the births according to this distribution are not available. Throughout the series, deaths among multigravidae predominate—inevitably, since births among multigravidae greatly outnumber births of primigravidae. The division of deaths between those bearing the first child and those having borne previous children shows that the proportion of multigravidae is greater among those attended by physicians at home (71.3 per cent to 27.9 per cent) than it is in the series as a whole (55.9 per cent to 43.6 per cent) and still greater among those attended by midwives (79.2 per cent to 20.8 per cent). What these figures indicate as to the hazards involved for the two groups with different attendants is, of course, not to be learned from such a table since the distribution of births by gravidity is prerequisite to any attempt at such an evaluation.

It is not unexpected to find (as Table 86 shows) that the midwife has a larger percentage of foreign-born women among her fatal cases than the series as a whole or the physician. Of the 48 women who died under care of a midwife, 29, or 58.7 per cent, were foreign born while in the whole series only 43.8 per cent were foreign born. The cases in this series delivered by physicians showed 43.6 per cent foreign women, while of those delivered by physicians at home 50.0 per cent

TABLE 85

DEATHS BY GRAVIDITY AND ATTENDANT AT DELIVERY

(Exclusive of deaths following abortion and ectopic gestation)

| | TOTAL | | PHYSICIAN | | | | MIDWIFE | | NONE OR OTHER | |
| | | | TOTAL | | HOME DELIVERY* | | | | | |
	Num- ber	Per cent	Num- ber	Per cent	Num- ber	Per cent	Num- ber	Per cent	Num- ber	Per cent
Total	1,564	*100.0*	1,442	*100.0*	136	*100.0*	48	*100.0*	74	*100.0*
Primigravidae	682	*43.6*	653	*45.3*	38	*27.9*	10	*20.8*	19	*25.7*
Multigravidae	874	*55.9*	784	*54.4*	97	*71.3*	38	*79.2*	52	*70.3*
Gravidity not reported	8	*.5*	5	*.3*	1	*.7*	—	—	3	*4.1*

*Included under "Physician, total."

TABLE 86

DEATHS BY NATIVITY AND ATTENDANT AT DELIVERY

(Exclusive of deaths following abortion and ectopic gestation)

| | TOTAL | | PHYSICIAN | | | | MIDWIFE | | NONE OR OTHER | |
| | | | TOTAL | | HOME DELIVERY* | | | | | |
	Num-ber	Per cent	Num-ber	Per cent	Num-ber	Per cent	Num-ber	Per cent	Num-ber	Per cent
Total deaths	1,564	100.0	1,442	100.0	136	100.0	48	100.0	74	100.0
Foreign-born	686	43.8	629	43.6	68	50.0	29	58.7	28	37.8
Native-born	878	56.2	813	56.4	68	50.0	19	41.3	46	62.2

*Included under "Physician, total."

were of foreign birth. The general puerperal death rate among foreign-born women is considerably higher than that among the native-born. We have no figures to show how many native and foreign-born women in all were attended by midwives, but it is generally accepted that the midwife attends more foreign-born than native-born women, and, if this is true, she is attending a group of women whose childbearing as a group is more hazardous than the average, with results better than average.

In Chapter V, page 148 *et seq.*, we have discussed the classification of our cases according to the economic status of the patient. Some of the data given there are repeated here for the light they throw on the present discussion. The general death rates for the various economic groups, presented in Table 87 (compare Table 62) should be kept in mind in the study of Table 88 (compare Table 64) which gives the distribution of deaths by economic group for each type of attendant.

Thus, while 17.6 per cent of all the deaths occurred in Group A, 43.8 per cent of the fatal cases delivered by midwives belonged to this group, 19.1 per cent delivered at home by physicians, and 16.3 per cent of all deaths delivered by physicians whether in home or hospital. Of all fatal cases delivered by midwives, 79.2 per cent came from Groups A and

TABLE 87

DEATHS BY ECONOMIC GROUP

(*Exclusive of deaths following abortion and ectopic gestation, and of non-resident births and deaths*)

	TOTAL	GROUP A	GROUP B	GROUP C	GROUP D
Total live births	341,879	56,019	155,457	125,241	5,162
Total deaths	1,520	275	653	572	20
Death rate per 1,000 live births	4.4	4.9	4.2	4.6	3.9

TABLE 88

DEATHS BY ECONOMIC GROUP AND ATTENDANT AT DELIVERY

(Exclusive of deaths following abortion and ectopic gestation)

| | TOTAL | | PHYSICIAN | | | | MIDWIFE | | NONE OR OTHER | |
| | | | TOTAL | | HOME DELIVERY* | | | | | |
	Number	Per cent	Number	Per cent	Number	Per cent	Number	Per cent	Number	Per cent
Total	1,564	100.0	1,442	100.0	136	100.0	48	100.0	74	100.0
Group A	275	17.6	235	16.3	26	19.1	21	43.8	19	25.7
Group B	653	41.8	600	41.6	65	47.8	17	35.4	36	48.6
Group C	572	36.6	547	37.9	41	30.1	10	20.8	15	20.3
Group D	20	1.3	20	1.4	1	.7	—	—	—	—
Non-resident	44	2.8	40	2.8	3	2.2	—	—	4	5.4

*Included under "Physician, total."

B, while of all live births during the period, only 61.9 per cent belonged in these two groups. It may be inferred that the midwife is working in homes where the surroundings are of the poorer and less well-equipped type. Forty-three and eight-tenths per cent of all the deaths following midwife deliveries were in definitely slum areas, with all that means in uncleanliness and overcrowding.

In Table 89 we show the results when preventability is indicated according to the attendant. This table shows a higher percentage of preventability (75.0 per cent) in the deaths among women attended by midwives than among the cases in general (62.9 per cent) or among those attended at home by a physician (61.0 per cent).

When the figures are further subdivided to show to whom the responsibility was ascribed, the division of those cases where delivery was by a physician shows the attending physician responsible in 74.2 per cent of the cases, the patient in 24.7 per cent, and the midwife in 1.1 per cent. Among the preventable deaths where delivery was attended at home by a physician, the responsibility was ascribed to the physician in 54.2 per cent of the deaths, to the patient in 44.6 per cent, and to the midwife in 1.2 per cent (one case). The division of the responsibility in the cases delivered by midwives shows the physician responsible in 19.4 per cent, the patient in 27.8 per cent, and the midwife in 52.8 per cent of the cases. Those instances in which midwives were held responsible for deaths following deliveries by physicians, and vice versa, were due to transfer of the cases from the midwife to the physician in the course of labor.

In forming a judgment as to preventability of death in the cases attended by midwives, the Advisory Committee has been inclined to ascribe the responsibility to the midwife except where it was clearly shown that such could not be the

TABLE 89

DEATHS BY PREVENTABILITY AND RESPONSIBILITY OF ATTENDANT AT DELIVERY

(Exclusive of deaths following abortion and ectopic gestation)

| | TOTAL | | PHYSICIAN | | | | MIDWIFE | | NONE OR OTHER | |
| | | | TOTAL | | HOME DELIVERY* | | | | | |
	Num-ber	Per cent	Num-ber	Per cent	Num-ber	Per cent	Num-ber	Per cent	Num-ber	Per cent
Total deaths	1,564	100.0	1,442	100.0	136	100.0	48	100.0	74	100.0
Not preventable	581	37.1	548	38.0	53	39.0	12	25.0	21	28.4
Preventable: total	983	62.9	894	62.0	83	61.0	36	75.0	53	71.6
Responsibility ascribed to										
Physician	678	69.0	663	74.2	45	54.2	7	19.4	8	15.1
Patient	276	28.1	221	24.7	37	44.6	10	27.8	45	84.9
Midwife	29	2.9	10	1.1	1	1.2	19	52.8	—	—

*Included under "Physician, total."

case. There is so little uniformity in the training of the midwife that there is no *a priori* assumption of her familiarity with the fundamentals of her work as is the case with the physician. The result represents the highest possible figure for the percentage of preventable cases among those attended by midwives.

Puerperal septicaemia is, of course, the most frequent cause of death in the whole series examined, as we have shown in Table 84. Death was caused by septicaemia in 50.0 per cent of the cases delivered by midwives, and in 32.6 per cent of all the cases. This is only an apparent preponderance of septicaemia in cases attended by midwives, as Table 90 indicates. This table shows the rate of fatal puerperal septicaemia per 1,000 live births classified according to the attendant. The general rate is 1.5 per 1,000 live births while the rates for those delivered at home by physicians and by midwives were both .8. This fact may be regarded as potentially very significant in relation to septicaemia, as these two groups are similar and comparable; the deliveries are non-operative and are conducted under home conditions which are not of the best.

The figure for total deliveries by physicians shows a rate nearly double that of the home deliveries. The operative in-

TABLE 90

SEPTICAEMIA DEATHS CLASSIFIED ACCORDING TO
ATTENDANT AT DELIVERY

| | TOTAL | PHYSICIAN | | MIDWIFE | NONE OR OTHER |
		TOTAL	HOME DELIVERY*		
Total live births	348,310	318,701	72,496	29,519	90
Septicaemia deaths	510	473	58	24	13
Septicaemia death rate per 1,000 live births	1.5	1.5	.8	.8	144.5

*Included under "Physician, total."

cidence in hospitals is perhaps chief among the manifold factors which may account for this. The home is not regarded as a suitable theatre for operative work and labor is allowed to proceed to its spontaneous conclusion. It is to be considered whether or not the facility with which interference can be undertaken in a properly equipped hospital does not tend to increase the incidence of such interference regardless of real indications—witness the term "prophylactic forceps," which name alone puts the indication for it, not in existing circumstances, but in future eventualities. As we have said, the circumstances of the home preclude that. The home is, moreover, less contaminated by virulent organisms; the patient has fewer attendants and is not in close proximity to other patients who may be a source of infection. There is, however, no possible way of arriving at a just figure for the septicaemia rate in spontaneous deliveries because the rate taken from deaths following spontaneous deliveries must be determined on a figure including all deliveries, no figure for the total incidence of spontaneous deliveries being available. It is evident that this lowers the rate in question in proportion to the percentage of operative deliveries in the total deliveries.

The highly trained specialist is not working in the home; that type of practice is largely confined to the general practitioner, so we may not ascribe the results to a higher degree of skill. It is rather to the combination of the circumstances to be met with in the home—spontaneous deliveries and uncontaminated surroundings with proper attendants—that we must look for an explanation. From the figures it would appear that domiciliary obstetrical practice must undergo further consideration and probable re-evaluation.

We have presented the data relating to the midwife with the results and conclusions which have been set out in their proper place. To the Committee it seems fair to say that contrary to the generally accepted opinion, the midwife is an acceptable attendant for properly selected cases of labor and delivery. There has never been a contention that she has any place except for the normal delivery at home, but we have seen that her results are as good as those obtained by the physician under what are justly regarded as comparable circumstances and for comparable cases.

Of the midwives seen and interviewed, it is significant and must be borne in mind that less than a third were judged to be competent and in the face of incompetence or only fair training and ability the results were by no means prejudicial to the midwife.

It is proper to consider what the desired end in midwife practice and control should be. Proper training is the first requisite and there is an increasing tendency among part of the medical profession to see that it is provided. Very recently a new school has been established under the supervision of a group of obstetricians for the purpose of training nurses as midwives. After proper training there must be suitable, adequate, and cooperative supervision and control of that practice.

The midwife should have a position in the scheme for providing maternity care. It remains for the medical profession to define what that position should be. She is able to supply attendance and nursing care for a smaller compensation than the costly training of a physician requires, but the necessity for every woman to have adequate care during pregnancy and at delivery, and to have the services of a physician if and when those services are needed, must be kept in mind.

It is necessary, first of all, to provide midwives who are properly trained. It would not seem absolutely necessary that a nurse's training be a prerequisite to training as a midwife, but in order to extend the practice of employing midwives as accoucheuses in normal parturition, a different type of woman must be brought into the field. The present type of non-nurse midwife would prove wholly unacceptable to certain classes of the community. While the only slightly educated woman with adequate training may be a capable midwife, the more educated patient will demand a different type of attendant. The two groups need not be mutually exclusive. There should be opportunities for both to receive the necessary training.

The standards met by such a school as that maintained by Bellevue Hospital would insure adequately trained women. Licensure should then follow an examination to prove the candidate's fitness for her work. The midwife should be encouraged and, if necessary, required to return for short courses at certain intervals. Her training must prepare her to understand the mechanisms of normal labor and delivery. She must be able to detect the signs of the abnormalities of pregnancy, and she must be able to measure the pelvis accurately. She must be thoroughly familiar with a simple method for maintaining asepsis. Finally, she must be equipped to give suitable care to both mother and infant during the puerperium.

It is to be desired that every woman be examined during pregnancy by a properly qualified obstetrician. In this way, abnormalities, constitutional defects, and possible sources of danger to the mother or foetus may be properly managed. This is essential; but if the inclination is to attempt to induce the patient to give up the services of a midwife for no better reason than that she is a midwife, it is impossible to expect the midwife to cooperate with a group who stand ready to undermine her practice. Such practices between physicians have met with violent denunciation; between the physician and midwife they are deserving of the same censure. If she is to be expected to cooperate with the physician, the physician must be ready to cooperate with her. If scrupulous fairness were exercised in the matter of judging the suitability of individual cases for midwife care, cooperation by the midwife would be forthcoming. It would be destructive of her own interests to withhold it and if she knew that she was to be held strictly accountable for the results if she failed to advise her patient to seek medical advice, there would be no difficulty.

Supervision should be extended and given some real meaning both as a check on the midwife and as an aid to her. She should be required to report births within forty-eight hours, and such reports should be followed by visits of an adequately trained supervisor. Nurse-midwives could no doubt be used admirably in this capacity with physicians directing them. In this way the disturbances of the puerperium could be guarded against and quickly treated.

A set of regulations concerning the conduct of labor would be necessary to a proper supervision. The requirement that a physician be called after a stipulated number of hours in labor would greatly assist the midwife in avoiding the difficulties of obstructed labors. Physicians must be ready to give her assistance when she needs it.

In many instances poorly trained, always inadequately supervised, the object of only faintly disguised and often open antagonism, lack of cooperation, and contempt, the midwife still attends almost 10 per cent of the deliveries of New York City with as good results both for mothers and babies as the physicians under similar circumstances. We believe she has proved her value in face of the pressing problem of assuring proper care for all women at an outlay that is not prohibitive.

Without her, those women who cannot afford physicians must become city charges, and we know that the municipal facilities could not stand this further strain.

The medical profession must accept the midwife as one of its adjuncts. Physicians must make themselves responsible for her proper training and supervision as such. They must regard her as an ally in the effort to reduce the morbidity and mortality associated with childbearing. Both officially and privately, there must be an alteration in the prevailing attitudes toward her. There must be a readiness to cooperate with her to insure the results both physician and midwife are anxious to achieve.

IX

CONCLUSIONS AND RECOMMENDATIONS

IN discussing in detail the various elements which have appeared relevant and significant to the study of puerperal mortality in New York City, we have pointed out what, in our opinion, were the factors which produced the result and where alteration might bring about an improvement.

It has seemed clear throughout that the rate of death was unnecessarily high. The high percentage of preventable deaths from each and all of the causes was ample proof of that fact. It was estimated that two-thirds of all the deaths studied could have been prevented if the care of the woman had been proper in all respects.

Where the lack of proper care was ascribed to failure on the part of the attendant, it is probable that this failure was not attributable to neglect or carelessness. Rather, the ignorance and insufficient training of the attendant prevented him from giving the high quality of care which he was attempting to provide for his patient and, further, prevented the understanding on his part of the fact that he was incapable.

The rate of deaths from puerperal causes is high, and unnecessarily so. It has shown no tendency to decrease during the last twelve years, in spite of progressive improvement in the methods of treatment and the increased hospitalization of the parturient. This fact is more striking when the falling rate for other types of conditions, such as infant mortality and the large groups of the communicable diseases, is considered.

Certain elements have been recurrently striking in relation

to every puerperal cause of death and seem to be contributory to the production and maintenance of the persistently high rate. They may be briefly reviewed, with suggestions for possible improvement.

First of all, it is evident that prenatal care was inadequate and improper. The patients repeatedly failed to seek prenatal care. Often if they did, it was very late in pregnancy and return visits were neglected. This was particularly true of patients from the lower economic groups.

It was plain that this arose out of the ignorance and misinformation still widespread among the lay public in spite of the persistent efforts which have been made to combat it. It was apparent that women did not know the necessity for prenatal care, and failed to understand just what constitutes proper prenatal care. Many patients were ignorant of the gravity of certain apparently mild symptoms which indicated the presence of serious abnormalities. Persistent vomiting was disregarded, repeated vaginal hemorrhage neglected, pain and bleeding early in pregnancy and the milder symptoms of toxaemia overlooked.

Many patients did attempt to obtain prenatal care. They consulted their physician early and returned regularly. But the attendant failed to give proper care. Physical examination was careless and incomplete. Contractions of the pelvis were overlooked. The severity of complications was repeatedly underestimated and they were improperly treated.

The high incidence of operative interference during labor was an important factor in the result. More than 45 per cent of the deaths in this series, exclusive of abortion and ectopic gestation, followed operative deliveries and the death rate per 1,000 live births for operative deliveries was greatly in excess of that for spontaneous deliveries.

Frequently the operation chosen was the wrong one. Often it was undertaken at an improper time. Manifestly obstructed labors were allowed to continue when it should have been clear that delivery could not be effected from below. Trial labors were frequently too greatly prolonged.

Special mention must be made of the situation in regard to caesarean section. Many sections were undertaken for improper indications. Many were done after long, exhausting labors. The classical type was repeatedly performed without due regard to the fact that the patient, after a long labor, when membranes had been ruptured and repeated vaginal examinations had been made, was potentially infected. There were many operations performed after previous attempts at instrumental delivery had failed. Frequently these attempts and the final operation were the result of the incapacity of the accoucheur properly to judge the patient's ability to deliver herself. Often the type of operation was one which demanded greater training and skill than the attendant could command.

The incapacity of the attendants, either in judgment or skill, contributed significantly to the large number of avoidable deaths. Their failure to provide proper prenatal care has already been pointed out. The prognosis of delivery was frequently incorrect. Labor was often improperly conducted. The physicians many times were apparently ignorant of indications and contra-indications for interference. Operative procedures were undertaken when there was no indication or a plain contra-indication. Labor was terminated by rapid traumatizing delivery when non-interference was called for. Operative procedures were performed on potentially infected patients. Attendants were tardy in obtaining proper consultations. There was failure to treat severe complication with all the means which should have been available. Difficult obstetrical operations were performed by physicians whose training and experience could not be considered adequate. At times the conclusion that proper asepsis had not been maintained could not be avoided.

Hospital standards were inadequate in many instances. The actual physical equipment was inadequate in some hospitals. Proper facilities for labor and delivery were lacking. Isolation was not always carried out promptly. In some proprietary hospitals, the operating room was also used as a delivery room. In some hospitals the resident staff was given too great responsibility. Resident physicians were permitted to perform major operative procedures unsupervised, after only telephonic consultation with the attending physician, whose responsibility it was to see the patient. Exacting and difficult obstetrical operations were performed by the junior members of attending staffs without consultation with the chiefs, when the ability of the former was not sufficient. Proprietary hospitals exercised no supervision over their staffs, each physician establishing his own standards.

Finally, midwife practice entered in as a contributory cause of the high rate. The training of these women was frequently insufficient. There is no attempt to evaluate the qualifications of candidates for license, graduation from an acceptable school being the only requirement.

RECOMMENDATIONS

To improve this situation and remove the causes out of which it arises, it is evident that there must be a determined effort to educate both the lay public and the medical profession to an understanding of the necessity for change in certain of the methods now employed. The profession itself must accept the responsibility for educating the lay public to a better understanding of the aims of obstetrics and the methods by which those aims may be realized. But prior to that must come increased education of the profession, that it in turn may wisely inform the lay public.

First, a prospective mother must have further instruction

in the necessity for prenatal care. She must be taught that prenatal care does not mean merely registering for confinement; that it is imperative to obtain that care as early as pregnancy is suspected; that one visit at which no abnormalities were discovered is no guarantee of continuing good health but that regular return for observation is vital if her attendant is to be enabled to give her the best possible care; that previous normal pregnancies and deliveries do not assure subsequent normal ones; that proper and sufficient prenatal care offers her the greatest assurance of an uneventful confinement.

Furthermore, some information must be made available to the patient as to the standards of such prenatal care. She should have some knowledge of the purposes of such care and what she may expect from her attendant as the minimum requirements of a proper prenatal supervision. She should know that the omission of urinalysis, blood pressure determination, or the measurement of her pelvis constitutes negligence; that a thorough physical examination is a necessary part of proper care. She must be informed of the possible gravity of symptoms that seem to her mild, and the fact that early treatment is the prerequisite to the prevention of later trouble.

The medical profession is obligated to inform the lay public that operative delivery undertaken merely to alleviate pain or shorten labor involves increased risk for both mother and baby.

The relative safety of delivery at home should be emphasized. Effort should be made to induce women who cannot obtain adequate medical or hospital care to avail themselves of the services of qualified midwives under the supervision of physicians.

To accomplish this education, the medical profession must assume a role which heretofore has been left to lay organizations. The confidence of the lay public in the medical profession enables this to be done with greater authority and increased chances of success. There are not lacking among lay writers those who are eager to inform or misinform their readers as to the proper conduct of the physician. Until now the medical profession has been content to ignore such outgivings. It is now time that the physician himself take the burden of giving to the lay public that authoritative and necessary information which he, best of all, can give. To do this well, the outstanding members of the profession in every community must actively interest themselves in the process. Obstetrical societies would do well to use the channels of the press and radio to broaden the sphere of their activities in this line. They would further increase their educational function by issuing authoritative pamphlets from time to time. They must assume responsibility for the teaching given through social service and lay organizations.

If the doctor is to be a useful teacher, he must himself be properly educated. The education must start with the medical student. It has been repeatedly asserted that medical schools do not now provide sufficient training in normal obstetrics. That they must do. But they have a further obligation: to inform the student that the training which he receives does not qualify him to practice as a specialist in obstetrics. His training is to enable him to conduct normal labors and to be able to recognize and evaluate the abnormalities requiring the services of a specially qualified obstetrician. The medical profession *must* insist that prolonged graduate study is necessary for specialization. So important is this element that it might be advisable to set up a legal barrier preventing any but those who had shown themselves specially qualified from doing any operative obstetrics.

The practitioner must avail himself of all opportunities

for further education. He should inform himself of the demands of proper prenatal care, not only for combating a toxaemia but for making the proper prognosis of delivery by an accurate evaluation of the pelvis. He must recognize the danger to his patient of undertaking operative procedures unless he is properly qualified by experience and training. The hazard associated with operative procedures undertaken as emergency measures must be emphasized. Indications for operative procedures must be re-stated, and adequate indications must be insisted on before operation is undertaken. The role of operation in predisposing to systemic or local infection must be stressed. It must be shown that the caesarean operation is undoubtedly subject to abuse; that the indications require careful examination and limitation; that such an operation is rightly within the province of only the highly skilled specialist.

If such education is to be demanded of the practitioner of medicine, facilities for obtaining it must be made available. Such facilities are strikingly lacking today. The graduate in medicine who wishes to further his study of any specialty meets with the greatest difficulty in doing so. Hospitals must be prepared to receive these men as internes in order that they may have the opportunity of using clinical material. Medical schools should offer courses to the practitioner.

If courses are offered and specialists are to be developed, there must be some way in which the public can inform itself as to the status of any given physician. Obstetrical societies or other qualified groups could prepare such lists, admitting candidates who had satisfactorily demonstrated their qualifications by examination. These lists should be made available to the public at request and the knowledge of their availability widely distributed.

With the establishment of such requirements for specialists, certain other correlative requirements will appear. If the practitioner is to confine his activities in obstetrics to normal deliveries, far more consultation will be required. Earlier and more frequent consultation with the highly trained specialist should be more freely resorted to. It must be made clear that consultation with the most highly trained specialists is always available to any patient for a minimum or nominal fee where circumstances demand it.

Hospitals, in order to qualify for recognition by the controlling authorities, must have qualified obstetricians as directors of their staffs. Thorough evaluation of the work of the attending staff should be made regularly. Certain other standards are to be regarded as necessary for such qualifications. Some of these have been outlined by the American Medical Association and the American College of Surgeons. The hospital must maintain a special clinic for prenatal care, in charge of a member of the visiting obstetrical staff. There must be a sufficient number of beds set aside for the hospitalization of clinic patients with complications. There must be a social service department adequate, as to training and personnel, to keep in touch with all patients; to insure early registration and regular attendance; to facilitate the patients' cooperation through home adjustments; to assist in the educational function of the hospital to the community.

All hospitals must maintain separate delivery rooms where only obstetrical cases are treated. The rules for the maintenance of asepsis must be rigid, including masking, the importance of which deserves re-emphasis. Labor rooms must be sufficient to insure their availability to all patients. Isolation must conform to the most stringent regulations and include proper technique on the part of the nursing staff. All nursing must be done by properly supervised nurses who should be especially trained in obstetrical nursing. The resident staffs must be under supervision at all times. There must be an invariable rule requiring the responsible attending physician to see patients promptly and supervise directly the residents who are assigned to them. Furthermore, the less experienced members of the staff must be under supervision of the responsible heads. No major operative procedure should be performed until the chiefs of the staff have been consulted and, unless they are confident of the capacity of the attending physician, the chiefs of staff should themselves perform or assist in the performance of such procedures. Where anaesthesia is required, the responsibility for the choice and proper administration must rest with the accoucheur.

Proprietary hospitals should be brought under the supervision of a responsible board of hospital control and unless they provide adequate facilities as described above, except for prenatal care and social service, they should not be permitted to accept obstetrical patients.

The situation in regard to midwives must be altered. More schools are needed for their training, including both women who have had previous training as nurses and those who have not; effort should be made to enroll types of women who would be acceptable to groups of the population now unwilling to employ a midwife, and the nurse-midwife is suitable for this purpose. Licensure should be based upon examination. Additional short courses, at stated intervals, should be compulsory. Supervision should be increased, and changed to include actual oversight of cases under care. With physicians in charge, appropriately trained nurse-midwives might make suitable supervisors. Midwives should be required to report births within forty-eight hours, to report immediately any abnormality during labor, and to call consultation if labor continues beyond a definite time-limit. The physician must be prepared to give the midwife unqualified cooperation.

Some hospitals might well make use of midwives to conduct the deliveries in their out-patient service, under the direction of the in-patient obstetrical department.

The hazards of childbirth in New York City are greater than they need be. Responsibility for reducing them rests with the medical profession.

APPENDIX

SUMMARY OF MATERNAL MORTALITY FOR THREE YEARS
1930-1931-1932
EXCLUSIVE OF ABORTION AND ECTOPIC GESTATION

	1930	1931	1932	TOTAL
Total maternal deaths	544	540	480	1,564
	DELIVERY			
Delivered in hospital	386	373	352	1,111
Delivered at home	70	70	49	189
Not delivered	88	97	79	264
	DEATH			
Died in hospital	490	483	448	1,421
Died at home	54	57	32	143
	DELIVERY AND DEATH			
Delivered and died in hospital	373	360	347	1,080
Delivered in hospital, died at home	13	13	5	31
Delivered and died at home	28	26	16	70
Delivered at home, died in hospital	42	44	33	119
Not delivered, died in hospital	75	79	68	222
Not delivered, died at home	13	18	11	42
	BOROUGH			
Manhattan	183	211	170	564
Brooklyn	246	195	181	622
Bronx	61	71	76	208
Queens	48	57	46	151
Richmond	6	6	7	19
	RACE			
White	492	465	435	1,392
Negro	51	74	45	170
Yellow	1	1	—	2
	NATIVITY			
Native-born	288	311*	279	878*
Foreign-born	256	229	201	686
	†FOREIGN-BORN, BY COUNTRY			
Armenia	1	—	1	2
Austria	17	8	16	41
Belgium	—	—	—	—
Bermuda	—	—	—	
Bohemia	—	1	—	1
Brazil	1	—	—	1
British Guiana	1	—	—	1
British West Indies	7	12	8	27
Canada	5	1	2	8
Central America	—	1	—	1

*Including one Chinese born in the U. S. A.

†For completeness the above list includes the names of all the countries of the foreign-born mothers who died during the three-year period. Where a blank appears (in the total column after the name of a country) the deaths are shown in the abortion or ectopic gestation summary.

EXCLUSIVE OF ABORTION AND ECTOPIC GESTATION (continued)

	1930	1931	1932	TOTAL
	FOREIGN-BORN, BY COUNTRY (*continued*)			
Chili	—	1	—	1
Colombia	—	1	1	2
Cuba	—	1	2	3
Czechoslovakia	2	3	1	6
Denmark	1	2	1	4
Dominican Republic	—	1	—	1
Egypt	—	1	—	1
England	8	5	4	17
Esthonia	—	1	—	1
Finland	—	1	—	1
France	1	2	3	6
French West Indies	—	—	1	1
Germany	13	15	14	42
Greece	3	2	3	8
Hungary	3	4	7	14
Ireland	32	28	36	96
Italy	79	56	32	167
Japan	1	—	—	1
Jugo-Slavia	—	1	—	1
Latvia	—	—	—	—
Lithuania	—	—	3	3
Luxemburg	—	—	1	1
Malta	—	1	—	1
Mexico	—	—	2	2
Newfoundland	2	—	1	3
Norway	4	—	4	8
Panama	—	—	2	2
Poland	20	15	13	48
Porto Rico	13	25	15	53
Roumania	1	2	3	6
Russia	30	19	11	60
Santo Domingo	—	—	—	—
Scotland	2	4	7	13
Serbia	1	—	—	1
South America	—	2	1	3
Spain	1	3	—	4
Sweden	3	3	2	8
Syria	1	2	3	6
Turkey	1	1	1	3
Venezuela	1	—	—	1
Virgin Isles	—	4	—	4
Wales	1	—	—	1
	AGE			
15 to 19 years	24	37	26	87
20 to 24 "	108	117	99	324
25 to 29 "	149	147	136	432
30 to 34 "	127	119	105	351
35 to 39 "	92	87	80	259
40 to 44 "	38	31	33	102
45 and over	6	2	1	9

EXCLUSIVE OF ABORTION AND ECTOPIC GESTATION (continued)

	1930	1931	1932	TOTAL
	PERIOD OF UTEROGESTATION			
Over 40 weeks	2	2	2	6
40 weeks	378	358	324	1,060
39 "	9	4	6	19
38 "	32	17	17	66
37 "	5	3	9	17
36 "	37	45	35	117
35 "	3	—	2	5
34 "	4	9	4	17
33 "	2	1	3	6
32 "	11	27	16	54
31 "	17	16	10	43
30 "	6	4	6	16
29 "	5	2	4	11
28 "	12	18	18	48
Not reported, over 28 weeks	—	—	—	—
27 "	—	3	—	3
26 "	—	1	2	3
25 "	2	1	2	5
24 "	3	1	—	4
23 "	—	1	4	5
22 "	7	6	2	15
21 "	—	—	—	—
20 "	2	3	1	6
19 "	—	—	—	—
18 "	2	5	4	11
17 "	—	1	—	1
16 "	—	—	—	—
15 "	1	—	1	2
14 "	—	2	1	3
13 "	3	1	2	6
12 "	—	5	2	7
11 "	—	1	—	1
10 "	—	—	—	—
9 "	—	1	1	2
8 "	1	2	—	3
7 "	—	—	1	1
6 "	—	—	1	1
Less than 6 weeks	—	—	—	—
Not reported, less than 28 weeks	—	—	—	—
	WASSERMANN			
No Wassermann, or not reported	426	378	292	1,096
Wassermann taken	118	162	188	468
	WASSERMANN REPORT			
Negative	105	149	172	426
Positive	9	13	16	38
Not reported	4	—	—	4

EXCLUSIVE OF ABORTION AND ECTOPIC GESTATION (continued)

	1930	1931	1932	TOTAL
POSITIVE WASSERMANN REPORT				
4+	3	7	12	22
3+	3	1	1	5
2+	—	—	1	1
1+	—	1	—	1
Not reported	3	4	2	9
GRAVIDITY				
Primigravidae	230	236	216	682
Multigravidae	312	300	262	874
Not reported	2	4	2	8
MULTIGRAVIDAE, BY GRAVIDITY				
Gravidae II	93	101	83	277
" III	67	66	59	192
" IV	56	40	32	128
" V	36	25	28	89
" VI	13	21	13	47
" VII	13	11	8	32
" VIII	11	6	14	31
" IX	8	14	10	32
" X	3	4	2	9
" XI	3	6	3	12
" XII	—	2	2	4
" XIII	3	—	3	6
" XIV	—	2	1	3
" XV	5	—	1	6
" XVI and over	1	—	1	2
Multigravidae, gravidity not reported	—	2	2	4
AUTOPSY				
With autopsy	76	106	90	272
No autopsy	468	434	390	1,292
BIRTHS (babies)				
Multiple births (all twins)	11	19	21	51
Total babies	555	559	501	1,615
Alive	324	339	301	964
Stillborn	141	122	118	381
Not delivered (including postmortem deliveries)	90	98	82	270
LEGITIMACY				
Legitimate (by number of mothers)	530	512	462	1,504
Legitimate (by babies)	539	530	483	1,552
Illegitimate (by number of mothers)	14	28	18	60
Illegitimate (by babies)	16	29	18	63

	1930	1931	1932	TOTAL
	PRESENTATION (babies)			
Vertex	406	409	372	1,187
Breech	29	31	30	90
Face	11	3	2	16
Transverse	12	9	9	30
Not reported	6	9	6	21
Not delivered	90	98	82	270
Excluded (abdominal pregnancy, 28 weeks or over)	1	—	—	1
	NOT DELIVERED PRESENTATIONS (babies)			
Vertex	29	31	22	82
Breech	1	2	2	5
Face	1	—	—	1
Transverse	2	1	—	3
Not reported	36	30	33	99
Excluded (abdominal pregnancy, 28 weeks or over)	—	—	1	1
Excluded (all less than 28 weeks)	21	34	24	79
	PRENATAL CARE			
Adequate	228	178	194	600
Inadequate	176	169	144	489
None	135	181	133	449
Excluded (all less than 16 weeks)	5	12	9	26
	PELVIS			
Normal	284	319	318	921
Abnormal	67	58	54	179
Not reported	172	129	84	385
Excluded (all less than 28 weeks)	21	34	24	79
	DELIVERY ATTENDANT			
Physician	365	298	279	942
Interne	63	106	102	271
Midwife	19	19	8	46
None	9	19	12	40
Not reported	—	1	—	1
Not delivered	88	97	79	264
	LABOR			
Spontaneous	408	390	351	1,149
Induced (includes attempted induced)	44	30	31	105
Forcé	1	2	3	6
None	91	113	95	299
Not reported	—	5	—	5

EXCLUSIVE OF ABORTION AND ECTOPIC GESTATION (continued)

	1930	1931	1932	TOTAL
	‡TYPE OF DELIVERY (mothers)			
Spontaneous	200	203	168	571
Operative	256	240	233	729
Not delivered	88	97	79	264
	TYPE OF DELIVERY (babies)			
Spontaneous	205	208	178	591
Operative	260	253	241	754
Not delivered	90	98	82	270
	§OPERATIVE DELIVERY (mothers)			
Low forceps	48	56	41(1)	145(1)
Mid forceps	29	30	32	91
High forceps	10	5	9	24
Version	7	1	1	9
Extraction	8	7	14(1)	29(1)
Version and extraction	46(1)	36(1)	31	113(2)
Craniotomy	11	4	11	26
Embryotomy	1	—	—	1
Caesarean (abdominal)	97(1)	106(7)	101(3)	304(11)
Others	3	1	1	5
Laparotomy for abdominal pregnancy	1	—	—	1
Operative attempt with spontaneous delivery	2	—	—	2
Vaginal caesarean	—	—	1	1
Not reported	—	1	—	1
	OPERATIVE ATTEMPTS ON DELIVERED CASES			
Number of mothers (all over 28 weeks)	15	10	14	39
Low forceps	1	—	—	1
Mid forceps	1	2	2	5
High forceps	10	6	10	26
Version	2	—	1	3
Extraction	1	2	—	3
Version and extraction	1	1	1	3
Craniotomy	—	—	1	1
Embryotomy	—	1	—	1

‡Two mothers who finally delivered spontaneously are included here under Operative because of an extensive attempt at operative delivery.

Two sets of twins where one baby was born spontaneously and the other by an operative procedure are counted here under Operative only.

§There were twenty-five sets of twins where both babies were born by operative procedures; fifteen of these, born by the same operative procedure, are shown by the figures in parentheses; these figures may be added to the main one to get the total procedures by babies. In the other ten sets each baby was born by a different operative procedure and both deliveries are counted.

Further differences in the total mothers with operative delivery and the total operative procedures are due to the fact that in a few instances two distinct procedures were employed on the same mother for the delivery of one baby.

EXCLUSIVE OF ABORTION AND ECTOPIC GESTATION (continued)

	1930	1931	1932	TOTAL
	OPERATIVE ATTEMPTS ON NOT DELIVERED CASES			
Number of mothers (all over 28 weeks)	14	2	1	17
Low forceps	1	1	—	2
Mid forceps	1	—	—	1
High forceps	3	1	1	5
Version	3	—	1	4
Version and extraction	4	—	—	4
Craniotomy	1	1	1	3
Caesarean	6	—	—	6
	POSTMORTEM DELIVERY			
Number of mothers (all over 28 weeks)	9	9	12	30
Number of babies	11	10	12	33
Forceps (1 twin) ¶	1	1	—	2
Extraction	2	—	1	3
Version and extraction	2	1	2	5
Caesarean	4(1)	7(1)	9	20(2)
Autopsy (other twin) ¶	1	—	—	1
	‖POSTMORTEM BIRTHS			
Born alive	1	1	2	4
Stillborn (includes autopsy) ¶	10	9	10	29
	COMPLICATIONS OF PREGNANCY			
With complications	209	176	169	554
No complications	310	318	263	891
Not reported	25	46	48	119
	COMPLICATIONS SPECIFIED			
Albuminuria	137	120	97	354
None	57	29	55	141
Not reported	15	27	17	59
Convulsions	54	57	38	149
None	155	119	131	405
Not reported	—	—	—	—
High blood pressure	115	114	93	322
None	75	43	61	179
Not reported	19	19	15	53
Oedema	88	97	96	281
None	113	74	73	260
Not reported	8	5	—	13
Prolonged headaches	48	32	34	114
None	149	126	130	405
Not reported	12	18	5	35

¶Includes one set of twins. One baby was delivered by forceps immediately postmortem (stillborn), the other baby was discovered later at autopsy.

‖All postmortem births are counted under the Not delivered babies.

EXCLUSIVE OF ABORTION AND ECTOPIC GESTATION (continued)

	1930	1931	1932	TOTAL
COMPLICATIONS SPECIFIED (*continued*)				
Pernicious vomiting	20	14	13	47
None	180	150	153	483
Not reported	9	12	3	24
Bleeding during pregnancy	56	16	37	109
None	147	148	129	424
Not reported	6	12	3	21
INTERCURRENT DISEASES OR ABNORMALITIES				
Number of diseases or abnormalities	88	90	112	290
Number of mothers with intercurrent diseases	72	85	98	255
Number of mothers without intercurrent diseases	444	437	371	1,252
Not reported	28	18	11	57
**INTERCURRENT OPERATIONS SPECIFIED				
Number of mothers with operation during pregnancy	8	7	13	28
Appendectomy	5	2	3	10
Cholecystectomy	—	—	1	1
Cholecystotomy	—	1	1	2
Colpotomy	—	1	—	1
Hemorrhoidectomy	1	—	—	1
Ileostomy	1	1	—	2
Incision and drainage: abscess of vulva	—	—	1	1
Incision and drainage: Bartholin's gland	1	—	1	2
Laparotomy: fibroids	2	—	—	2
Laparotomy: exploratory	—	1	3	4
Mastoidectomy	—	1	—	1
Myringotomy	—	—	1	1
Myomectomy	—	1	—	1
Sinus: drainage, nasal	—	—	1	1
Splenectomy	—	—	1	1
PREVENTABILITY				
Not preventable	184	204	193	581
Preventable:				
Responsibility ascribed to physician	251	225	202	678
Responsibility ascribed to patient	97	95	84	276
Responsibility ascribed to midwife	12	16	1	29
CAUSE OF DEATH				
Puerperal causes	455	398	367	1,220
Extra-puerperal causes	89	142	113	344

**Abnormalities requiring operation are counted under Intercurrent disease also.

EXCLUSIVE OF ABORTION AND ECTOPIC GESTATION (continued)

	1930	1931	1932	TOTAL
	††PUERPERAL CAUSE OF DEATH SPECIFIED			
144: Hemorrhage	68	65	64	197
145: Puerperal septicemia	183	163	164	510
146: Albuminuria and eclampsia	91	80	60	231
147: Pernicious vomiting	1	6	7	14
148: Phlegmasia alba dolens and embolus	25	37	27	89
149: Accidents of labor	87	39	45	171
150: Accidents of puerperium	—	8	—	8
	††EXTRA-PUERPERAL CAUSE OF DEATH SPECIFIED			
92: Chronic cardiac disease	28	43	28	99
108: Lobar pneumonia	14	22	16	52
11: Influenza	2	4	15	21
107: Bronchopneumonia	3	12	5	20
131: Chronic nephritis	4	7	7	18
23: Tuberculosis (respiratory)	5	5	6	16
91: Acute cardiac disease	4	4	2	10
121: Appendicitis	3	3	3	9
122: Intestinal obstruction	3	2	3	8
200: Cause ill-defined or unspecified	—	4	4	8
36: Septicaemia, non-puerperal	—	2	4	6
125: Acute yellow atrophy and other diseases of liver	—	4	2	6
133: Other diseases of kidneys and annexa	2	3	1	6
178: Accidental absorption of poison, etc.	2	4	—	6
179: Other acute accidental poisonings	3	1	2	6
194: Other accidents	5	1	—	6
82: Cerebral hemorrhage	3	1	1	5
111: Congestion, oedema of lung, etc.	1	4	—	5
34: Syphilis	2	1	—	3
59: Diabetes mellitus	1	2	—	3
130: Acute nephritis	—	1	2	3
18: Meningococcus meningitis	1	1	—	2
79: Meningitis (simple)	1	—	1	2
85: Epilepsy	—	—	2	2
115: Diseases of buccal cavity and annexa	—	2	—	2
129: Peritonitis, cause not specified	—	2	—	2
8: Scarlet fever	—	—	1	1
10: Diphtheria	—	1	—	1
15: Erysipelas	1	—	—	1
16: Poliomyelitis	—	1	—	1
17: Lethargic encephalitis	—	1	—	1
56: Acute rheumatic fever	—	1	—	1
66: Diseases of the thyroid gland	—	1	—	1
72: Leukemia	—	1	—	1

††The figure appearing before each cause of death is the code number as taken from the *Manual of the International List of Causes of Death.*

SUMMARY OF MATERNAL MORTALITY FOR THREE YEARS
1930-1931-1932
EXCLUSIVE OF ABORTION AND ECTOPIC GESTATION (*continued*)

	1930	1931	1932	TOTAL
	††EXTRA-PUERPERAL CAUSE OF DEATH SPECIFIED (*continued*)			
73: Diseases of the spleen	—	—	1	1
78: Encephalitis (non epidemic)	1	—	—	1
81: Other diseases of the spinal cord	—	—	1	1
89: Mastoiditis	—	1	—	1
94: Angina pectoris	—	1	—	1
112: Asthma	—	—	1	1
117: Gastric ulcer	—	—	1	1
120: Enteritis	—	1	—	1
139: Mastitis	—	1	—	1
166: Suicide by drowning	—	1	—	1

††The figure appearing before each cause of death is the code number as taken from the *Manual of the International List of Causes of Death.*

SUMMARY OF MATERNAL MORTALITY FOR THREE YEARS
1930-1931-1932
ABORTIONS

	1930	1931	1932	TOTAL
Total maternal deaths following abortion	91	129	137	357
	DELIVERY			
Delivered in hospital	24	35	40	99
Delivered at home	67	94	97	258
	DEATH			
Died in hospital	84	119	131	334
Died at home	7	10	6	23
	DELIVERY AND DEATH			
Delivered and died in hospital	23	35	40	98
Delivered in hospital, died at home	1	—	—	1
Delivered and died at home	6	10	6	22
Delivered at home, died in hospital	61	84	91	236
	BOROUGH			
Manhattan	31	53	51	135
Brooklyn	40	54	56	150
Bronx	12	11	13	36
Queens	8	11	14	33
Richmond	—	—	3	3
	RACE			
White	82	105	112	299
Negro	9	24	25	58
	NATIVITY			
Native-born	51	86	84	221
Foreign-born	40	43	53	136
	FOREIGN-BORN, BY COUNTRY			
Austria	2	4	2	8
British West Indies	2	4	6	12
Canada	—	1	2	3
Czechoslovakia	1	—	—	1
England	2	1	3	6
Finland	2	1	1	4
Germany	2	4	3	9
Greece	1	—	—	1
Hungary	1	—	—	1
Ireland	4	4	7	15
Italy	10	8	10	28
Jugo-Slavia	—	—	1	1
Latvia	1	—	—	1
Newfoundland	—	1	—	1
Norway	1	1	—	2
Poland	—	—	3	3
Porto Rico	6	6	7	19

ABORTIONS (*continued*)

	1930	1931	1932	TOTAL
	FOREIGN-BORN, BY COUNTRY (*continued*)			
Roumania	—	1	—	1
Russia	3	3	3	9
Santo Domingo	—	1	—	1
Scotland	—	—	3	3
Sweden	—	2	2	4
Syria	—	1	—	1
Turkey	2	—	—	2
	AGE			
15 to 19 years	6	10	4	20
20 to 24 "	19	38	28	85
25 to 29 "	25	32	39	96
30 to 34 "	23	18	23	64
35 to 39 "	13	26	34	73
40 to 44 "	5	5	9	19
45 and over	—	—	—	—
	PERIOD OF UTEROGESTATION			
27 weeks	—	1	—	1
26 "	1	5	5	11
25 "	2	2	1	5
24 "	3	1	3	7
23 "	2	5	9	16
22 "	4	4	5	13
21 "	—	1	—	1
20 "	2	3	5	10
19 "	—	1	—	1
18 "	8	7	9	24
17 "	1	2	1	4
16 "	1	3	—	4
15 "	3	4	2	9
14 "	1	4	2	7
13 "	11	27	28	66
12 "	3	11	12	26
11 "	1	2	6	9
10 "	8	4	5	17
9 "	17	9	13	39
8 "	9	10	8	27
7 "	1	5	4	10
6 "	8	5	6	19
Less than 6 weeks	—	2	3	5
Not reported	5	13	8	26
	WASSERMANN			
No Wassermann, or not reported	87	103	112	302
Wassermann taken	4	26	25	55
	WASSERMANN REPORT			
Negative	4	23	25	52
Positive	—	3	—	3

ABORTIONS (continued)

	1930	1931	1932	TOTAL
POSITIVE WASSERMANN REPORT				
4+	—	1	—	1
3+	—	1	—	1
Not reported	—	1	—	1
GRAVIDITY				
Primigravidae	30	57	47	134
Multigravidae	56	62	79	197
Not reported	5	10	11	26
MULTIGRAVIDAE, BY GRAVIDITY				
Gravidae II	14	19	14	47
" III	10	12	11	33
" IV	14	10	13	37
" V	6	6	10	22
" VI	3	1	11	15
" VII	4	5	6	15
" VIII	4	2	1	7
" IX	—	1	2	3
" X	1	1	2	4
" XI	—	—	1	1
" XII	—	—	1	1
" XIII	—	—	2	2
" XIV	—	—	—	—
" XV	—	—	1	1
" XVI and over	—	1	—	1
Multigravidae, gravidity not reported	—	4	4	8
AUTOPSY				
With autopsy	57	84	82	223
No autopsy	34	45	55	134
BIRTHS (babies)				
Multiple births (all twins)	2	—	1	3
Total babies	93	129	138	360
Alive	1	2	—	3
Stillborn (includes incomplete abortions)	92	127	138	357
LEGITIMACY				
Legitimate (by number of mothers)	78	101	116	295
Legitimate (by babies)	79	101	117	297
Illegitimate (by number of mothers)	13	28	21	62
Illegitimate (by babies)	14	28	21	63

ABORTIONS (continued)

	1930	1931	1932	TOTAL
PRENATAL CARE				
Adequate	5	8	9	22
Inadequate	4	2	5	11
None	15	23	26	64
Excluded (all less than 16 weeks)	67	96	97	260
DELIVERY ATTENDANT				
Physician	24	19	23	66
Interne	2	10	11	23
Midwife	6	7	6	19
None	52	74	86	212
Not reported	7	19	11	37
LABOR				
Spontaneous	52	66	80	198
Induced (includes attempted induced)	33	47	34	114
None	6	14	12	32
Not reported	—	2	11	13
***TYPE OF DELIVERY**				
Spontaneous	50(1)	64	78(1)	192(2)
Operative	8(1)	16	17	41(1)
Induced	33	47	34	114
Not reported	—	2	8	10
***OPERATIVE DELIVERY SPECIFIED**				
Dilatation and curettage (when used to deliver)	4	13	10	27
Version and extraction	—	1	3	4
Vaginal hysterotomy	2(1)	—	2	4(1)
Abdominal hysterotomy	2	2	2	6
***THERAPEUTIC ABORTIONS SPECIFIED**				
Induced	4	1	3	8
Dilatation and curettage	4	13	8	25
Version and extraction	—	1	3	4
Vaginal hysterotomy	2(1)	—	2	4(1)
Abdominal hysterotomy	2	2	2	6
COMPLICATIONS OF PREGNANCY				
With complications	30	24	23	77
No complications	51	83	86	220
Not reported	10	22	28	60

*Delivery tables: Incomplete abortions are included in all of these tables. The figures in parentheses indicate twin births and may be added to the main figure to get the total number of babies.

ABORTIONS (continued)

	1930	1931	1932	TOTAL
	COMPLICATIONS SPECIFIED			
Albuminuria	6	12	6	24
None	22	11	15	48
Not reported	2	1	2	5
Convulsions	1	1	2	4
None	29	23	21	73
Not reported	—	—	—	
High blood pressure	4	6	4	14
None	25	17	17	59
Not reported	1	1	2	4
Oedema	2	5	4	11
None	27	19	19	65
Not reported	1	—	—	1
Prolonged headaches	3	1	2	6
None	26	22	21	69
Not reported	1	1	—	2
Pernicious vomiting	6	13	7	26
None	23	11	16	50
Not reported	1	—	—	1
Bleeding during pregnancy	21	8	13	42
None	9	16	10	35
Not reported	—	—	—	—
	INTERCURRENT DISEASES OR ABNORMALITIES			
Number of diseases or abnormalities	7	19	27	53
Number of mothers with intercurrent diseases	6	17	25	48
None	77	102	101	280
Not reported	8	10	11	29
	†INTERCURRENT OPERATIONS SPECIFIED			
Appendectomy	2	2	1	5
	PREVENTABILITY			
Not preventable	16	33	37	86
Preventable:				
Responsibility ascribed to physician	21	21	27	69
Responsibility ascribed to patient	54	75	72	201
Responsibility ascribed to midwife	—	—	1	1
	CAUSE OF DEATH			
Puerperal causes	87	114	117	318
Extra-puerperal causes	4	15	20	39

†Abnormalities requiring operation are counted under Intercurrent disease also.

ABORTIONS (continued)

	1930	1931	1932	TOTAL
	PUERPERAL CAUSE OF DEATH SPECIFIED			
Abortions: with septic conditions	70	97	95	262
Abortions: without septic conditions	17	17	22	56
Above abortions: specified				
Hemorrhage	10	7	10	27
Pernicious vomiting	3	7	4	14
Albuminuria and eclampsia	3	—	6	9
Phlegmasia alba dolens and embolus	—	2	1	3
Accidents of labor	1	1	—	2
Not reported (non septic)	—	—	1	1
	‡EXTRA-PUERPERAL CAUSE OF DEATH SPECIFIED			
108: Lobar pneumonia	1	6	5	12
11: Influenza	—	—	6	6
92: Chronic cardiac	—	4	2	6
23: Tuberculosis (respiratory)	1	—	2	3
91: Acute cardiac	—	1	1	2
121: Appendicitis	—	2	—	2
131: Chronic nephritis	1	—	1	2
130: Acute nephritis	—	1	—	1
139: Cysts, tumors, etc.	—	1	—	1
178: Accidental absorption of poison, etc.	1	—	—	1
118: Uncontrollable vomiting	—	—	1	1
125: Acute yellow atrophy of liver	—	—	1	1
163: Suicide by corrosive substance	—	—	1	1

‡The figure appearing before each cause of death is the code number as taken from the *Manual of the International List of Causes of Death.*

SUMMARY OF MATERNAL MORTALITY FOR THREE YEARS
1930-1931-1932

ECTOPIC GESTATIONS

	1930	1931	1932	TOTAL
Total maternal deaths following ectopics	40	39	41	120
*DELIVERY				
Delivered in hospital	28	30	33	91
Not delivered	12	9	8	29
DEATH				
Died in hospital	36	38	41	115
Died at home	4	1	—	5
DELIVERY AND DEATH				
Delivered and died in hospital	27	30	33	90
Delivered in hospital, died at home	1	—	—	1
Not delivered, died in hospital	9	8	8	25
Not delivered, died at home	3	1	—	4
BOROUGH				
Manhattan	16	15	18	49
Brooklyn	19	17	18	54
Bronx	1	3	4	8
Queens	4	3	1	8
Richmond	—	1	—	1
RACE				
White	29	36	32	97
Negro	11	3	9	23
NATIVITY				
Native-born	26	26	22	74
Foreign-born	14	13	19	46
FOREIGN-BORN, BY COUNTRY				
Austria	1	2	—	3
Belgium	—	1	—	1
Bermuda	—	—	1	1
British West Indies	2	—	1	3
Canada	1	—	—	1
Czechoslovakia	—	—	1	1
England	1	—	—	1
France	1	—	—	1
Germany	4	3	2	9
Greece	—	1	—	1
Ireland	2	—	1	3
Italy	—	2	6	8
Norway	1	—	—	1
Poland	—	2	—	2
Porto Rico	—	1	—	1
Roumania	—	1	—	1
Russia	1	—	6	7
Santo Domingo	—	—	1	1

*The terms "delivered" and "not delivered" are used, in connection with ectopic gestations, to signify those cases in which a laparotomy was or was not performed.

ECTOPIC GESTATIONS (continued)

	1930	1931	1932	TOTAL
AGE				
15 to 19 years	—	1	—	1
20 to 24 "	9	8	3	20
25 to 29 "	12	8	11	31
30 to 34 "	9	9	16	34
35 to 39 "	8	10	8	26
40 to 44 "	2	3	3	8
45 and over	—	—	—	—
PERIOD OF UTEROGESTATION				
27 weeks	—	—	—	—
26 "	—	—	—	—
25 "	—	1	—	1
24 "	—	1	—	1
23 "	1	1	—	2
22 "	—	—	—	—
21 "	—	—	—	—
20 "	—	1	1	2
19 "	—	—	—	—
18 "	1	1	—	2
17 "	—	—	—	—
16 "	1	—	—	1
15 "	1	1	—	2
14 "	—	—	—	—
13 "	3	5	6	14
12 "	—	2	3	5
11 "	—	1	1	2
10 "	2	2	1	5
9 "	4	6	8	18
8 "	11	6	3	20
7 "	2	—	4	6
6 "	12	5	5	22
Less than 6 weeks	—	6	9	15
Not reported	2	—	—	2
WASSERMANN				
No Wassermann, or not reported	39	37	34	110
Wassermann taken	1	2	7	10
WASSERMANN REPORT				
Negative	1	1	5	7
Positive	—	1	2	3
POSITIVE WASSERMANN REPORT				
4+	—	1	1	2
1+	—	—	1	1

ECTOPIC GESTATIONS (*continued*)

	1930	1931	1932	TOTAL
GRAVIDITY				
Primigravidae	16	18	17	51
Multigravidae	23	19	23	65
Not reported	1	2	1	4
MULTIGRAVIDAE, BY GRAVIDITY				
Gravidae II	9	8	10	27
" III	7	3	1	11
" IV	4	4	3	11
" V	1	1	2	4
" VI	—	—	2	2
" VII	1	1	2	4
" VIII	—	—	—	—
" IX	—	1	—	1
" X	—	—	—	—
" XI	1	—	—	1
Over XI	—	—	—	—
Multigravidae, gravidity not reported	—	1	3	4
AUTOPSY				
With autopsy	11	9	13	33
No autopsy	29	30	28	87
LEGITIMACY				
Legitimate	33	34	37	104
Illegitimate	7	5	4	16
PRENATAL CARE				
Adequate	—	—	—	—
Inadequate	—	1	—	1
None	3	4	1	8
Excluded (all less than 16 weeks)	37	34	40	111
DELIVERY ATTENDANT				
Physician	27	29	32	88
Interne	1	1	1	3
Not delivered	12	9	8	29
COMPLICATIONS OF PREGNANCY				
With complications	24	17	18	59
No complications	13	19	21	53
Not reported	3	3	2	8

ECTOPIC GESTATIONS (*continued*)

	1930	1931	1932	TOTAL
	COMPLICATIONS SPECIFIED			
Albuminuria	1	—	—	1
None	22	14	17	53
Not reported	1	3	1	5
Convulsions	—	—	—	—
None	24	17	18	59
Not reported	—	—	—	—
High blood pressure	—	—	—	—
None	23	14	16	53
Not reported	1	3	2	6
Oedema	—	—	—	—
None	24	16	18	58
Not reported	—	1	—	1
Prolonged headaches	—	—	—	—
None	24	17	18	59
Not reported	—	—	—	—
Pernicious vomiting	—	—	—	—
None	24	17	18	59
Not reported	—	—	—	—
Bleeding during pregnancy	24	17	18	59
None	—	—	—	—
Not reported	—	—	—	—
	INTERCURRENT DISEASES OR ABNORMALITIES			
Number of diseases or abnormalities	5	7	11	23
Number of mothers with intercurrent diseases	4	7	10	21
None	35	32	30	97
Not reported	1	—	1	2
	†INTERCURRENT OPERATIONS SPECIFIED			
Number of mothers operated during pregnancy	2	4	9	15
Colpotomy	—	1	3	4
Dilatation and curettage	2	3	6	11
Instrumental attempt to induce an abortion	—	—	1	1
	PREVENTABILITY			
Not preventable	14	12	5	31
Preventable:				
Responsibility ascribed to physician	20	20	33	73
Responsibility ascribed to patient	6	7	3	16

†Abnormalities requiring operation counted under intercurrent disease also.

ECTOPIC GESTATIONS (continued)

	1930	1931	1932	TOTAL
	CAUSE OF DEATH			
Puerperal causes	36	36	38	110
Extra-puerperal causes	4	3	3	10
	PUERPERAL CAUSE OF DEATH SPECIFIED			
Hemorrhage and shock	23	22	27	72
Septicaemia	12	13	10	35
Phlegmasia alba dolens and embolus	1	1	1	3
	‡ EXTRA-PUERPERAL CAUSE OF DEATH SPECIFIED			
107: Bronchopneumonia	—	2	2	4
122: Intestinal obstruction	1	1	1	3
131: Chronic nephritis	1	—	—	1
179: Other acute accidental poisonings	1	—	—	1
194: Spinal anaesthesia	1	—	—	1

‡The figure appearing before each cause of death is the code number as taken from the *Manual of the International List of Causes of Death.*

CAUSE OF DEATH, BY AGE GROUPS

(Exclusive of deaths following abortion and ectopic gestation)

	TOTAL		15 TO 19 YEARS		20 TO 24 YEARS		25 TO 29 YEARS		30 TO 34 YEARS		35 TO 39 YEARS		40 YEARS AND OVER	
	Number	Per cent	Number	Per cent	Number	Per cent	Number	Per cent	Number	Per cent	Number	Per cent	Number	Per cent
Total	1,564	100.0	87	100.0	324	100.0	432	100.0	351	100.0	259	100.0	111	100.0
Per cent	*100*		*5.6*		*20.7*		*27.6*		*22.4*		*16.6*		*7.1*	
Hemorrhage	197	12.6	5	5.8	31	9.6	47	10.9	54	15.4	43	16.6	17	15.3
Per cent	*100*		*2.5*		*15.7*		*23.9*		*27.4*		*21.8*		*8.6*	
Puerperal septicaemia	510	32.6	30	34.5	128	39.5	143	33.1	106	30.2	70	27.0	33	29.7
Per cent	*100*		*5.9*		*25.1*		*28.0*		*20.8*		*13.7*		*6.5*	
Albuminuria and eclampsia	231	14.8	21	24.1	48	14.8	66	15.3	42	12.0	43	16.6	11	10.0
Per cent	*100*		*9.1*		*20.8*		*28.6*		*18.2*		*18.6*		*4.6*	
Pernicious vomiting	14	.9	3	3.4	2	.6	4	.9	3	.9	2	.8	—	—
Per cent	*100*		*21.4*		*14.3*		*28.4*		*21.4*		*14.3*			
Phlegmasia alba dolens and embolus	89	5.7	3	3.4	13	4.0	27	6.3	27	7.7	12	4.6	7	6.3
Per cent	*100*		*3.4*		*14.6*		*30.3*		*30.3*		*13.5*		*7.9*	
Accidents of labor	171	10.9	5	5.8	30	9.3	48	11.1	34	9.7	35	13.5	19	17.1
Per cent	*100*		*2.9*		*17.5*		*28.1*		*19.9*		*20.5*		*11.1*	
Accidents of puerperium	8	.5	2	2.3	—	—	2	.5	2	16.0	1	.4	1	1.0
Per cent	*100*		*25.0*				*25.0*		*25.0*		*12.5*		*12.5*	
Extra-puerperal causes	344	22.0	18	20.7	72	22.2	95	22.0	83	23.6	53	20.5	23	20.7
Per cent	*100*		*5.2*		*20.9*		*27.6*		*24.1*		*15.4*		*6.7*	

CHART G

PERCENTAGE DISTRIBUTION OF DEATHS BY AGE, FOR PRINCIPAL CAUSES OF DEATH AND ALL CAUSES

———— SPECIFIED CAUSE   ••••••ALL CAUSES

HEMORRHAGE

SEPTICAEMIA

ALBUMINURIA AND ECLAMPSIA

PHLEGMASIA ALBA DOLENS AND EMBOLUS

ACCIDENTS OF LABOR

EXTRA-PUERPERAL CAUSES

247

CAUSE OF DEATH, BY GRAVIDITY

(Exclusive of deaths following abortion and ectopic gestation)

	TOTAL		PRIMIGRAVIDAE		MULTIGRAVIDAE		GRAVIDITY UNKNOWN	
	Number	Per cent	Number	Per cent	Number	Per cent	Number	Per cent
Total	1,564	100.0	682	100.0	874	100.0	8	100.0
Per cent	*100*		*43.6*		*55.8*		*.5*	
Hemorrhage	197	12.6	68	10.0	127	14.5	2	25.0
Per cent	*100*		*34.5*		*64.5*		*1.0*	
Puerperal septicaemia	510	32.6	230	33.7	280	32.0	—	—
Per cent	*100*		*45.1*		*54.9*		—	
Albuminuria and eclampsia	231	14.8	122	17.9	106	12.1	3	37.5
Per cent	*100*		*52.8*		*45.9*		*1.3*	
Pernicious vomiting	14	.9	8	1.2	6	.7	—	—
Per cent	*100*		*57.1*		*42.9*		—	
Phlegmasia alba dolens and embolus	89	5.7	43	6.3	46	5.3	—	—
Per cent	*100*		*48.3*		*51.7*		—	
Accidents of labor	171	10.9	75	11.0	96	11.0	—	—
Per cent	*100*		*43.9*		*56.1*		—	
Accidents of puerperium	8	.5	4	.6	4	.5	—	—
Per cent	*100*		*50.0*		*50.0*		—	
Extra-puerperal causes	344	22.0	132	19.4	209	23.9	3	37.5
Per cent	*100*		*38.4*		*60.8*		*.9*	

CHART H

PERCENTAGE DISTRIBUTION OF DEATHS
BY GRAVIDITY, FOR EACH CAUSE OF DEATH

☐ PRIMIGRAVIDAE   ▨ MULTIGRAVIDAE

Cause	Primigravidae	Multigravidae
ALL CAUSES	43.6	55.8
HEMORRHAGE	34.5	64.5
SEPTICAEMIA	45.1	54.9
ALBUMINURIA AND ECLAMPSIA	52.8	45.9
PERNICIOUS VOMITING	57.1	42.9
PHLEGMASIA ALBA DOLENS AND EMBOLUS	48.3	51.7
ACCIDENTS OF LABOR	43.9	56.1
ACCIDENTS OF PUERPERIUM	50.0	50.0
EXTRA-PUERPERAL CAUSES	38.4	60.8

EXCLUSIVE OF CASES IN WHICH GRAVIDITY WAS UNRECORDED

GRAVIDITY, BY AGE GROUPS

(Exclusive of deaths following abortion and ectopic gestation)

	TOTAL		15 TO 19 YEARS		20 TO 24 YEARS		25 TO 29 YEARS		30 TO 34 YEARS		35 TO 39 YEARS		40 YEARS AND OVER	
	Number	Per cent	Number	Per cent	Number	Per cent	Number	Per cent	Number	Per cent	Number	Per cent	Number	Per cent
Total	1,564	100	87	5.6	324	20.7	432	27.6	351	22.4	259	16.6	111	7.1
Primigravidae	682	100	78	11.4	212	31.1	216	31.7	111	16.3	46	6.7	19	2.8
Multigravidae	874	100	9	1.0	112	12.8	215	24.6	238	27.2	209	23.9	91	10.4
Gravidity not reported	8	100	—	—	—	—	1	12.5	2	25.0	4	50.0	1	12.5
Gravidae II	277	100	9	3.3	60	21.7	94	33.9	74	26.7	33	11.9	7	2.5
" III	192	100	—	—	26	13.5	59	30.7	58	30.2	43	22.4	6	3.1
" IV	128	100	—	—	17	13.3	34	26.6	41	32.0	26	20.3	10	7.8
" V	89	100	—	—	5	5.6	13	14.6	23	25.8	32	36.0	16	18.0
" VI	47	100	—	—	3	6.4	6	12.8	18	38.3	17	36.2	3	6.4
" VII	32	100	—	—	—	—	5	15.6	10	31.3	10	31.3	8	21.9
" VIII	31	100	—	—	1	3.2	—	—	7	22.6	15	48.4	8	25.8
" IX	32	100	—	—	—	—	3	9.4	4	12.5	16	50.0	9	28.1
" X and over	42	100	—	—	—	—	1	2.4	2	4.8	15	35.7	24	57.1
Multigravidae, gravidity not reported	4	100	—	—	—	—	—	—	1	25.0	2	50.0	1	25.0

SUMMARY OF DATA OBTAINED FROM SIXTY-SEVEN HOSPITALS ANSWERING QUESTIONNAIRE*

SERIES A—HOSPITALS WITH 4,000 OR MORE DELIVERIES DURING THE YEARS 1930, 1931, AND 1932

HOSPITAL BY CODE	TOTAL PUERPERAL DEATHS	DEATH RATE†	CORRECTED DEATHS‡	CORRECTED DEATH RATE‡	DEATHS FROM PUERPERAL SEPTICAEMIA	PREVENTABLE DEATHS FROM PUERPERAL SEPTICAEMIA	OPERATIVE DELIVERIES		CAESAREAN DELIVERIES		CAESAREAN DEATHS		PREVENTABLE DEATHS	
							Number	Per cent of all deliveries	Number	Per cent of all deliveries	Number	Per cent of caesarean deliveries	Number	Per cent of corrected deaths
Total	629	8.1	490	6.3	153	85	19,802	25.5	2,043	2.6	98	4.8	201	41.0
A	29	3.9	26	3.5	12	8	2,396	32.2	200	2.7	6	3.0	11	42.3
B	29	7.0	28	6.8	8	4	2,723	66.0	187	4.5	6	3.2	16	57.1
C	41	8.4	34	7.0	6	4	590	12.1	40	0.8	4	10.0	9	26.5
D	83	11.7	52	7.3	14	2	870	12.3	169	2.4	9	5.3	12	23.1
E	33	6.3	32	6.1	11	7	1,543	29.2	178	3.4	12	6.7	17	53.1
F	16	2.8	14	2.4	2	1	2,160	37.4	202	3.5	2	1.0	4	28.6
G	36	8.9	31	7.7	11	7	1,545	38.3	133	3.3	6	4.5	12	38.7
H	91	16.4	51	9.2	19	7	721	13.0	80	1.4	5	6.3	15	29.4
I	44	5.1	41	4.8	9	6	1,725	20.2	320	3.7	17	5.3	25	61.0
J	114	28.1	83	20.4	24	10	414	10.2	47	1.2	7	14.9	27	32.5
K	32	5.5	28	4.8	12	9	1,208	20.8	82	1.4	8	9.8	14	50.0
L	41	9.0	32	7.0	8	6	861	19.0	73	1.6	5	6.8	18	56.3
M	28	4.3	27	4.2	12	9	2,242	34.6	303	4.7	7	2.3	12	44.4
N	12	2.9	11	2.7	5	5	804	19.7	29	0.7	4	13.8	9	81.8

*See copy of questionnaire on page 257.
†Per 1,000 total births.
‡Cases delivered in hospital regardless of place of death, and cases dying in hospital without being delivered.

SUMMARY OF DATA OBTAINED FROM SIXTY-SEVEN HOSPITALS ANSWERING QUESTIONNAIRE*

SERIES B—HOSPITALS WITH 3,000 TO 4,000 DELIVERIES DURING THE YEARS 1930, 1931, AND 1932

HOSPITAL BY CODE	TOTAL PUERPERAL DEATHS	DEATH RATE†	CORRECTED DEATHS‡	CORRECTED DEATH RATE‡	DEATHS FROM PUERPERAL SEPTICAEMIA	PREVENTABLE DEATHS FROM PUERPERAL SEPTICAEMIA	OPERATIVE DELIVERIES Number	OPERATIVE DELIVERIES Per cent of all deliveries	CAESAREAN DELIVERIES Number	CAESAREAN DELIVERIES Per cent of all deliveries	CAESAREAN DEATHS Number	CAESAREAN DEATHS Per cent of caesarean deliveries	PREVENTABLE DEATHS Number	PREVENTABLE DEATHS Per cent of corrected deaths
Total	388.	8.7	333	7.4	117	68	7,612	17.0	621	1.4	64	10.3	143	42.9
A	41	12.7	39	12.1	13	7	431	13.4	100	3.1	16	16.0	17	43.6
B	13	4.2	9	2.9	1	1	831	26.8	36	1.2	2	5.6	5	55.6
C	17	5.6	16	5.2	8	4	1,280	41.8	58	1.9	3	5.2	9	50.3
D	10	2.7	11	3.0	5	2	646	17.5	17	0.5	3	17.6	6	54.5
E	29	7.4	30	7.7	11	8	1,148	29.4	72	1.8	6	8.3	12	40.0
F	25	7.4	19	5.6	9	4	612	18.1	50	1.5	3	6.0	5	26.3
G	30	8.3	23	6.4	6	3	173	4.8	15	0.4	3	20.0	10	43.5
H	15	4.4	13	3.8	2	2	758	22.2	82	2.4	2	2.4	6	46.2
I	42	13.8	32	10.5	9	5	208	6.9	30	1.0	2	6.7	13	40.6
J	46	14.9	39	12.7	19	11	471	15.3	36	1.2	6	16.7	16	41.0
K	32	8.6	32	8.6	11	8	553	14.8	48	1.3	5	10.4	15	46.9
L	40	10.5	31	8.1	12	6	323	8.5	41	1.1	8	19.5	16	51.6
M	48	13.0	39	10.6	11	7	178	4.8	36	1.0	5	13.9	13	33.3

*See copy of questionnaire on page 257.

†Per 1,000 total births.

‡Cases delivered in hospital regardless of place of death, and cases dying in hospital without being delivered.

SUMMARY OF DATA OBTAINED FROM SIXTY-SEVEN HOSPITALS ANSWERING QUESTIONNAIRE*

SERIES C—HOSPITALS WITH 2,000 TO 3,000 DELIVERIES DURING THE YEARS 1930, 1931, AND 1932

HOSPITAL BY CODE	TOTAL PUERPERAL DEATHS	DEATH RATE†	CORRECTED DEATHS‡	CORRECTED DEATH RATE‡	DEATHS FROM PUERPERAL SEPTICAEMIA	PREVENTABLE DEATHS FROM PUERPERAL SEPTICAEMIA	OPERATIVE DELIVERIES Number	OPERATIVE DELIVERIES Per cent of all deliveries	CAESAREAN DELIVERIES Number	CAESAREAN DELIVERIES Per cent of all deliveries	CAESAREAN DEATHS Number	CAESAREAN DEATHS Per cent of caesarean deliveries	PREVENTABLE DEATHS Number	PREVENTABLE DEATHS Per cent of corrected deaths
Total	186	7.0	154	5.8	46	28	6,526	24.6	502	1.9	31	6.2	66	42.9
A	33	12.2	31	11.5	6	6	587	21.7	49	1.8	9	18.4	18	58.1
B	24	9.4	18	7.1	4	3	851	33.5	71	2.8	4	5.6	7	38.9
C	23	8.7	18	6.8	4	2	927	35.1	59	2.2	2	3.4	6	33.3
D	12	5.7	10	4.7	3	2	789	37.4	30	1.4	2	6.7	3	30.0
E	7	3.3	6	2.9	1	1	990	47.3	112	5.3	3	2.7	3	50.0
F	9	4.3	5	2.4	5	4	301	14.4	49	2.3	2	4.1	4	80.0
G	23	9.6	20	8.3	5	—	177	7.4	23	1.0	2	8.7	4	20.0
H	12	5.1	13	5.6	10	5	367	15.7	18	0.8	2	11.1	5	38.5
I	5	1.7	7	2.4	1	1	656	22.2	20	0.7	1	5.0	3	42.9
J	20	8.6	14	6.1	3	2	532	23.0	42	1.8	4	9.5	8	57.1
K	18	7.7	12	5.1	4	2	349	14.9	29	1.2	—	—	5	41.7

*See copy of questionnaire on page 257.
†Per 1,000 total births.
‡Cases delivered in hospital regardless of place of death, and cases dying in hospital without being delivered.

SUMMARY OF DATA OBTAINED FROM SIXTY-SEVEN HOSPITALS ANSWERING QUESTIONNAIRE*

SERIES D—HOSPITALS WITH 1,000 TO 2,000 DELIVERIES DURING THE YEARS 1930, 1931, AND 1932

HOSPITAL BY CODE	TOTAL PUERPERAL DEATHS	DEATH RATE†	CORRECTED DEATHS‡	CORRECTED DEATH RATE†	DEATHS FROM PUERPERAL SEPTICAEMIA	PREVENTABLE DEATHS FROM PUERPERAL SEPTICAEMIA	OPERATIVE DELIVERIES		CAESAREAN DELIVERIES		CAESAREAN DEATHS		PREVENTABLE DEATHS	
							Number	Per cent of all deliveries	Number	Per cent of all deliveries	Number	Per cent of caesarean deliveries	Number	Per cent of corrected deaths
Total	179	7.6	152	6.4	47	29	7,527	37.9	539	2.3	30	5.6	82	54.0
A	17	11.3	9	6.0	4	4	444	29.6	15	1.0	2	13.3	6	66.7
B	8	4.0	9	4.5	2	2	316	15.8	28	1.4	—	—	5	55.6
C	18	12.8	15	10.7	5	3	355	25.3	29	2.1	3	10.3	9	60.0
D	13	8.8	11	7.5	4	3	298	20.2	44	3.0	2	4.5	6	54.5
E	9	7.2	7	5.6	3	3	845	68.0	33	2.7	1	3.0	5	71.4
F	10	5.2	10	5.2	3	2	909	47.7	80	4.2	6	7.5	6	60.0
G	8	5.4	7	4.8	2	—	485	33.0	48	3.3	1	2.1	1	14.3
H	8	4.3	9	4.8	3	—	729	38.7	52	2.8	1	1.9	4	44.4
I	14	9.8	10	7.0	1	1	454	31.8	22	1.5	1	4.5	4	40.0
J	18	9.4	15	7.8	6	1	560	29.2	22	1.1	4	18.2	12	80.0
K	7	3.9	8	4.5	—	4	743	41.7	47	2.6	1	2.1	2	25.0
L	13	7.5	15	8.7	6	—	225	13.0	23	1.3	4	17.4	10	66.7
M	6	5.9	6	5.9	2	4	304	29.8	16	1.6	—	—	3	50.0
N	5	3.0	3	1.8	—	2	262	15.6	48	2.9	1	2.1	1	33.3
O	25	21.7	18	15.6	6	—	598	51.9	32	2.8	3	9.4	8	44.4

*See copy of questionnaire on page 257.

†Per 1,000 total births.

‡Cases delivered in hospital regardless of place of death, and cases dying in hospital without being delivered.

254

SUMMARY OF DATA OBTAINED FROM SIXTY-SEVEN HOSPITALS ANSWERING QUESTIONNAIRE*

SERIES E—HOSPITALS WITH LESS THAN 1,000 DELIVERIES DURING THE YEARS 1930, 1931, AND 1932

HOSPITAL BY CODE	TOTAL PUERPERAL DEATHS	DEATH RATE†	CORRECTED DEATHS†	CORRECTED DEATH RATE†	DEATHS FROM PUERPERAL SEPTICAEMIA	PREVENTABLE DEATHS FROM PUERPERAL SEPTICAEMIA	OPERATIVE DELIVERIES Number	OPERATIVE DELIVERIES Per cent of all deliveries	CAESAREAN DELIVERIES Number	CAESAREAN DELIVERIES Per cent of all deliveries	CAESAREAN DEATHS Number	CAESAREAN DEATHS Per cent of caesarean deliveries	PREVENTABLE DEATHS Number	PREVENTABLE DEATHS Per cent of corrected deaths
Total	100	11.7	80	9.4	17	11	2,555	29.9	258	3.0	17	6.6	39	48.8
A	9	12.1	9	12.1	4	4	338	45.5	33	4.4	3	9.1	6	66.7
B	4	9.0	1	2.2	—	—	96	27.6	11	2.5	—	—	1	—
C	16	17.9	14	15.7	2	1	51	5.7	6	0.7	2	33.3	4	28.6
D	4	6.7	4	6.7	—	—	69	11.6	10	1.7	1	10.0	—	—
E	12	37.6	6	18.8	—	—	77	24.1	11	3.4	1	9.1	5	83.3
F	4	5.0	2	2.5	—	—	340	42.7	41	5.1	1	2.4	2	100.0
G	4	5.2	2	2.6	—	—	122	15.8	5	0.6	1	20.0	2	100.0
H	5	30.1	4	24.1	4	2	58	34.9	10	6.0	2	20.0	3	75.0
I	2	2.2	2	2.2	1	1	322	36.2	49	5.5	—	—	2	100.0
J	—	—	—	—	—	—	18	8.0	—	—	—	—	—	—
K	12	19.8	10	16.5	2	1	233	38.4	24	4.0	2	8.3	5	50.0
L	5	6.6	4	5.3	1	1	310	40.7	8	1.1	1	12.5	3	75.0
M	11	12.4	10	11.2	2	1	386	43.4	41	4.6	1	2.4	5	50.0
N	12	26.5	12	26.5	1	—	135	29.8	9	2.0	2	22.2	2	16.7

*See copy of questionnaire on page 257.

†Per 1,000 total births.

‡Cases delivered in hospital regardless of place of death, and cases dying in hospital without being delivered.

SUMMARY OF DATA OBTAINED FROM SIXTY-SEVEN HOSPITALS ANSWERING QUESTIONNAIRE*

HOSPITAL BY CODE	TOTAL PUERPERAL DEATHS	DEATH RATE†	CORRECTED DEATHS‡	CORRECTED DEATH RATE‡	DEATHS FROM PUERPERAL SEPTICAEMIA	PREVENTABLE DEATHS FROM PUERPERAL SEPTICAEMIA	OPERATIVE DELIVERIES		CAESAREAN DELIVERIES		CAESAREAN DEATHS		PREVENTABLE DEATHS	
							Number	Per cent of all deliveries	Number	Per cent of all deliveries	Number	Per cent of caesarean deliveries	Number	Per cent of corrected deaths
Grand total	1,482	8.2	1,209	6.7	380	221	44,022	24.3	3,963	2.2	240	6.1	531	43.9
A	629	8.1	490	6.3	153	85	19,802	25.5	2,043	2.6	98	4.8	201	41.0
B	388	8.7	333	7.4	117	68	7,612	17.0	621	1.4	64	10.3	143	42.9
C	186	7.0	154	5.8	46	28	6,526	24.6	502	1.9	31	6.2	66	42.9
D	179	7.6	152	6.4	47	29	7,527	37.9	539	2.3	30	5.6	82	54.0
E	100	11.7	80	9.4	17	11	2,555	29.9	258	3.0	17	6.6	39	48.8

*See copy of questionnaire on page 257.
†Per 1,000 total births.
‡Cases delivered in hospital regardless of place of death, and cases dying in hospital without being delivered.

QUESTIONNAIRE SENT EACH YEAR TO ALL HOSPITALS DOING OBSTETRICS

1. Number of Mothers delivered (exclusive of abortions)
    . . . .
2. Number of Mothers delivered *without* operative inter-ference . . . .
3. *Number of Mothers delivered *with* operative interfer-ence . . . .
4. *Classification of *operative* interference:
    (a) Forceps deliveries . . . .
        High . . . .
        Medium . . . .
        Low . . . .
    (b) Caesarean deliveries (abdominal) . . . .
    (c) Version and extraction (both on same case) . . . .
    (d) Others (specify) . . . .
    . . . .

* These should not include episiotomies or induced labors.

PROPOSED SCHEDULE FOR STUDIES
IN PUERPERAL MORTALITY

The following schedule is adapted freely from the one used in this survey, which was supplied by the Children's Bureau of the Department of Labor. The revisions represent those which were found to be necessary in the course of the survey. The schedule can be arranged in a four-page folder.

MATERNAL MORTALITY STUDY

MOTHER (information from death certificate)   1. Serial No. ....

2. Registered No. ....

3. PLACE OF DEATH:

     Boro (etc.) .... City............................

     Died at ....(write word HOME or name of hospital)

4. Full name .... (a) Resident (b) Non-resident

     Address ....

5. Length of residence in city or town of DEATH ....years ....months ....days

     Length of residence in U.S.A. (if foreign-born) ....years ....months ....days

PERSONAL AND STATISTICAL DATA

6. Age	7. Color	8. Marital status

9. Occupation of deceased—Housewife, Other (specify) ....

10. Birthplace of deceased ....

11. National origin:

     Paternal ....

     Maternal ....

12. Interval between birth and mother's death:

     ....days ....hours ....mins.—Not reported, Not

     delivered (truly) (ectopic)

13. Number of children of this mother including this birth (or births) ....
    (a) Born alive and now living ....
    (b) Born alive and now dead ....
    (c) Stillborn .... Not born ....

14. Date of final hospital admission ....

MEDICAL CERTIFICATE OF DEATH

15. Date of death (month, day, year) ...., 19......
16. I HEREBY CERTIFY, that I attended deceased from
    ...., 19......, to ...., 19......
    that I last saw her alive on ...., 19......
    and that death occurred on the above date at ....m.
    The CAUSE OF DEATH or DIAGNOSIS DURING THE LAST ILLNESS was as follows:
....
....
....
....
duration................... years.......... mos.......... days..........
Contributory (secondary) ....
....
....
....
duration................... years.......... mos.......... days..........
             Signed ....
             Address ....
             ....

17. Autopsy— Examination, None
18. Pathologist, Medical examiner, Other ....
19. AUTOPSY REPORT:
....
....
....
....
             Signed ....

20. INTERNATIONAL CODE CAUSE OF DEATH:
    (a) Health Dept. ....
    (b) Study ....

21. No birth certificate — (a) Not required ....

   (b) Required but not registered ....

   Date of search and notes ....

BABY (information from birth certificate)

22. PLACE OF BIRTH:

   Boro (etc.) .... City......................

   Born at .... (write word HOME or name of hospital)

23. Sex of child (or children if plural birth)—Male, Female, Not reported, Not
   determined (because of immaturity, etc.), Not delivered

24. Plural births—Twins, Triplets, Other (specify) .... 25. Legitimate, N.

CERTIFICATE OF ATTENDING PHYSICIAN OR MIDWIFE*

26. I HEREBY CERTIFY, that I attended the birth of this child who was born on the

   date above stated at ......m. o'clock. Alive, Stillborn, Not delivered

   { * When there was no attending physician
   or midwife, then the father, householder, etc.,   Signed ....
   should make this return. A stillborn child
   is one that neither breathes nor shows other   Address ....
   evidence of life after birth. }

27. Postmortem deliveries (counted under 26 as "not delivered")—State here the
   result: Postmortem alive, Postmortem stillborn. Type of postmortem delivery ....

   ....

28. CONDITIONS IN MOTHER, NONE, NOT KNOWN

   (a) Cardiac ....   (d) Tumors, etc. ....   (g) Others (specify) ....

   (b) Chronic nephritis ..   (e) Uterine displ. ....

   (c) Tuberculosis ......   (f) Syphilis (specify) ....

                              ....

29. PAST MEDICAL OR SURGICAL HISTORY, NONE, NOT KNOWN

   Specify ....

   ....

30. INTERCURRENT DISEASES, OPERATIONS, ABNORMALITIES, ETC., NONE, NOT REPORTED

   Specify ....

   ....

31. Treatment by physician, None. Specify and describe ....

   ....

32. COMPLICATIONS OF PREGNANCY, NONE, NR
33. Albuminuria, N. Began or first noted ....wk.
34. Convulsions, N. Began ....wk.
35. Oedema, N. Where and when began or noted ....
36. High blood pressure, N. Began or first noted ....wk.
    Normal........... Lowest........... Highest...........
37. Prolonged headache, N. Began or first noted ....wk.
    Duration...........
38. Pernicious vomiting, N. Began ....wk. Duration ....
39. Bleeding during pregnancy, N. Began ....wk. Scanty, Moderate, Profuse
    Once only, Recurred: daily, monthly, irregular
40. Treatment by physician, N. Specify ....
    ....

41. Abnormal conditions at onset of labor (not otherwise stated), N. Specify ....
    ....
    ....

42. PRENATAL CARE: Given by ....
43. Summary—Adequate, Inadequate, None, Excluded, NR
44. Visits

	Month of pregnancy											
	1	2	3	4	5	6	7	8	9			
									1	2	3	4
(a) Saw patient, N.												
(b) Urine exam., N.												
(c) Abdom. exam., N.												
(d) Blood pressure, N.												

45. Physical examination during pregnancy, N
    (a) Heart, N — Normal, Abnormal (specify) ....
    (b) Lungs, N — Normal, Abnormal (specify) ....
    (c) Pelvis, N — Normal, Abnormal (specify) ....
    (d) Wassermann or Kahn, N — Negative, Positive........+, NR
46. Abnormalities not observed by examining physician, N. Specify ....
    ....

47. Abnormalities affecting delivery and third stage, N
    (a) Placenta—Adherent, Retained, Praevia, Premature separation, ...
    (b) Hemorrhages—Antepartum, Intrapartum, Postpartum, Amount (estimate) ...
    (c) Ruptured uterus—Spontaneous, Instrumental, During labor, During delivery,
        Before labor, Not known. Describe ....
    (d) Others (specify) ....
    (e) Treatment ....

261

48. ABORTION—Complete, Incomplete, Missed
 Spontaneous, Induced (self), Questionable
 Therapeutic, N, Consultation, N, Indications for ....

49. ECTOPIC— Delivered, Not delivered (attempted)
 Notes ....

---

50. NOT DELIVERED: (a) In labor, N, No attempt at delivery
 (b) Attempted delivery
 1. Attempt to induce labor (a) Medical (b) Packing, etc.
 2. Attempted operative delivery ....

DELIVERY DATA:

51. Attendant at actual delivery — Physician, Interne, Midwife, Student, Other, None,
 NR, Not delivered

52. Assisted, N (specify by whom) ....

53. Technique—(a) Vaginal examinations, N, Number .... (b) Rectal examinations,
 N, Number .... (c) Gloves, N (d) Shaved, N (e) Sterile goods, N
 (f) Preparation method and agents used ....

54. Others attempting delivery (specify) ....
 Technique (a).......(b).......(c).......(d).......(e).......(f).......

55. Presentation—Vertex (ROA) (ROP) (LOA) (LOP) ....
 Transverse (specify) ....
 Face (specify) ....
 Other (specify) ....
 Breech (specify) ....
 ....
 Prolapsed (cord) (arm) (arms) (leg) (legs) etc. ....

56. Membranes—Ruptured, Not ruptured, Excluded (a) Spontaneous, Artificial (b)
 Length of time before delivery ....hours

57. Labor—In labor, N, Excluded, Spontaneous, Induced (method used for induction)
 ....
 Describe labor.........................Duration....hours....mins.

58. Delivery—Spontaneous, Operative (specify) ....
 Operative attempts (specify) ....

59. Third Stage—None, Normal, Abnormal (specify) ....
 Management of third stage (if abnormal) and how long after delivery ....
 ....

60. Tears—N (a) Episiotomy, N (b) Perineal, N, Degree ....
 (c) Repaired, N (d) Cervical, N, NR (e) Repaired, N

61. Anaesthetic—N (specify kind used) ....
 Given by Attendant, Assistant ....

62. MATERNAL HISTORY: Times pregnant .... Para ...... Gravida ......

No.	Interval between	Uterogestation (weeks)	Alive or stillborn (write the word)	Abnormalities that would affect pregnancy	Delivery (if operative, specify)
1					
2					
3					
4					
5					
6					
7					
8					
9					
10					
11					
12					
13					
14					
15					

63. Operation preceding death (only if other than shown under 58), N. Specify .....
....
....

(State how long after delivery or if not delivered how long before death.)

HOSPITAL CASE, N: **64.** Delivered in hospital, No.   Planned, Emergency
65. Entered hospital—Before labor, During labor, After delivery ....days
66. Total hospital days...... Days in hospital of delivery...... Days in hospital of death...... Days in other hospitals...... Home......days

(These refer only to hospitals connected with delivery and puerperium.)

67. If septic—(a) Developed in hospital, N   (b) Others in hospital at time, N

Notes:
....
....

140 : *Abortion with Septic Condition*

SPECIFY: ....
....
....

(Enter details under 48)

141 : *Abortion without mention of Septic Condition*

SPECIFY: ....
....
....

(Enter details under 48)

142 : *Ectopic Gestation*

(a) Symptoms began ....week. Describe ....
(b) Interval between recognition of first symptom and operation ....
(c) No operation .... (d) Sepsis ....
....

(Enter details under 49)

143 : *Other Accidents of Pregnancy* (not to include hemorrhages)

SPECIFY: ....
....
....
....

144 : *Puerperal Hemorrhages*

1. Placenta praevia — Premature separation of the placenta
   (a) When recognized ....
   (b) Specify method of control ....
   (c) Method of delivery (enter details under 58) ....
   ....
2. Ante, Intra, Postpartum hemorrhages, N. See entries under 47, 58, 59 ....
   Inspection of placenta at delivery, N   Left patient after delivery, N, ...hours
   Patient's condition satisfactory with dropping pulse, N
3. Other causes under 144 (specify) ....
   ....

TREATMENT (describe fully) ....
....

TRANSFUSION (state definitely the time given, etc., in relation to hemorrhage, delivery,
    operative interference) ....

1. Operative delivery (enter the details under 58)   2. Spontaneous   3. Not delivered
4. Care after delivery: (a) First call ....hours after, ...days after
   (b) Nursing care ....   5. Symptoms appeared ....hours before
   delivery, ...hours after delivery (describe) ....
6. Intra-uterine manipulation, N—Before symptoms, After symptoms
7. Duration of sepsis: ......days 8. Spreading peritonitis, N
9. Blood culture, Smear, etc., N—Negative, Positive (give organism) ....
10. Specify treatment, transfusion, etc. ....
   ....
   ....

146 : Puerperal Albuminuria and Eclampsia

(See prenatal care) 1. Medical supervision before convulsions, N, Duration ....
2. Conditions when first seen ....   3. Symptoms began ....before death
Convulsions, N. Began ....hours Before labor, During labor, ...hours
After delivery
4. Cooperation of patient—Good, Poor, None (reason) ....
5. Home case: Bed at first symptoms ....
6. Hospital case: Hospital at first symptoms or when in a serious condition ....
   ....

Notes:
   ....
   ....

, 147 : Other Toxaemias of Pregnancy

1. Pernicious vomiting (a) Duration ....
                        (b) Operation, N.   Refused by patient, N ....
2. Others (specify) ....
   ....

148 : Phlegmasia Alba Dolens, Embolus, Sudden Death (not specified as septic)

1. Embolus (specify) ....   (a) Respiratory distress, N   (b) Cyanosis, N
   (c) Cough, N (d) Pain, N (e) Other (specify) ....
2. Other causes, under 148, Remarks ....
   ....

149 : Other Accidents of Childbirth

1. Caesarean section: (a) Specify type of operation ....
   (b) Indications for ....
   (c) Elective, Emergency
   (d) Vaginal examination immediately before, N ....
   (e) Membranes ruptured, N (......hours)
   (f) Patient in labor, N (......hours). Type ....
   (g) Temperature (specify) ....
   (h) Operative interference before caesarean, N ....

2. Instrumental delivery and other operative procedures (enter the details under 58) ....
   ....

3. Ruptured uterus, N (a) Spontaneous, Instrumental (b) Treatment ....
4. Operative shock
5. Other causes under 149, Remarks, Treatment ....
   ....
   ....

---

150 : Other and Unspecified Conditions of the Puerperal State

Specify: ....
....

NON-PUERPERAL CAUSES OF DEATH *either Primary or Contributing*
Give number as coded in the Manual of the International List of Causes of Death
with the cause written after (as 121-Appendicitis)

A + Primary: B + Contributory:
....
....
....
....

Remarks: ....
....
....

Accoucheur ....
Field worker ....   Informant ....
                                           ....
                                           Dates of visits to following: (check if
                                              visited)
                                              1. Hospital ....
                                              2. Doctor ....
                                              3. Medical examiner ....
                                              4. Midwife ....
                                              5. Family ....
                                              6. Others (specify) ....
                                              ....

DIRECTIONS FOR FILLING IN SCHEDULE

General: If item is applicable to the case, check it; if not, check *N* or *None;* if information is not available, check *NR* or *Not known.*

1. Enter number assigned to the case in this study.
2. Enter number from death certificate.
3. If patient died at home, write "Home"; if she died in hospital, give name of institution.
4. As given on death certificate. If patient was non-resident, give city in addition to street.
5. Copy from death certificate.
6. Age at death.
7. Enter "White," "Black," or "Yellow."
8. Enter "Married," "Single," "Widowed," or "Divorced."
9. Specify if other than housewife.
10. Copy from death certificate. Give state in addition to city.
11. Birthplaces of parents.
12. In undelivered cases of 28 weeks' gestation or over, check *Not delivered;* in undelivered cases of less than 28 weeks' gestation, check also *(truly)* or *(ectopic).*
13. Enter postmortem deliveries under *Not born.*
14. Enter date patient was admitted to hospital in which she died. If she died at home, enter "None."
15. Copy from death certificate.
16. Copy from death certificate.
17. Check proper item.
18. Check proper item and give name of person who performed autopsy.
19. Enter autopsy report in detail.
20. (a) As given on death certificate.
    (b) As determined by Advisory Committee or director of study.
21. Check proper item.

22. Copy from birth certificate.

23. In case of plural births, check for each child.

24. Check proper item.

25. Check proper item.

26. Enter time and check proper item. In case of plural births of different sexes, indicate by numerals the order of delivery. Postmortem deliveries should be entered as not delivered.

27. Check proper item and enter type of postmortem delivery.

28. Check proper item. Where history is vague, check probable conditions and write "Doubtful" in space beside *Not known*.

29. Check proper item.

30. Include here any conditions arising during pregnancy, except those properly considered complications of pregnancy.

31. Specify in some detail.

32. If any complications were present, check *Complications of pregnancy*; if none were present, check *None*; if there is no record, check *NR*.

33–39. If *None* or *NR* is checked in item 32, no further entries are required. Check proper items and make entries called for. Give date of onset or time it was first noted if condition was present at first examination. In item 34, give part affected.

40. Give treatment in detail.

41. This item calls for conditions which appeared at onset or during the course of labor, not those present during pregnancy.

42. Give name of physician, midwife, or clinic to whom patient went for prenatal care.

43. Check proper item according to classification given on page 271, as follows: Adequate, Grade IA only; Inadequate, Grades IB, II, and III; Excluded, all cases in which death occurred at or prior to fifteenth week of gestation.

44. Enter check in proper monthly column for each item if examination was made. If examination was not made at any time, check *N*.

45. Check proper items and enter data asked for, for all grades including "excluded" where such is available. If no examinations were made until admission or visit during labor, check examinations made at that time and write "On admission" across findings.

46. Specify conditions such as contracted pelvis, etc., not discovered by physician during prenatal period.
47. Check proper item and specify where necessary.
48. Check proper item. If abortion was self-induced, check both (*self*) and *Induced*; if it was induced by another, cross out (*self*).
49. Check proper item. If operation was attempted, give details.
50. This item applies only to cases of 28 weeks' gestation or over. Check proper items.

Items 51 through 61 are to be filled in for all cases. If information is not available, check *NR*.

51. Check proper item.
52. Check proper item. Specify as physician, interne, nurse, midwife, or other. Do not include anaesthetist.
53. Check proper items. Under (f) give antiseptic or antiseptics used on field.
54. Specify. Check proper items as for *Technique*.
55. Check proper items.
56. Check proper items and enter time. If membranes were ruptured in the course of actual delivery, write in "At delivery."
57. Check proper items. Give type as normal, slow, ineffective, or intermittent.
58. Check proper item. Enter after *Operative attempts*, delivery maneuvers aimed at delivery but failing to effect it. In case of plural births, enter procedure used for each child, numbering procedure according to baby. Two consecutive maneuvers resulting in delivery are to be counted as one, i.e., version and extraction with forceps. For version and extraction, give interval between the version and extraction or indicate that it was version and immediate extraction. Enter after *Operative attempts* those performed on not delivered cases as well as attempts made prior to delivery.
59. Check and specify. In case of abortion, if D & C was done, enter here and in item 63. In cases of caesarean where placenta was delivered through abdominal incision, check *None*.

60. Check proper item. Check *N* if there was episiotomy, unless there was an extension, then check *Tears*, *Episiotomy*, and *Perineal* and give degree.
61. Check proper item; give type or types and administrator.
62. After *Para*, enter number of viable births; after *Gravida*, enter number of viable and non-viable births. If gravidity is not known, write "NR" or "NR multigravida."
63. Enter any operation after delivery or, in undelivered case, prior to death. Give interval between delivery and death.
64. Check proper items. If delivery had been arranged for, check *Planned* even if admission was an emergency.
65. Check proper items.
66. Give total time in days, including all admissions to any hospital relative to this delivery.
67. Check proper items.

Numbers 140 through 150 are the code numbers of puerperal causes of death as given in the *Manual of the International List of Causes of Death*. Check all conditions which were present, whether primary or contributory cause of death. The condition determined on by the Advisory Committee as the true cause of death will be checked in red and entered in item 20 (b) when decision is made. Answer all questions here whether or not they have been answered before.

Under *Non-puerperal causes of death*, enter name of condition and code number. Include all conditions not specified in items 140 through 150. Indicate whether the condition was considered primary or contributory cause of death.

Under *Remarks*, give an inclusive summary of the case, including any relevant data not properly included in the schedule itself.

Informant. Enter name of the person giving information. In case of a hospital, give chief of staff and name of the responsible visiting physician, not name of interne.

Dates of visits. Check proper items and give dates of all visits.

For the purposes of classification, the prenatal care that these patients received is divided into grades. Certain groups of cases—the self-induced and criminal abortions and cases where pregnancy terminated before the third month—are excluded from those for which prenatal care is studied. The phrase "Prenatal care inapplicable" is used to describe this group. The others are classified as follows:

Grade IA: Those who had prenatal care as described in *Standards of Prenatal Care*, Children's Bureau publication No. 153. This is the only grade that can be considered adequate. It may be summarized as follows: The physician at the first visit should take and record a careful history, medical, surgical, gynecological, and obstetrical. He should make a complete physical examination, including the examination of heart, lungs, and abdomen; pelvic measurements, both internal and external; and the taking of blood for a Wassermann reaction. Minute instructions in the hygiene of pregnancy should be given. The patient should be examined by a physician at least once a month during the first six months, then oftener as indicated, preferably every week in the last four weeks. (For the purpose of this study the first visit is allowed to take place during the second month.) At each visit to the physician the patient's general condition must be investigated, blood pressure taken and recorded, urinalysis done, pulse and temperature recorded, and the weight of the patient taken if possible. Abdominal examination should be made at each visit and the height of the fundus determined at this examination.

Grade IB: Those who had: first, a general physical examination, including examination of heart, lungs, and abdomen; second, pelvic measurements external and internal (except in pregnancies terminating before the eighth month and for multiparae who have had a previous normal delivery); third, regular monthly visits to physician beginning with or before the fifth month, with examination of urine and blood pressure at each visit.

Grade II: Those who had: first, a general physical examination, including examination of heart, lungs, and abdomen; and, second, regular monthly visits to physician beginning not later than the seventh month, with examination of urine and blood pressure at each visit.

Grade III: Those who had some prenatal care, but not care meeting the requirements of Grade II. It may have consisted of only a single visit.

LITERATURE CITED

1. Maternal Mortality in Fifteen States. Children's Bureau Publication No. 223. Washington: Government Printing Office, 1933.

2. SCOTTISH BOARD OF HEALTH. Report on Maternal Mortality in Aberdeen, 1918–1927, with Special Reference to Puerperal Sepsis. By J. Parlane Kinloch, J. Smith, and J. A. Stephen. Edinburgh: His Majesty's Stationery Office, 1928.

3. MAYES, H. W. The Development of the Mercurochrome Technique in Obstetrics. A Report of Ten Thousand Cases, Five Thousand of Which Were Studied during the Experimental Stage. Surgery, Gynecology and Obstetrics, 54: 529–539 (March, 1932).

4. WATSON, BENJAMIN P. Puerperal Infection and Thrombophlebitis. Chapter XXXIX of Obstetrics & Gynecology, Vol. 2. Edited by Arthur Hale Curtis, M.D. Philadelphia and London: W. B. Saunders Company, 1933.

5. PLASS, E. D. The Relation of Forceps and Cesarean Section to Maternal and Infant Morbidity and Mortality. American Journal of Obstetrics and Gynecology, 22: 176–199 (August, 1931).

6. HAWKS, E. M. Maternal Mortality in 582 Abdominal Cesarean Sections. American Journal of Obstetrics and Gynecology, 18: 393–406 (September, 1929).

7. SACKETT, NELSON B. Cesarean Section at the New York Lying-In Hospital. A Preliminary Report for the Years 1928 to 1931 Inclusive. Reprinted from the Bulletin of the Lying-In Hospital of the City of New York (February, 1932).

8. DAVIDSON, A. H. Caesarean Section: Its History and Present Status. Irish Journal of Medical Science, Sixth series, No. 72: 642–654 (December, 1931).

9. ACKEN, HENRY S., JR. Report of 535 Consecutive Cases of Mid and High Forceps. American Journal of Obstetrics and Gynecology, 23: 538–545 (April, 1932).

10. MILLER, JAMES RAGLAN. Caesarean Sections at the Hartford Hospital, 1904–1927. New England Journal of Medicine, 199: 651–656 (October 4, 1928).

11. SMITH, DAVID L. A Study of Caesarean Section Mortality in Indianapolis. Journal of the Indiana State Medical Association, 22: 141–145 (April, 1929).

12. MILLER, C. JEFF. A General Consideration of Caesarean Section. Surgery, Gynecology and Obstetrics, 48: 745–750 (June, 1929).

13. THOMPSON, WILLIAM BENBOW. An Analysis of Cesarean Sections Performed in Los Angeles from 1923 to 1928 Inclusive. American Journal of Obstetrics and Gynecology, 19: 392–405 (March, 1930).

14. HIRSCH, MAX. Zur Frage der geburtshilflichen Neuordnung. Missverständnisse, Fehldeutungen, Klärungen. Zentralblatt für Gynäkologie, 53: 2019–2031 (August 10, 1929).

15. WINTER, G. Die allgemeine deutsche Kaiserschnittsstatistik von 1928. Zentralblatt für Gynäkologie, 53: 1874–1883 (July 27, 1929).

16. MARTIN, ED., and SPIECKHOFF, K. Die "neuen Wege" in der Geburtshilfe von M. Hirsch. Monatschrift für Geburtshülfe, 81: 154–163 (February, 1929).

17. KRUKENBERG, HEINZ, and BODEWIG, HANNS. Ein Beitrag zur Kaiserschnittfrage. Monatschrift für Geburtshülfe und Gynäkologie, 83: 57–63 (September, 1929).

18. SCHRÖDER, HANS. Zur Frage des Kaiserschnittes bei unreinen Fällen. Zeitschrift für Geburtshülfe und Gynäkologie, 95: 328–339 (1929).

19. HORNUNG, R. Die Stellung des Kaiserschnittes in der Modernen Geburtshilfe. Archiv für Gynäkologie, 137: 825–829 (1929).

20. GREENHILL, J. P. An Analysis of 874 Cervical Cesarean Sections Performed at the Chicago Lying-In Hospital. American Journal of Obstetrics and Gynecology, 19: 613–623 (May, 1930).

21. DANFORTH, W. C., and GRIER, R. M. An Analysis of 124 Cases of Low Cervical Cesarean Sections. American Journal of Obstetrics and Gynecology, 20: 405–410 (September, 1930).

22. STEELE, KYLE B. Extraperitoneal Cesarean Section; an Analytic Study of 59 Cases Done by the Latzko Method. American Journal of Obstetrics and Gynecology, 19: 747–759 (June, 1930).

23. Homes by Tenure and Value of Monthly Rental, by Health Areas, New York City, 1930. New York: Welfare Council of New York City, 1933.

INDEX

MATERNAL MORTALITY

IN

PHILADELPHIA

1931 - 1933

REPORT OF
COMMITTEE ON MATERNAL WELFARE

PHILIP F. WILLIAMS, M.D.
CHAIRMAN

PHILADELPHIA COUNTY MEDICAL SOCIETY
1934

THIS REPORT of the survey conducted by the Committee on Maternal Welfare of The Philadelphia County Medical Society is printed through the resources and under the auspices of the Doctor I. P. Strittmatter Award of The Philadelphia County Medical Society. The Award for the year 1933 was presented to Philip F. Williams, M. D., Chairman of the Committee on Maternal Welfare, in recognition of his conduct of the survey and the preparation of the report.

CONTENTS

————

Contents

4

May 23, 1934.

The President and Board of Directors,
The Philadelphia County Medical Society,
S. E. Corner 21st and Spruce Streets,
Philadelphia, Pennsylvania.

Gentlemen:

We have the honor to present the Report of a Survey and Analysis of Maternal Mortality in Philadelphia, made by your Committee on Maternal Welfare.

The Report considers the 717 deaths occurring in 1931, 1932 and 1933.

STATEMENT REGARDING THIS SURVEY

In 1929 a Survey of the Hospital and Health Facilities of Philadelphia was conducted by Dr. Haven Emerson under the auspices of a Citizens' Survey Committee sponsored by the Philadelphia Chamber of Commerce. The report,[1] published in 1930, dealt at length with the local problems of maternity, a section of some 75 pages being devoted to maternity and to child hygiene. Significant comments were made on various phases of maternity service. In regard to maternity hygiene, Dr. Emerson stated (page 37), "In this field Philadelphia gives a service of superiority, due to the excellence of plan and performance by both official and volunteer agencies," hence a rating of 98. This rating was based on the appraisal form for city health work of the American Public Health Association.

In regard to Philadelphia, it was shown (page 243) that over a period of nine years, 1919 to 1927 inclusive, the maternal mortality rate, according to the figures published by the United States Bureau of the Census, ranged almost constantly ten deaths greater per 10,000 live births than the figures published by the Philadelphia Bureau of Vital Statistics. In 1919, the Census Bureau showed 73 as against 63, and in 1927, 76 as against 67. It was suggested, from the printed parallel rates, that Philadelphia would seem to be crediting itself with more favorable maternal death rates than that to which it was entitled. This difference in degree was explained by the greater accuracy and thoroughness with which the Bureau of the Census searches for and discovers deaths related to pregnancy and the puerperium, which are sometimes hidden under other and less significant certifications of death.

In a striking manner, the report called attention, by means of a graph (page 231), to a reduction in the number of septic deaths from 1919 to 1928, and an opposingly great increase in the number of deaths

[1] Philadelphia Health and Hospital Survey, 1929. Published by The Survey Committee, Chamber of Commerce, Philadelphia, Pa.

due to "other accidents of pregnancy."[1] The increased hospitalization of maternity patients and the marked reduction in midwife deliveries was also noted. The apparent discrepancies in the number of patients cared for by the clinics reporting to the Child Health Society, the number delivered and the maternal mortality rate in this group received consideration. It was recommended (page 299) that the termination of the "lost" cases, that is, the excess of cases cared for in the prenatal period over the number delivered, should be discovered, in order to exclude a possibility of error in a seemingly more favorable maternal mortality rate.

Attention was called (page 318) to the fact that Philadelphia was a community with a falling birth rate and a stationary maternal death rate from childbirth for the previous ten years. It was pointed out that this death rate remained the same in spite of a reduction in the percentage of septic deaths and deaths due to convulsions. It was recommended that a study of some of these problems should be made.

The various recommendations were brought to the attention of Dr. George P. Muller, President of the Health League of Philadelphia, on his assuming the Presidency of the Philadelphia County Medical Society in May, 1930, and as a consequence a Committee on Maternal Welfare was appointed by him and requested to conduct a survey and analysis of the maternal deaths in Philadelphia. This committee included the following members: Jesse O. Arnold, M.D., Charles S. Barnes, M.D., P. Brooke Bland, M.D., George M. Boyd, M.D., Collin Foulkrod, M.D., Clifford B. Lull, M.D., Harriet L. Hartley, M.D., William R. Nicholson, M.D., Richard C. Norris, M.D., Edmund B. Piper, M.D., James L. Richards, M.D., E. A. Schumann, M.D., Alice W. Tallant, M.D., Norris W. Vaux, M.D., and Philip F. Williams, M.D., Chairman. This committee has been continued, by appointment, by the succeeding Presidents, Dr. Jay F. Schamberg, Dr. Charles F. Nassau, and Dr. Walter S. Cornell.

After some preliminary discussion, it was determined to follow the line of survey and analysis then in progress by the Committee on Public Health Relations of the New York Academy of Medicine,[2] in order that the reports of the two committees might be comparable. To Dr. Ransom S. Hooker, Director of the New York Study, we here acknowledge our deep appreciation of his many courtesies.

ACKNOWLEDGMENT OF ASSISTANCE

The material assistance of Mrs. John C. Martin and Mr. Joseph Wassermann, whose generosity has made the survey possible, is gratefully noted, and their deep and continued interest in the survey has been a measure of their public spiritedness. The Philadelphia Child Health Society made a very substantial grant toward the survey, which was

---

[1] For earlier Philadelphia statistics see "The Real Risk-Rate of Death to Mothers from Causes Connected with Childbirth." W. T. Howard, Jr., Amer. Jour. Hygiene, 1921, Vol. I, p. 197.
[2] "Maternal Mortality in New York City." New York Academy of Medicine. R. S. Hooker, M.D., Director of the Study. Commonwealth Fund, New York, 1933.

deeply appreciated. The Officers of the Health League of Philadelphia, The Philadelphia Child Health Society, the Community Council, the Coroner's Office, the Division of Child Hygiene of the Department of Health, the Bureau of Vital Statistics of the State Department of Health, and the Philadelphia County Medical Society, have tirelessly aided in the details of the survey. To them our thanks are rendered, especially to Mr. Alexander Fleisher of the Child Health Society, Miss Amy D. Swift of the Division of Child Hygiene, and Mr. Ewan Clague and Miss Blanche Hamer of the Community Council. The Committee also wishes to thank many other individuals and organizations who have co-operated in the work of the survey. Much of the statistical work was done through the courtesy of the Philadelphia Technical Service Committee. The Committee is also obligated to Mrs. Berthold Strauss and Dr. P. Brooke Bland for their personal help and good offices. Dr. Ruth H. Weaver has been a splendidly efficient and tactful Recorder, and has rendered inestimable assistance in the preparation of the report. The collection of the necessary data has been facilitated by the hearty co-operation of the physicians and hospitals concerned. In no single instance has there been any objection either by an institution or an individual in the search or interview for information desired.

METHOD OF SURVEY

The survey has been conducted by using, as a basic report, the standard form for Maternity Mortality surveys published by the Children's Bureau, United States Department of Labor. This form,[4] originally suggested by Dr. Robert L. De Normandie, has been slightly revised to meet certain needs. On the first page there appeared a copy of the certificate of each maternal death as received in the Bureau of Vital Statistics, City Hall, together with the birth certificate if a birth had occurred. These forms were sent by the Bureau of Vital Statistics to the office of the Committee at the County Medical Society building. If the death occurred in a hospital, the Recorder of the Committee, Dr. Ruth H. Weaver, through the courtesy of the hospitals throughout the city, made a visit to the record room to abstract the particular history and autopsy record. Additional information was obtained by personal interview with each physician connected with the case; the midwife where such a connection was shown; and the family, when necessary. If the death occurred at home, the information was obtained by personal interview with the physicians. As a check on the data, the maternal mortality records for Philadelphia were forwarded to the Committee quarterly from the Bureau of Vital Statistics of the Pennsylvania Department of Health. Further, the maternal mortality records for Philadelphia from the Bureau of the Census, United States Department of Commerce for 1931 and 1932, were checked against our own records for possible omission. Finally, through the Bureau of Vital Statistics at City Hall, for certain trial months, birth certificates were checked against

4 See Appendix, No. 1.

GRAPH 1

BIRTHS AND MATERNAL DEATHS IN PHILADELPHIA 1921-1933

Showing Percent of Deliveries by Physicians at Home and in Hospitals and by Midwives Compared with the Births by 1000's and Mortality Rate per 10,000 Live Births. Percent of Deliveries Calculated on Total Live Births.

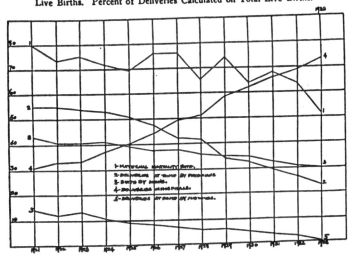

1. Maternal Mortality Rate in Philadelphia per 10,000 live births each year beginning with 80 in 1921.
2. Percentage of Deliveries at Home by Physicians. Percentages expressed in the left hand column by 55 percent in 1921.
3. The Number of Births by Thousands in Philadelphia. The number in thousands expressed by the figures in the left hand column. 43,000 in 1921.
4. Percentage of Deliveries in Hospitals. Percentages are expressed by the figures in the left hand column having been 32 percent in 1921.
5. Percentage of Deliveries by Midwives. Percentages are expressed as in lines 2 and 4 by the figures in the left hand column.

the death certificates of women in the childbearing age for overlapping periods. This single method of obtaining the maternal deaths must fail of necessity in deaths from abortions and deaths in pregnant women dying undelivered. While this method should be ideal for ascertaining the numbⅇr of deaths of women recently delivered, yet it would be inadequate in some instances, because of the large number of unregistered births of children stillborn or dying soon after birth in the earlier months. A birth certificate is required in Pennsylvania for every fetus born after the fourth month, but it is evident that this requirement is not fulfilled in many cases. This fact is another reason why the maternal mortality rate is figured by the Bureau of the Census against the live births rather

TABLE 1

BIRTH AND DEATH RATES FOR PHILADELPHIA 1920-1932

Year	Per 1000 Population		Per 1000 Live Births	Per 1000 Living and Still Births		
	Birth Rate	General Death Rate	Infant Mortality	Total Maternal Mortality	Puerperal Septicæmia	Other Puerperal Causes
1920	23.80	14.49	88.57	6.23	2.28	3.95
1921	23.58	12.87	77.84	6.98	2.79	4.19
1922	21.93	13.53	82.07	6.56	2.39	4.17
1923	21.89	14.28	78.63	6.87	2.31	4.56
1924	22.00	13.45	74.98	6.44	2.47	3.97
1925	20.65	13.77	76.58	6.30	2.88	3.42
1926	20.29	14.54	77.27	6.54	2.29	4.25
1927	20.10	12.94	64.24	6.46	1.79	4.67
1928	19.13	13.96	70.06	5.99	1.48	4.51
1929	18.14	13.05	61.49	5.37	1.90	3.47
1930	18.19	12.56	63.91	4.95	1.35	3.60
1931	17.17	12.82	64.13	5.75	1.81	3.94
1932	16.22	12.02	55.63	6.29	1.88	4.41
1933	14.8	12.01	....	4.4	1.79	2.61

Source: Bureau of Vital Statistics, Philadelphia.

than the total births. By means of these various methods of obtaining cases it is doubted if an appreciable number of maternal deaths have been overlooked.

The assembled data, after being charted and tabulated, was reviewed month by month, by an Analysis Committee consisting of Doctors Collin Foulkrod, Edward A. Schumann, Alice Weld Tallant and Norris W. Vaux. This Analysis Committee endeavored to determine whether the deaths were due to puerperal causes or were non-obstetrical in nature, also whether or not there was any preventability, and if so, upon whom responsibility for the prevention of the death rested, and what avoidable factors were concerned. They also decided whether the death certificate agreed with the evident cause of death. If, in their opinion, it did not agree, then it became necessary to make changes in order to group the case properly. At these discussions of the deaths the identity of the physicians signing the death certificates has not been disclosed to the Committee and the decisions have thus been made in an impersonal manner. The Recorder has been present at all of the meetings to supply any further necessary details obtained in her personal interviews. In this work the Analysis Committee had the frequent advice and judgment of other members of the Committee. In 1931, 269 cases were studied;

TABLE 2

BIRTH AND DEATH RATES FOR PENNSYLVANIA EXCLUSIVE OF PHILADELPHIA: 1920-1932

Year	Live Births	Birth Rates*	Infant Deaths	Infant Death Rates*	Total Puerperal Deaths	Puerperal Death Rates*	Puerperal Septicemia		Other Puerperal Causes	
							Deaths	Rates*	Deaths	Rates*
1920	176,820	25.5	17,459	99	1,378	7.4	485	2.6	893	4.8
1921	186,000	26.5	16,725	90	1,222	6.3	520	2.7	702	3.6
1922	174,094	24.6	15,535	89	1,037	5.7	394	2.2	643	3.5
1923	176,378	24.6	16,388	93	1,127	6.1	494	2.7	633	3.4
1924	181,564	25.1	14,414	79	1,111	5.8	439	2.3	672	3.5
1925	175,946	24.0	14,633	83	1,109	6.0	460	2.5	649	3.5
1926	169,057	22.9	14,115	83	1,032	5.9	398	2.3	634	3.6
1927	171,505	23.0	12,025	70	1,051	5.9	438	2.5	613	3.4
1928	163,694	21.7	11,857	72	978	5.7	374	2.2	604	3.5
1929	154,426	20.3	11,202	73	974	6.1	411	2.6	563	3.5
1930	153,640	20.0	10,605	69	911	5.7	349	2.2	562	3.5
1931	144,909	18.6	9,745	67	932	6.2	394	2.6	538	3.6
1932	136,355	17.4	8,443	62	810	5.7	351	2.5	459	3.2
1933	127,277	12.8	6,882	54	668	5.0	225	1.7	443	3.3

*Birth rates are per 1,000 population.
Infant death rates are per 1,000 live births.
Puerperal death rates are per 1,000 total births.
Source: Bureau of Vital Statistics, State of Pennsylvania.

TABLE 3
BIRTH AND DEATH RATES FOR THE UNITED STATES BIRTH REGISTRATION AREA 1920-1932

Year	Per 1,000 Population		Per, 1,000 Live Births			
	Birth Rate	General Death Rate	Infant Mortality	Total Maternal Mortality	Puerperal Septicæmia	Other Puerperal Causes
1920	23.7	13.1	85.8	8.0	2.7	5.3
1921	24.2	11.7	75.6	6.8	2.7	4.1
1922	22.3	11.8	76.2	6.6	2.4	4.2
1923	22.2	12.3	77.1	6.7	2.5	4.1
1924	22.4	11.7	70.8	6.6	2.4	4.1
1925	21.5	11.8	71.7	6.5	2.4	4.0
1926	20.7	12.2	73.3	6.6	2.4	4.1
1927	20.6	11.4	64.6	6.5	2.5	4.0
1928	19.8	12.0	68.7	6.9	2.5	4.4
1929	18.9	11.9	67.6	7.0	2.6	4.3
1930	18.9	11.3	64.6	6.7	2.4	4.3
1931	18.0	11.1	61.6	6.6	2.5	4.1
1932	17.4	10.9	57.6	6.3	2.3	4.0

Source: United States Bureau of the Census.

in 1932, 267; in 1933, 181; making a total of 717. For convenience and for the purpose of classifying the cases according to viability of the fetus they were divided into two groups according to the time of uterogestation. There were 425 cases over 28 weeks pregnant, and 292 cases under 28 weeks pregnant. The conclusions of the Analysis Committee appear in the correlations of the various puerperal and non-obstetrical causes of death.

THE MATERNAL MORTALITY RATE IN PHILADELPHIA AND OTHER VITAL STATISTICS.

The stationary maternal mortality rate and the falling birth rate for the city of Philadelphia may be seen from a study of Table No. 1 and Graph 1. These figures were furnished by the Bureau of Vital Statistics, Philadelphia. In ten years ending with 1933 the number of births has dropped from 41,343 in 1924 to 30,753 in 1933. Over an even longer period there was no reduction in the maternal death rate; there has been, however, an appreciable reduction in the septicemia rate. Unfortunately this is offset by increases in other categories.

The State of Pennsylvania, exclusive of Philadelphia, has shown an appreciable decline in the maternal death rate when compared to the Philadelphia figures, as shown in Table No. 2. The tabulation was furnished through the courtesy of Dr. Emlyn Jones, Director of the Bureau of Vital Statistics, Department of Health of Pennsylvania. In both these tables the rates for maternal deaths have been calculated upon the total births. The maternal mortality rates for Pennsylvania as a whole for the first two years of the survey, 1931 and 1932, as calculated by the Bureau of the Census, were 65 and 61 per 10,000 live births. The urban rates were 81 and 73, the rural rates 44 and 45. In 1933, Pennsylvania lost 874 mothers from causes associated with childbirth. One maternal death occurred in approximately every 187 deliveries. The deaths and the death rate of 5.4 per 1,000 total births were slightly lower than in preceding years.

The figures for the United States as a whole are seen in Table No. 3. This has been furnished by the Bureau of the Census, U. S. Department of Commerce. In this table the maternal death rate has been calculated upon live births. There has been no appreciable decline in the maternal death rate in the original birth registration of the United States since its inception in 1915. Nor has there been any appreciable decline from the figures of the original area in 1915 to the latest figures for the present expanded area. The needless sacrifice of mothers continues at an apparently fixed level locally, regionally and nationally.

The differences in data regarding the maternal mortality rate in Philadelphia when collected from different sources are shown in Table No. 4 and Chart No. 1.

TABLE 4

MATERNAL MORTALITY RATES FOR PHILADELPHIA 1924-1933
AS PUBLISHED BY THREE OFFICIAL SOURCES

1924	1925	1926	1927	1928	1929	1930	1931	1932	1933
7.2*	7.0	7.6	7.6	6.6	7.4	6.4	6.8	6.2	..
6.9†	6.7	7.2	7.3	6.4	7.0	6.1	6.3	6.4	5.0
6.4‡	6.3	6.5	6.5	6.0	5.4	5.0	5.8	6.3	4.4

*Bureau of the Census, U. S. Department of Commerce, Washington, D. C.
    (Rate per 1,000 live births)
†Bureau of Vital Statistics, Department of Health, State of Penna., Harrisburg, Penna.
    (Rate per 1,000 total births)
‡Bureau of Vital Statistics, Department of Health, City of Philadelphia.
    (Rate per 1,000 total births)

In this table the figures in the first line are from the Bureau of the Census, the second line represents the local rate as calculated by the Pennsylvania State Bureau of Vital Statistics, and the last line the local rate as calculated by the Philadelphia Bureau of Vital Statistics. It is evident that the more stringent check on questionable death certificates at the state office has resulted in developing a higher rate than is shown by the figures from the local registrar. The figures from the Bureau of the Census are still higher. This is due to the more diligent and persistent effort on the part of the trained vital statisticians of the Bureau of the Census in following by query the certificates which might mask a puer-

CHART 1

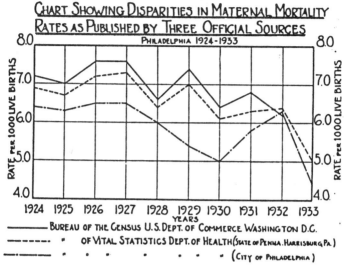

CHART SHOWING DISPARITIES IN MATERNAL MORTALITY RATES AS PUBLISHED BY THREE OFFICIAL SOURCES
PHILADELPHIA 1924-1933

——————— BUREAU OF THE CENSUS U.S. DEPT. OF COMMERCE WASHINGTON D.C.
– – – – – – " OF VITAL STATISTICS DEPT. OF HEALTH (STATE OF PENNA. HARRISBURG PA.)
–·–·–·– " • " • " • " (CITY OF PHILADELPHIA)

Bureau of the Census computes figures per 1000 live births, while Pennsylvania and Philadelphia compute figures per 1000 total births.

peral connection or cause. This diligence is not always possible in state or local offices, nor are the methods of calculation the same.

CALCULATION OF MATERNAL MORTALITY RATE

The method adopted by the Bureau of the Census is based upon the ratio of puerperal deaths to live births rather than total births. As expressed by Woodbury,[1] live births as a basis for calculating the maternal mortality rate yield approximately the same result as would be secured by using the number of confinements, and when only live births are used, comparisons between states and countries are not subject to error arising from differences in definition of still birth. Deaths from puerperal causes, in the Census figures, include all those of which pregnancy and confinement are the only and decisive cause. In the past few years surveys on puerperal mortality in different states have shown increases ranging from five to thirty percent when birth certificates and death certificates for women from 15 to 44 years of age were compared.

In the present survey all maternal deaths in Philadelphia have been

---

[1] "Maternal Mortality." R. M. Woodbury. Children's Bureau Publication No. 158, 1926.

studied regardless of whether the cause of death was obstetrical or non-obstetrical. They have been divided as to cause of death in several tables for purposes of correlation. In addition, all cases of criminal abortion, abortions induced by a person other than the deceased, usually coded as "Homicides," Title No. 175, have been included. This inclusion is supported by the opinion of R. A. Boldt,[•] who states, "So-called criminal abortion should no longer be classified as manslaughter or homicide, as it is impossible to draw a clear distinction. They are definitely under the puerperal state and the effects on the mother may be the same whoever induces the abortion."

Table No. 5 shows the difference in maternal mortality rates for the past three years between the Bureau of Vital Statistics, Philadelphia, and those of this study.

TABLE 5

PUERPERAL MORTALITY RATES AS ESTABLISHED BY THIS
SURVEY COMPARED WITH RATES BY PHILA-
DELPHIA BUREAU OF VITAL STATISTICS

PER 1000 LIVE BIRTHS				
PHILADELPHIA BUREAU VITAL STATISTICS	SURVEY—THE PUERPERAL STATE			SURVEY
All Puerperal Causes	All Puerperal Causes	Puerperal Septicæmia[*]	Other Puerperal Causes	Total Maternal Mortality[**]
1931 — 5.75	7.35	3.38	3.97	7.8
1932 — 6.29	7.44	2.71	4.75	8.3
1933 — 4.4	5.17	2.67	2.50	6.1

[*]Includes 140, Abortion with septic conditions specified.
142, Ectopic Pregnancy, with septic condition specified and
145, Puerperal Septicæmia not specified as due to abortion.
[**]Includes Non-Obstetrical Cases.

CODING IN JOINT CAUSES OF DEATH

There are very definite rules in use by the Bureau of the Census for separating puerperal deaths from deaths from associated or complicating causes, and these rules, with one exception, already noted, have been followed in this report. Briefly they may be expressed as follows: (1) Most acute infectious diseases (*e. g.*, diphtheria, small-pox) and external causes, including criminal abortion, are preferred to any other puerperal cause. (2) Puerperal Septicemia is generally preferred to any other cause excepting some acute infectious diseases, cancer, syphilis or external causes. (3) A serious disease (*e. g.*, pulmonary tuberculosis) is preferred to any puerperal cause except puerperal septicemia. The full list of such exceptions and preferences is given in the Manual of

[•] "Maternal Mortality and Morbidity." Report of R. A. Boldt, p. 439. D. Appleton-Century Co., New York, 1933.

the Joint Causes of Death.[7] Further discussion of the measurement and definition of puerperal mortality is a matter of involved vital statistics not relevant to this report, but which may be found in Woodbury's article.

Until there is a complete registration of all births, stillbirths and maternal deaths under uniform standards, definitions and rules for preference in joint causes, comparisons between states and countries as to maternal death rates will prove unsatisfactory. This is exemplified above in Table No. 4, showing the varying rates of maternal mortality for Philadelphia as calculated by the local, state and federal bureaus. This difficulty would be solved easily if universal birth and stillbirth registration was practiced and if death certificates required a statement as to the association of the puerperal state. The Province of Alberta, Canada, however, is the only local governmental sub-division on this continent, so far as it is known, which has appearing on the death certificate such a printed question as to associated pregnancy. The question reads as follows: "If deceased was a woman of childbearing age, was she pregnant, and if so, was this a contributing factor to the cause of death?" The standard death certificate of the United States Birth Registration Area has no such question.

MORTALITY RATES IN FOREIGN COUNTRIES

In many discussions, printed and otherwise, on Maternal Mortality[8] during the past few years, it has been repeatedly stated that the maternal mortality rate in the United States is unusually high, especially when contrasted and compared with the rates of various foreign countries, those of Europe in particular. The factors leading to misinterpretations of maternal mortality rates have been well set forth by Dr. Haven Emerson.[9] The lack of uniformity in procedure of national registration offices in classifying certificates which present multiple or joint causes of death is largely the cause of such misinterpretation. Emerson shows that in such joint cause certificates, the United States rules could classify 88 percent as puerperal causes; England and Norway under their present rules would classify only 64 percent as a puerperal cause; while only one country out of sixteen refers a larger proportion of joint causes of death to the puerperal list than does the United States. According to Runnels,[10] only Chili, Spain and the Argentine are as strict in classifying puerperal deaths as the United States. He feels "that the very unfavor-

[7] Manual of the Joint Causes of Death, Showing Assignment to the Preferred Title of the International List of Causes of Death When Two Causes Are Simultaneously Reported. Third edition. U. S. Government Printing Office, Washington, D. C., 1933.

[8] "Maternal Mortality," Monthly Epidemiological Report, League of Nations. Geneva. July 15, 1930.

[9] "Factors Leading to Misinterpretation of Maternal Mortality Rates." Haven Emerson. American Journal of Obstetrics and Gynecology. 1932. XXIII, p. 605.

[10] "Maternal Mortality." S. C. Runnels. J. Am. Inst. Homœ, 1932, XXV, 1408.

able light in which American Obstetrics has been thrown is a false one, being about 40 percent too high." He makes an excellent point in declaring that we should differentiate between puerperal and obstetrical mortality. Anyone studying the rules for preference in puerperal death in the Manual for Joint Causes of Death in connection with a series of maternal deaths, will be inclined to agree with this statement.

The Final Report of the Departmental Committee on Maternal Mortality and Morbidity, Ministry of Health, London, 1932, gives the details o. the report of a Committee sent to the Netherlands, Denmark and Sweden, to investigate the factors leading to a lower maternal mortality rate in those countries as compared to England and Wales. The rate for England in 1929 was 4.3, for the Netherlands, 3.3. It is admitted that the procedure of defining and calculating the maternal mortality was practically identical in these two countries. The factors favoring the Netherlands were found to be a sound training of physician and midwife, extensive antenatal supervision, early hospitalization of all but the simplest abnormalities of pregnancy and parturition—in short, the excellence of the obstetric service of the country and the rarity of severe degrees of pelvic deformity.

In regard to the difference of the official figures for Denmark as compared with England and Wales, it is noted (page 73) that the statistical procedure in Denmark was adopted in 1860, and has been changed comparatively little since then. On account of the differences in the classification of cause of death and the preference practiced, when two or more causes have contributed to the death, published statistics of maternal mortality of the two countries are not comparable. A cardiac case in Denmark dying from antepartum hemorrhage is usually recorded by the physician as a death from cardiac disease. It is noted, however, that a new system of nomenclature and procedure is being instituted, and it will be of interest to observe the death rate from puerperal causes in Denmark during the next decade.

In regard to Sweden, the English report stated (page 89) that the Swedish method of recording maternal death connected with childbirth differs from that used in the British Isles and tends to yield a lower recorded maternal mortality rate than that which would be obtained if the English method were employed. Very striking is the comment on the report of the maternal deaths in the Gothenburg Maternity Hospital for the year 1930. Fifteen maternal deaths occurred, and only two of these, a case of chronic nephritis and uremia at the fourth month, and a case of tuberculosis of the lungs and peritoneum complicating pregnancy, could have been eliminated from the list as non-puerperal. Yet, when the officially reported deaths for Gothenburg for 1930 were printed, only seven appeared. Such a method of definition and calculation which produces almost a fifty percent reduction, if nation-wide, would necessarily produce a favorable national rate of maternal mortality for Sweden.

In discussing the differences in practice of classifying joint causes in puerperal deaths, Woodbury (page 130) states that if the United

States rules for classification had been used in England and Wales in 1920 their rate of maternal mortality would have been raised fourteen and eight-tenths percent. Until a uniform procedure for preference in joint causes found in maternal deaths is adopted, any comparisons between countries will be useless and futile. As a matter of fact, the stationary maternal death rate is not confined to the United States, it is discernible in most civilized countries. In England and Wales, Sweden, Denmark and the Netherlands the rate has actually been rising since 1910.[1]

COMPARISON OF PUERPERAL AND OTHER DISEASE RATES, BIRTH AND STILLBIRTH RATES.

The objective of this survey has not been a study of comparative rates, but rather an examination as to why Philadelphia loses so many mothers each year. The seriousness of this problem has a medical aspect, for it reflects on the ability of our physicians and hospitals to care properly for maternity patients. From a public health standpoint, it involves the relation of the falling birth rate and the diminishing marriage rate in the United States. From a social view the advancing age of marriage, the increase of abortions and the limitation of family, bear a distinct relation to the question. The breaking up of families and the dependency of orphaned children presents one of the greatest social problems, since the women dying, after pregnancies of twenty-eight weeks duration or over, leave an average of over two living children.[2] From the economic side, it has been estimated that the maternal mortality in Philadelphia causes annually a loss in productive value of four million dollars.[3]

The Department of Labor and Industry of the State of Pennsylvania reports that in Philadelphia for the three years of this survey there were 405 industrial accidents. This number may be contrasted with the 717 fatalities of the puerperal state in the same period. It would appear that childbirth is a more hazardous undertaking than industry. Possibly the workers and employers used more safeguards, relatively, than do the maternity patients and their attendants.

From a study of the practically stationary maternal mortality rate, it is obvious that the advantages of modern surgical technic and increased hospital facilities for specialized obstetrical practice have brought no definite decrease in the number of maternal deaths. In the past decade the maternal mortality rate has dropped only from 8 per 1,000 live births in 1921, to 6.6 in 1932, although the birth rate fell from 23.8 per 1,000 population to 16.22.

In contrast to this, one illogically but inevitably compares the steadily declining death rate from many communicable diseases. It is seen that

[1] Statistical Bulletin, Metropolitan Life Insurance Co., December, 1933.
[2] "Orphans and Maternal Mortality." Alexander Fleisher, Weekly Roster and Medical Digest. Phila. Co. Med. Soc. October 22, 1932.
[3] "The Economic Loss in a Maternal Death." Blanche Hamer, Weekly Roster and Medical Digest. Phila. Co. Med. Soc. May 13, 1933.

the death rate from diphtheria was reduced from 17.53 per 100,000 population in 1921 to 0.86 in 1932; the infant mortality rate from 77.84 per 1,000 living births to 51.63; the tuberculosis death rate from 103.78 per 100,000 population to 62.35; the typhoid death rate from 73 per 100,000 in 1906 to 6. in 1917; and the general death rate dropped from 14.49 per 1,000 population to 12.01 in 1933. The stillbirth rate for Philadelphia in 1924 was 46.6 per 1,000 live births; in 1933 the rate was 41.4.[4] The advances of modern medicine evidently do not give the fetus a much more favorable chance than the mother.

Since it is realized that a comparison of the maternal death rate with the death rates from causes affecting various elements of the population as a whole cannot be made logically, the death rates from important causes in women in the ages from 15 to 44 have been contrasted with the maternal mortality rates. Chart 2 shows a comparison of the death rates from various causes with the maternal mortality rates in the years 1926 to 1932. Deaths from diseases of the heart and from cancer have shown a notable increase, and deaths from puerperal causes have shown practically no decrease. The figures refer to Philadelphia and have been obtained from the Bureau of the Census.

It is not without interest to compare the percentage distribution of deaths from all puerperal causes with other important causes in the five cities in the United States which have over a million population. Thus we find over the period from 1926 to 1932 inclusive, the percentage distribution of deaths from all puerperal causes, in women from 15 to 44 years of age, compared with all other deaths in that group, was 11.3 percent in Detroit; 9.9 percent in Philadelphia; 8.8 percent in New York; 8.6 percent in Los Angeles, and 8.5 percent in Chicago.[5]

DEATHS INACCURATELY AND INCOMPLETELY CERTIFIED

In reviewing the tabulated data on the series of cases here reported, it was evident a number of times, in the opinion of the Analysis Committee, that the cause of death as certified did not express correctly the true cause. In some instances bronchopneumonia or embolus occurring late in a septic puerperium was given as the cause of death; or secondary anemia was given as the cause of death following a postpartum hemorrhage, as described in the history; or chronic nephritis was given as the cause in a convulsive toxemia of pregnancy. In some cases the cause of death as stated upon the certificate did not correspond with the facts found on the hospital record. In such instances, a note of the difference of opinion was placed on the record and the ostensible true cause added in order to group the case more properly under the appropriate title of the International List. The number of times in which disparity between the stated and actual cause of death occurred is shown in Table No. 6.

---

[4] Source: Department of Health, Philadelphia.
[5] Source: U. S. Bureau of the Census.

CHART 2

PERCENTAGE OF DEATHS FROM IMPORTANT CAUSES AMONG WOMEN
15 TO 44 YEARS OF AGES

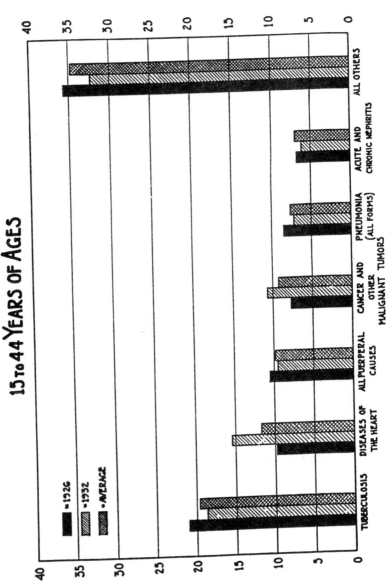

TABLE 6
ERRORS ON DEATH CERTIFICATES
PREVENTING CORRECT CODING

CAUSES OF DEATH AS DETERMINED BY ANALYSIS COMMITTEE	TOTAL DEATHS	ERRORS ON DEATH CERTIFICATES	
		Number	Percent
TOTAL	717	155	21.6
Septic Abortion	162	25	15.4
Abortion	26	3	11.5
Ectopic Gestation	33	10	30.3
Hemorrhage	62	12	19.4
Puerperal Septicæmia	119	43	36.1
Albuminuria and Eclampsia	85	8	9.4
Pernicious Vomiting	24	7	29.2
Embolus and Sudden Death	44	13	29.5
Accidents of Labor	79	23	29.1
Accidents of Puerperium	5	1	20.0
Non-Obstetrical Causes	78	10	12.8

DISCUSSION OF CERTIFICATION OF SEPTICEMIA

Dr. Emlyn Jones, Director of the Bureau of Vital Statistics, Department of Health of the State of Pennsylvania, in a communication to the Committee, wrote regarding the compulsory notification of puerperal sepsis, "The reports of this disorder are so incomplete that they are practically useless from a statistical standpoint. In the past twenty-seven years, 2,167 cases of puerperal fever have been reported, while 15,269 deaths from the disease are on record for the same period. It is possible that puerperal fever will be dropped from the list of notifiable diseases." Evidently the recognition of puerperal sepsis before death is a more difficult problem than the certification of it as a cause of death.

In this connection reference may be made to an article by Dr. Harriet L. Hartley.[6] Commenting on Goodall's remarks[7] on patients alleged to have died from lobar pneumonia during a septic puerperium, Dr. Hartley states, "The remedy for our inaccurate figures is an easy one and necessitates only a little thoughtful and conscientious care on the part of the individual filling out the original certificate of death. He should record complete information and state honestly the real cause of death." What proportion of these evidently incorrectly certified causes of death was due to self-delusion or to lack of knowledge cannot be measured. Possibly some of the evident errors in certification of death referred to above

[6] "Maternal Mortality Statistics." Harriet L. Hartley. Weekly Roster and Medical Digest, Phila. Co. Med. Soc. September 10, 1932.
[7] "Puerperal Infection." James R. Goodall. Murray Pr. Co., Toronto, 1932.

arise from the fact that in some hospitals internes sign the death certificates. This violation of the Pennsylvania Department of Health regulations became so obvious that in February, 1932, a notice was sent to all the hospitals in the state calling attention to the ruling, "The attending physician must sign all birth and death certificates." This ruling was made in order to avoid the development of any legal difficulty following the issuance of certified copies of the records.

In many cases no mention was made of the puerperal state being associated with the given cause of death. The List of the Causes of Death issued by the Bureau of the Census, under the definition of a puerperal death, states: "The fact that childbirth occurred within a month of death should always be stated, even though it may not have been a cause of death."

Confusion between the primary and secondary cause of death has in many instances obscured the correct cause of death. It would facilitate the work of the bureaus of vital statistics if the International List and the Manual of the Joint Causes of Death were consulted more frequently in filling out of maternal death certificates. It seems inexcusable that "forceps delivery" should be given as a primary cause and "sepsis" as a secondary cause, even though the infection may have been introduced at the time of operation, but this and similar mistakes were frequently made. Hysterectomy may have been an appropriate treatment but was not a cause of death from rupture of the uterus following version and craniotomy on the aftercoming head.

CHANGES IN CODING BY THE ANALYSIS COMMITTEE

For the first two years of the study the transcripts of the death certificates relating to puerperal deaths in Philadelphia, as defined by the Bureau of the Census, were obtained and checked against the file and code numbers of the records of the Committee. It was found that for the year 1931 the Committee obtained 29 puerperal death certificates which apparently had not come to the attention of the Bureau of the Census. These deaths were coded by the Committee as follows: 13 under 140; 3 under 141; 2 under 144; 8 under 146; and 1 each under 147, 148 and 149. They were all included in the study here reported and a list of these file numbers was furnished by the Bureau.[*] Conversely, there appeared in the transcript numbers of the list furnished by the Bureau of the Census, 8 certificates which the Analysis Committee rejected after careful consideration. The reasons for rejecting these certificates were as follows: one was found to be a woman of 81 years; another a 9 months old infant; a third, a certificate of a male; four were decided not to have been pregnant after the history had been reviewed in detail, and in the last one the cause of death was not considered related to the pregnancy. It is probable that the statisticians in the Bureau of the Census did not have such detailed reports on these deaths as did the Committee.

[*] Title numbers will be found in Table No. 14.

TABLE 7

CLASSIFICATION OF DEATHS IN RELATION TO EFFECT OF PREGNANCY

	TOTAL			PREGNANCY AND LABOR		
	Deaths	28 Weeks and Over	Under 28 Weeks	Directly Responsible for Death	A Contributing Cause	Not a Contributing Cause
TOTAL	717	425	292	543	129	45
1931 TOTAL	269	...	...	212	47	10
28 Weeks and Over ..	...	155	...	119	28	8
Under 28 Weeks	...	...	114	93	19	2
1932 TOTAL	267	...	...	195	54	18
28 Weeks and Over ..	...	169	...	118	39	12
Under 28 Weeks	...	...	98	77	15	6
1933 TOTAL	181	...	...	130	28	17
28 Weeks and Over ..	...	101	...	71	21	9
Under 28 Weeks	...	...	80	65	7	8

For the year 1932, the Committee added in the study 33 deaths not included in the list of Philadelphia's transcript numbers furnished by the Bureau of the Census. The deaths were coded by the Analysis Committee for the cause of death as follows: 11 under 140; 3 under 141; 2 under 142; 3 under 144; 1 under 145; 4 under 146; 4 under 148; 3 under 149, and 2 under 150. Probably most of these deaths did come to the attention of the Bureau of the Census, but may have been filed under other mentioned joint causes according to the rules of preference. Nevertheless, the Analysis Committee felt justified in including these cases. Seven deaths included by the Bureau of the Census in 1932 were rejected by the Committee, after hearing detailed histories and autopsy reports. There were two coded as abortions, two coded as septicemia, two coded as eclampsia, and one coded as obscure toxemia of pregnancy. The Committee changed the coding to one suppurating fibroid, one to intestinal obstruction, two to non-puerperal pelvic disease, one to diabetes, and two to arsphenamin shock.

One of the factors leading to the increase in the number of abortions, with mention of septic conditions (Title No. 140), was the decision of the Committee to include those septic abortions which had been induced by a person other than the patient, and which are usually coded as homicides (Title No. 175) by the various departments of vital statistics.

Dame Louise McIlroy,[*] in discussing the prevention of maternal mortality, states: "The proper definition of a maternal death is one which is directly due to pregnancy, labor or the puerperium." This brings up

---

[*] "The Prevention of Maternal and Infantile Mortality." Louise McIlroy. J. State Med., 1932, XI, 188.

two other groups, which have been suggested by Runnels in his classification: second, those cases in which pregnancy and labor were a contributing cause, but in which there was another primary cause; and third, those deaths in which pregnancy and labor had no contributing effect. The Committee reviewed the data from this angle and tabulated the deaths as shown in Table No. 7 (page 21).

HOSPITAL OBSTETRICAL DATA

In order to develop a basic table for use in specific correlations, the hospitals were asked, each year of the survey, for various data. The totals are presented in Table No. 8, and graphically in Chart No. 3. The yearly calculations of the Bureau of Vital Statistics, City Hall, Philadelphia, showed that in 1931, 22,186 or 65.7% of the total live births occurred in hospitals; in 1932, 21,949 or 69.1% of the live births occurred in hospitals; and in 1933, 21,491 or 73.5% of the live births occurred in hospitals. In the three years of the survey 65,626 or 69.2% of all live births in the city occurred in hospitals. The progressive increase of hospital over the home as a place for delivery is shown in Graph No. 1.

The apparent discrepancies in the number of deaths reported by the hospitals (not shown in the table) and the total deaths studied by the Analysis Committee, arose from the fact that the latter included all deaths, puerperal and non-puerperal in cause. Miller says, "I believe that all these 'non-puerperal' deaths should be shown in our reports just as much as the truly puerperal causes, whether or not they be included in a mortality ratio, for it is quite evident that skill in obstetrics is shown at its best in the management of these complicated cases."[10] Many of the puerperal cause deaths occurred in pregnancies of under 28 weeks duration in medical and surgical wards and in private room departments. Some became "lost" to the maternity department through transfer to other services. Often they were not reported as true maternal deaths because of a faulty preference in joint causes.

The puerperal death rate of a general hospital is frequently out of proportion to the delivery death rate of its maternity division. A hospital puerperal death rate may be influenced by an active gynecological and surgical service admitting all types of complicated cases in early pregnancy together with an active emergency service. When this situation is contrasted with the almost irreducible rate of a maternity hospital or service admitting only "booked" cases, the comparison will appear misleading, unless the situation is clearly explained.

Skeel in discussing this phase of the problem of maternal mortality calculation gave a classification of deaths used in the continuous study being conducted by the Cleveland Hospital Obstetrical Society. This classification may be used by a single hospital, or by a group, for suitable interval studies.

---

[10] "The Use of Mortality Statistics in Rating Maternity Service." J. R. Miller. Amer. Jour. Obs. and Gyn. 1933, XXV, 577.

HOSPITAL DELIVERIES BY TYPE OF DELIVERY

HOSPITAL NUMBER	1000	2000	3000	4000	5000	6000	7000	PERCENT SPONTANEOUS	PERCENT OPERATIVE	DEATH RATE PER 1000 DELIVERIES
1								34.5	65.5	8.0
2								87.7	12.3	8.4
3								87.9	12.1	18.9
4								87.6	12.4	5.8
5								83.2	16.8	7.4
6								56.4	43.6	11.7
7								58.2	41.8	6.3
8								63.5	36.5	7.7
9								85.4	14.6	5.7
10								79.3	20.7	6.7
11								62.5	37.5	8.7
12								66.2	33.8	9.9
13								52.3	47.7	16.4
14								82.5	17.5	12.4
15								74.8	25.2	4.7
16								73.7	26.3	9.7
17								91.7	8.3	0.6
18								83.6	16.4	11.9
19								69.1	30.9	12.4
20								62.3	37.7	4.8
21								83.5	16.5	7.3
22								76.5	23.5	3.3
23								81.3	18.7	7.6
24								62.6	37.4	15.1
25								75.8	24.2	4.3
26								68.4	31.6	8.1
27								85.1	14.9	8.6
28								76.7	23.3	3.3
29								80.2	19.8	11.8
30								82.5	17.5	12.0
31								72.9	27.1	6.2
32								57.0	43.0	10.4
* 33 to 55								75.8	24.2	18.2

ALL HOSPITALS
PERCENT SPONTANEOUS 72.0
· OPERATIVE 28.0
DEATH RATE PER 1000 DELIVERIES 9.1

■ - SPONTANEOUS   ▧ - FORCEPS   ▨ - OTHER OPERATIVE

* TOTAL OF 22 HOSPITALS WITH LESS THAN 500 DELIVERIES EACH

HOSPITAL DELIVERY STATISTICS
1931-1932-1933

Hospital	Total Deliveries	Spontaneous Deliveries	Operative Deliveries	Operative Incidence	Cesarean Section	Cesarean Section Incidence	Forceps	Version	Breech Extraction	Craniotomy
1	6354	2193	4161	65.5%	308	4.8%	3307	315	231	0
2	4850	4254	596	12.3	90	1.9	309	44	153	0
3	4614	4057	557	12.1	81	1.8	302	48	122	4
4	3965	3472	493	12.4	37	.9	294	29	133	0
5	3252	2705	547	16.8	96	3.0	347	37	67	0
6	2817	1590	1227	43.6	48	1.7	1072	14	93	0
7	2815	1639	1176	41.8	78	2.8	983	40	73	0
8	2723	1728	995	36.5	61	2.2	901	12	21	2
9	2637	2250	387	14.6	39	1.5	252	29	66	0
10	2519	1998	521	20.7	98	3.9	320	30	65	1
11	2413	1509	904	37.5	70	2.9	702	34	98	0
12	2036	1348	688	33.8	44	2.2	566	15	62	0
13	1896	992	904	47.7	80	4.2	725	68	76	1
14	1858	1532	326	17.5	47	2.5	235	22	22	0
15	1711	1280	431	25.2	58	3.4	311	19	43	0
16	1644	1212	432	26.3	64	3.9	316	10	42	0
17	1583	1452	131	8.3	13	.8	30	18	70	0
18	1423	1189	234	16.4	22	1.5	151	19	39	3
19	1295	895	400	30.9	17	1.3	321	18	44	0
20	1244	775	469	37.7	23	1.8	385	8	53	0
21	1231	1028	203	16.5	4	.3	155	13	31	0
22	1198	916	282	23.5	21	1.8	190	13	57	1
23	1183	962	221	18.7	47	4.0	110	24	40	0
24	1126	705	421	37.4	75	6.7	291	25	30	0
25	1113	844	269	24.2	9	.8	102	12	44	2
26	1106	756	350	31.6	32	2.9	280	15	23	0
27	1047	891	156	14.9	6	.3	98	16	36	0
28	952	730	222	23.3	3	.3	188	12	19	0
29	678	544	134	19.8	23	3.4	93	4	14	0
30	664	548	116	17.5	17	2.6	58	12	29	0
31	646	471	175	27.1	9	1.4	127	18	21	0
32	575	328	247	43.0	64	11.1	156	15	12	0
Total	65168	46793	18375	24.2 Av.	1684	2.6	13677	1008	1929	14
33-55*	3565	2703	862		91	2.6 Av.	615	42	110	4
Total	68733	49496	19237	28.0 Av.	1775	2.6 Av.	14292	1050	2039	18

*Total of 22 hospitals with less than 500 deliveries each.

TABLE 9

DEATHS FOLLOWING HOSPITAL AND HOME DELIVERIES

	Total	Hospital Delivery	Home Delivery
TOTAL	717*	587	80
VIABLE	375	320	55
Septic	119	98	21
Non-Septic	256	222	34
PREVIABLE	292	267	25

*50 Cases Undelivered; 41 in hospital, 9 at home.
20 Cases Delivered after death; 18 in hospital, 2 at home.

HOSPITAL VIABLE BIRTHS

TOTAL 320

SEPTIC 98

   Intra Hospital Infection 77

   Extra Hospital Infection 21

NON-SEPTIC 222

   Admitted to Hospital with pathologic condition known or recognized on admission 168

   Admitted as normal case 54

	TOTAL	ADMISSION	
		Planned	Emergency
SEPTIC	98	77	21
Intra Hospital Infection	77	66	11
Extra Hospital Infection	21	11	10

The deaths from puerperal causes in this survey have been grouped in Table No. 9, according to Skeel's Classification.[1] In fairness to the hospitals the next to last heading has been changed from "Sent to hospital with known pathologic condition," to read: "Admitted to hospital with pathological condition known or recognized on admission." This change was made to cover the occasional unregistered maternity case whose abnormal condition is discovered at the first or admission examination. In this respect Kerr and McLannan say: "The organization of institutions should be judged by the adequacy with which the emergency obstetrical complications are dealt with, and by the precautions taken to prevent infection."[2] Routine staff conference discussions should clear up such matters for each hospital.

[1] "New Methods of Study Applied to Maternal Mortalities in the Hospital." R. J. Skeel. Am. Jour. Obst. and Gyn., 1933, XXV, 187.
[2] "An Investigation Into the Mortality in Maternity Hospitals." J. M. M. Kerr and H. R. McLannan. Lancet, London, 1932, 1, 633.

PREVENTABILITY OF MATERNAL DEATHS

In considering the cases studied during the three years the Analysis Committee has endeavored to determine what deaths might be regarded as preventable. The term "preventable" in regard to maternal deaths has been selected instead of certain similarly sounding words and phrases, such as "avoidable" or "associated with controllable causes," because in its derivation it signifies the ultimate aim of the study. "To stop or hinder from happening by means of previous measures" would be a more potent method of lessening the number of maternal deaths than "by exercising a directing, restraining or governing influence over" such deaths. The factors governing the decisions in each individual death have been debated amply and discussed unhurriedly in order to render a thoughtful judgment in each decision. In determining this theoretical preventability of deaths the Analysis Committee felt that the standard adopted by the New York Committee (1.c) was too rigid and inflexible. Their standard was: "In judging whether or not the death was inevitable, the criterion has always been that of the best possible skill, both in diagnosis and treatment, which the community could make available." The Philadelphia Analysis Committee used as a basis in this survey the standard[3] which the courts of the nation have always held sufficient, namely: "A reasonable degree of learning and skill, and the use of reasonable care and diligence in the exercise of that skill and the application of that learning."

The preventability, when determined to be present, has been assigned either to a physician in charge of the case at some period, or to the patient, provided her conduct has been determined to be the preventable element. In cases where there was no avoidance of the death, under the usual and accepted mode of practice, the decision has been that it was non-preventable. When an error of omission or commission, occurring at some period in the care of the case, was determined to have been the deciding factor, then the responsibility for the death has been assigned to the physician, at times a referring physician, a member of a hospital staff or the attending physician in a home delivery.

PREVENTABILITY DUE TO THE PHYSICIAN

The physician was considered responsible for a preventable death under certain conditions. If, because of insufficient training, instruction, or experience, the physician failed to recognize early in pregnancy the signs and symptoms pointing to complications later in pregnancy or in labor, then the responsibility of the death in such a case was attributed to him. It is his duty to be thoroughly familiar with the accepted standards of prenatal care.[4]

---

[3] "Courts and Doctors." L. P. Stryker. MacMillan Company, New York, 1932.
[4] "Standards of Prenatal Care." U. S. Department of Labor, Children's Bureau Publication No. 153, 1925.

If a patient died from a long complicated labor through failure to recognize, by means of pelvimetry, the presence of pelvic deformity, the physician was considered responsible for that death.

The physician should make a vaginal examination in the early months in order to diagnose, if possible, the presence of abnormal pregnancy (ectopic). In cases where he failed to do this and the patient died of hemorrhage or shock, the responsibility for the death was assigned to the physician.

The physician should be able to recognize the presence of disproportion between the fetus and the pelvis. He should know if there is a mal-position or mal-presentation before the onset of labor. It is essential that he inquire into the past maternal history very carefully so as to learn if there were any complications in the previous deliveries. It is in his province, too, to impress upon the patient the need for early and regular examinations in order to recognize as soon as possible any signs, symptoms or abnormalities, such as early toxemia.

If the physician failed to carry out any of the procedures just mentioned, and as a result of this inadequate prenatal care the patient died from some condition that could have been avoided, then the death was attributed directly to the physician.

The physician was considered responsible for deaths in another group of cases, namely, where the abnormality was recognized but the treatment was inadequate. For instance, if the physician failed to have consultation, either through the clinics or by other individual physicians, for patients whose general condition warranted more careful study, especially in renal, cardiac, or pulmonary complications, he was held responsible for the deaths. He was considered at fault when he failed to have the patient hospitalized promptly for serious complications that could not be treated adequately at home, such as cases of placenta previa, eclampsia, or disproportion. The only exception to this rule being when there was absolute refusal on the part of the patient or her family to agree to hospitalization.

The physician was thought responsible if he failed to recognize that long labor and loss of blood tend to lower tissue vitality and as a consequence increase the possibility of infection.. He was also considered responsible if he failed to realize that the use of both vaginal and rectal examinations during labor is injudicious, in cases where there is a question of possible operative delivery, because of the danger of infection. .

The physician should be able to determine the proper time to terminate labor. Unnecessary or ill-timed operations, that is, too early or too late, were regarded as the physician's responsibility.

Where there was too free use of operative interference by a physician untrained in the indications for interference or unskilled in the procedure required, the responsibility rested upon the physician in question. If he retained charge of the case when he was incapable of giving the patient reasonable care, the Committee regarded him as blameworthy.

Following operative interference in emergency cases, the physician should be alert to recognize threatening shock and to combat it. In cases where he failed to do this, he was considered responsible.

He was considered responsible for death if he delayed in emptying the uterus in cases of placenta previa, or premature separation of the placenta, or if he delayed in operating on cases of ectopic gestation with evident severe hemorrhage, unless transfusion was needed and was available immediately. If he failed to pack the uterus following delivery in cases complicated by placenta previa, premature separation of the placenta, or inverted uterus, he was thought to be responsible.

In women who had lost considerable blood either antenatally or during labor, it was considered the duty of the physician to see that preparations were made for transfusions before such cases were submitted to operative interference. His failure to do this rendered him responsible in the deaths of such patients.

Deaths following rupture of the uterus in version or in forceps deliveries; deaths following proven mistakes in diagnosis; and deaths from infection following operations in clean cases, were all considered the responsibility of the physician.

In cases where students, internes, or residents handled complicated labors without supervision or where they resorted to operative interference even under supervision, the death was attributed to the physician in charge of the case. The Analysis Committee felt that no responsibility could be assigned to a hospital through its equipment, rules or nursing. In certain instances, where it might have been said that a hospital was at fault, it was plainly evident that the responsibility for any errors must be borne by the physician, whether a private doctor in charge of the case or a chief of a public service.

If a physician failed to handle cases of abortion conservatively he was regarded as being responsible in case of death, no matter whether the abortion was threatened, incomplete, inevitable or complete, septic or not. In septic abortions it was accepted as the rule that such cases should be treated expectantly, and interference instituted only for excessive hemorrhage or for proven sapremia with an open cervix.

In cases where death was considered due to anesthesia, the physician was thought to be at fault. Such cases included deaths from spinal anesthesia, or from experimentation with new drugs as anesthetics, as well as cases in which the anesthetic was administered by an untrained person.

PREVENTABILITY DUE TO PATIENT

Responsibility for the prevention of death has been assigned to the patient under certain conditions:

When an abortion was induced, whether by the patient or some one else, and resulted in septic or other fatal termination of the case.

When the patient received inadequate prenatal care, due to late registration, particularly in multipara with known complications in previous pregnancies; or when she failed to co-operate with clinics and physicians; or when she showed lack of appreciation of her responsibility.

When the negligence or ignorance of the individual led her to assume responsibility of complications occurring during pregnancy without reporting to the physician or clinic.

When the individual failed to report sufficiently early in pregnancy, at which time medical complications could be more satisfactorily met. Such responsibility has been mitigated frequently by the Committee due to the fact that education of the public regarding the advantages of proper prenatal care is as yet admittedly insufficient.

When the individual refused to accept hospital care promptly, if advised to do so by the physician. The economic situation offered as an excuse in some instances, has not been accepted by the Committee in the refusal of a patient to be hospitalized when necessary.

When there was refusal of the patient or her family to permit interruption of pregnancy in toxic vomiting or in other grave diseases, with the single exception of a religious belief interfering with the compliance of advice.

NON-PREVENTABLE OR UNAVOIDABLE DEATHS

Deaths have been regarded as non-preventable under the following circumstances:

Cases of hemorrhage, either ante or post-partum, when treated promptly and in the accepted fashion, such as placenta previa, accidental hemorrhage or post-partum hemorrhage.

Spontaneous rupture of the uterus, unless caused by drugs and due to a previous section, if in a hospital and promptly handled.

Certain cases of ectopic gestation if prompt and adequate treatment given.

Toxemic bleeding which has been carefully evaluated from the standpoint of the recognition and the treatment of the toxemia.

Chronic infections lighted up by pregnancy.

Acute infections complicating pregnancy or the puerperium, such as pneumonia and influenza.

Some forms of cardiac and renal disease; some forms of metabolic disease; some anemias; carcinomas; organic diseases of the nervous system complicating pregnancy.

ASSIGNING RESPONSIBILITY

The assigning of responsibility by the Analysis Committee was a difficult task and at times the conclusions may not have been correct. The routine procedure was to assign the responsibility to the physician if there had been an infection, and to lay the infection to an error in technic. It is probable, however, that in the majority of these cases the physician used the same aseptic precautions as in many of his other cases which did not become infected. There was also the possibility that in a hospital delivery the technic of some person other than the physician may have been at fault. In home deliveries among certain classes there is always the chance that the patient may become infected in some way, as by intercourse, or self-examination shortly before the beginning of labor. Yet there seemed to be no other way to classify these deaths due to infection except to place them under the heading, "Physician's Responsibility," even though the Committee did not feel that they were all necessarily the fault of the physician.

Many cases were classified as an error in judgment on the part of the physician. This was correct enough when the error was a gross one and the management of the situation clearly open to censure. Yet there was often room for difference of opinion in the choice of treatment, and frequently, where the physician's treatment was debatable, it was the fatal outcome which made it easy to say that he must have been wrong. It is quite another thing to be faced with the problem beforehand and to view it with hindsight. It was often said in the meetings of the Analysis Committee that a particular patient should have been hospitalized earlier, yet there was no guarantee that hospital treatment would have saved her.

It is probable that the physician was held responsible in a greater number of maternal deaths than should have been laid at his door. It was necessary to err on that side, however, to avoid being accused of shielding the profession. The Committee being wholly obstetrical might otherwise appear to be finding too many excuses for the physician. Nevertheless, it is confidently believed that there has been very little distortion in the results, since every factor materially influencing the reliability of the decisions has been given fullest weight.

In the following Tables Nos. 10, 11, 12, 13, the decisions of the Analysis Committee are recorded.

TABLE 10

CLASSIFICATION OF DEATHS BY PREVENTABILITY

CAUSE OF DEATH	TOTAL	NOT PREVENTABLE		PREVENTABLE	
		Number	Percent	Number	Percent
TOTAL DEATHS	717	310	43.2	407	56.7
Septic Abortions	162	39	24.1	123	75.9
Abortions	26	13	50.0	13	50.0
Ectopic Gestation	33	11	33.3	22	66.7
Hemorrhage	62	33	53.2	29	46.8
Puerperal Sepsis	119	20	16.8	99	83.2
Albuminuria and Eclampsia	85	37	43.5	48	56.5
Vomiting of Pregnancy	24	19	79.2	5	20.8
Embolus and Sudden Death	44	32	72.7	12	27.3
Accidents of Labor	79	37	46.8	42	53.2
Accidents of Puerperium	5	5	100.0	...	....
Non-Obstetrical Causes	78	64	82.1	14	17.9

TABLE 11

CLASSIFICATION OF PREVENTABLE DEATHS BY RESPONSIBILITY

Cause of Death	Total	Ascribed to Physician		Ascribed to Patient	
		Number	Percent	Number	Percent
TOTAL DEATHS	407	230	56.5	177	43.5
Septic Abortion	123	15	12.2	·108	87.8
Abortion	13	6	46.2	7	53.8
Ectopic Gestation	22	16	72.7	6	27.3
Hemorrhage	29	21	72.4	8	27.6
Puerperal Sepsis	99	97	98.0	2	2.0
Albuminuria and Eclampsia	49	19	38.8	30	61.2
Vomiting of Pregnancy	5	..	....	5	100.0
Embolus and Sudden Death	12	10	83.3	2	16.7
Accidents of Labor	42	37	88.1	5	11.9
Accidents of Puerperium	..	..	....	..	....
Non-Obstetrical Causes	13	8	69.2	5	30.8

TABLE 12

ANALYSIS OF PREVENTABLE DEATHS FOR WHICH RESPONSIBILITY WAS ASCRIBED TO THE PHYSICIAN

(Exclusive of deaths following abortion)

Cause of Death	Total	Error in Judgment		Error in Technic	
		Number	Percent	Number	Percent
TOTAL	208	135	64.9	73	35.1
Ectopic Gestation	16	16	100.0	..	....
Hemorrhage	21	20	95.2	1	4.8
Puerperal Sepsis	97	38	39.2	59	60.8
Albuminuria and Eclampsia	19	12*	63.2	7	36.8
Embolus and Sudden Death	10	10	100.0	..	....
Accidents of Labor	37	33	89.2	4	10.8
Non-Obstetrical Causes	8	6	75.0	2	25.0

*Inadequate prenatal care in seven cases.

TABLE 13

ANALYSIS OF PREVENTABLE DEATHS FOR WHICH RESPONSIBILITY WAS ASCRIBED TO THE PATIENT

(Exclusive of deaths following abortion)

CAUSE OF DEATH	TOTAL	FAILURE TO OBTAIN SUITABLE CARE		IGNORANCE OR LACK OF COOPERATION	
		Number	Percent	Number	Percent
TOTAL	63	21	33.3	42	66.7
Ectopic Gestation	6	1	16.7	5	83.3
Hemorrhage	8	2	25.0	6	75.0
Puerperal Sepsis	2	..	....	2	100.0
Albuminuria and Eclampsia	30	15	50.0	15	50.0
Vomiting of Pregnancy	5	0	....	5	100.0
Embolus and Sudden Death	2	0	....	2	100.0
Accidents of Labor	5	1	20.0	4	80.0
Non-Obstetrical Causes	5	2	40.0	3	60.0

THE AVOIDABLE FACTORS

After having assigned the responsibility in the various cases, there arose the question of the "avoidable factor," in other words, how could the death have been prevented? This has been an even more difficult problem, and erroneous speculation as to the effects of treatment other than that demonstrated, may have led to incorrect conclusions at times.

The avoidable factors, the primary basic errors, have been adopted, with modification, from the Interim Report of the Departmental Committee on Maternal Morbidity and Mortality, Ministry of Health, London, 1930. This English Committee drew up a standard of acceptable practice for physician and patient in a maternity case. While arbitrary, this standard certainly could not be considered unduly high in any urban area in the United States. The first deviation from this standard was considered the original break in the conduct of the case, or the basic error. The four primary avoidable factors of the English report were:

A. Omission or inadequacy of antenatal examination.

B. Error in judgment in the management of the case.

C. Lack of reasonable facilities.

D. Negligence of the patient or her friends.

It will be observed that the first factor, lack of, or inadequacy of care, may operate either through the physician or the patient. It is hardly conceivable that a death in which this was the primary avoidable factor could occur in Philadelphia when our prenatal clinics received a rating of 98 by the Haven Emerson Survey, and when medical education is featured by five Class "A" medical schools. As stated above, it was clearly recognized by the Analysis Committee that the education of the public as to adequate maternity care is still woefully incomplete or ineffective. This is not altogether the fault of the medical profession, but is due in great part to the indifference of the laity. In 1932 letters were sent to 836 lay organizations in Philadelphia, offering the services of a medical speaker on the subject, "What Constitutes Adequate Maternity Care?" Less than fifty organizations responded requesting speakers.

The second factor of the English Committee refers to "Errors in Judgment." This factor, already discussed under preventability, has been well expressed by Kerr:[8] "Obstetric surgery is in marked contrast to general surgery. In the latter, when operation is deemed necessary, the procedure is well defined; only occasionally has the surgeon any difficulty in deciding between alternative procedures. Technical skill is all-important. In obstetric surgery, on the other hand, while technical skill is equally important, judgment in choice of procedure and in the time to interfere may make all the difference as regards success or failure. This can only be learned by long experience, accurate observation and constant practice." The Committee has added here an additional factor, "Error in Technic," which has been used to include various deaths from infection in presumably clean cases, evident unskillful performance of operative deliveries, and other apparent and often admitted mistakes.

The third factor, "Lack of Reasonable Facilities," has been found very few times in the series of deaths studied. It should not be operable at all in a city so well hospitalized as Philadelphia, where there is available a hospital bed for every maternity patient at the time of her confinement. Ambulance transportation is also available.

The fourth factor, "Negligence of the Patient or Her Friends," has been expressed in an earlier paragraph in the detailed reasons for placing the responsibility for the death upon the patient or her family.

In many instances more than one avoidable factor was apparent. Under these circumstances, the Committee endeavored to determine which one factor most certainly influenced the fatal outcome. The relationship of these factors to the preventable deaths may be seen in Tables Nos. 12 and 13.

DEATHS FROM PUERPERAL CAUSES

The International List of the Causes of Death,[9] Section XI, page 143, lists the Diseases of Pregnancy, Childbirth and the Puerperal State under eleven headings, 140-150. The purpose of this group of titles is to include all causes of death of women which are due, more or less directly, to childbearing. These are as follows:

---

[8] "Maternal Mortality and Morbidity." J. M. Munro Kerr. P. 109. William Wood and Co., Baltimore. 1933.

[9] Manual of the International List of the Causes of Death. Fourth Revision. U. S. Government Printing Office, Washington, D. C. 1931.

140. Abortion with septic conditions.
141. Abortion without mention of septic conditions (to include hemorrhages).
142. Ectopic gestation.
143. Other accidents of pregnancy (not to include hemorrhages).
144. Puerperal hemorrhage.
145. Puerperal septicemia (not specified as due to abortion).
146. Puerperal albuminuria and eclampsia.
147. Other toxemias of pregnancy.
148. Puerperal phlegmasia alba dolens, embolus, sudden death (not specified as septic).
149. Other accidents of childbirth.
150. Other and unspecified conditions of the puerperal state.

In following our idea of making this report comparable to the New York Report, the same terminology has been adopted. It has been found in this Survey, as in the New York Study, that almost every cause of death listed under Title Number 143 showed an error in certification. Consequently this category has been dropped and the cases assigned to the proper coding. A chart, Table No. 14, has been prepared to show the total number of cases under each puerperal title number for the three years, and under each primary cause will be found the International List number of the contributing causes of death. The make-up of this chart reflects the complex background of the pathology which plays a part in rendering so many pregnancies abnormal and stresses the importance of early detection and prompt treatment of complications. There were many other intercurrent diseases and complicating conditions present, but not certified, in these pregnancies. Had these been added to this table, the need for intensive care of the expectant mother would have been made more insistent. The tragedies these complications helped to produce might then have been averted. The percentage distribution of puerperal causes appears in Chart No. 4.

FACTORS INFLUENCING MATERNAL MORTALITY

There are other factors which play a part in causing maternal mortality. Some of them can be assessed as to their influence, others are doubtedly potential factors, yet their specific influence cannot be measured. The latter include such general conditions as the character of the population of a given area, the type of housing and overcrowding, the economic status, the nature of attendance, general health of the community, personal hygiene and mode of life of the individual. It has not seemed relevant to discuss these factors in full in this report. They have been considered fully in the literature[7] and recently at length by Kerr.

---

[7] "Maternal Mortality in Aberdeen, 1918-1927." Scottish Board of Health. J. Parlane Kinloch, J. Smith, and J. A. Stephen. His Majesty's Stationary Office, Edinburgh, 1928.

CHART 4

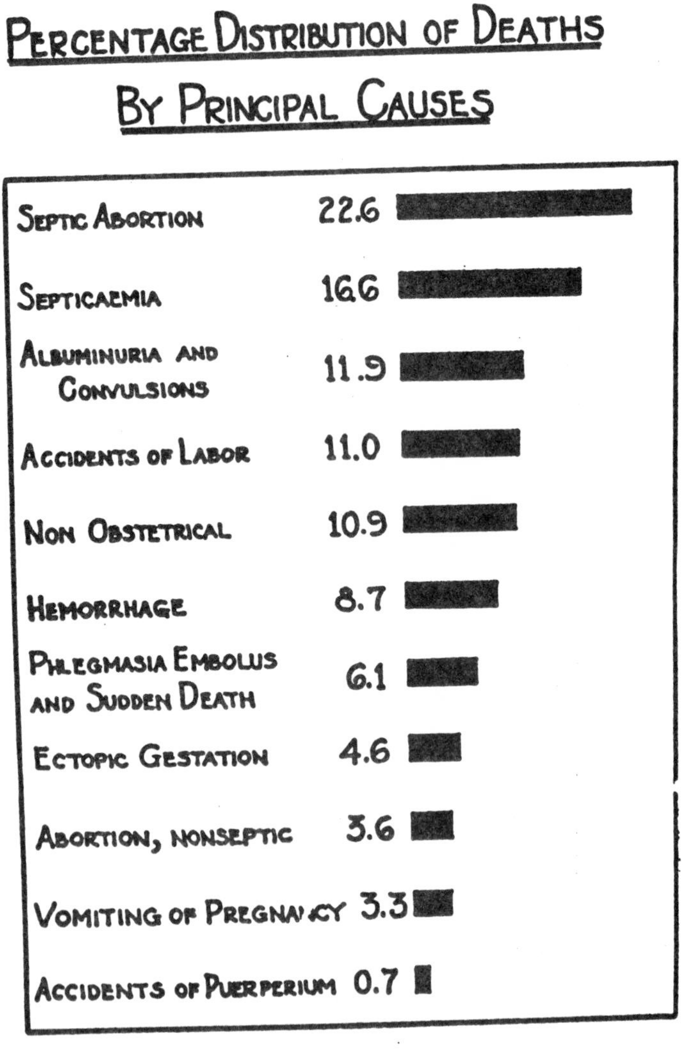

PERCENTAGE DISTRIBUTION OF DEATHS

BY PRINCIPAL CAUSES

SEPTIC ABORTION	22.6	████████████
SEPTICAEMIA	16.6	█████████
ALBUMINURIA AND CONVULSIONS	11.9	██████
ACCIDENTS OF LABOR	11.0	█████
NON OBSTETRICAL	10.9	█████
HEMORRHAGE	8.7	████
PHLEGMASIA EMBOLUS AND SUDDEN DEATH	6.1	███
ECTOPIC GESTATION	4.6	██
ABORTION, NONSEPTIC	3.6	██
VOMITING OF PREGNANCY	3.3	██
ACCIDENTS OF PUERPERIUM	0.7	█

TABLE 14

PUERPERAL DEATHS
AND
CONTRIBUTING AND NON-OBSTETRICAL CAUSES
PHILADELPHIA — 1931 — 1932 — 1933

International List No.	Primary Cause of Death	Total Deaths	%
0	Total Deaths	717	100
0	Septic Abortion	162	22.6
	Abortion no mention of Sepsis	26	3.6
	Abortion Extractena	33	4.6
2	Hemorrhage of Pregnancy	62	8.7
45	Puerperal Septicemia	119	16.6
46	Albuminuria and Eclampsia	85	11.9
7	Vomiting of Pregnancy	24	3.3
8	Embolus and Sudden Death	44	6.1
9	Accidents of Labor	79	11.0
0	Accidents of Puerperium	5	0.7
	TOTALS OF CONTRIBUTING CAUSES	349	*
	NON-OBSTETRICAL CAUSES	78	10.9

Column categories (contributing and non-obstetrical causes) across the table:
Ectopic Pregnancy; Hemorrhage of Pregnancy; Albuminuria Eclampsia; Vomiting of Pregnancy; Embolus Sudden Death; Accidents of Labor; Accidents of Puerperium; Scarlet Fever; Influenza; Lethargic Encephalitis / Epidemic Meningitis; Tuberculosis; Syphilis; Gonorrhea; Cancer; Cancer of the Uterus; Fibroid of Uterus; Tumors of other Organs; Tumors of Brain; Acute Rheumatic Fever; Diabetes; Goitre; Addisons Disease; Purpura Hemorrhagic Condition; Meningitis; Cerebral Hemorrhage; Cerebral Embolism; Epilepsy; Diseases of Nervous System; Pericarditis; Acute Endocarditis; Chronic Endocarditis; Myocarditis; Other Heart Diseases; Diseases of Arteries; Essential Hypertension; Abscess of Frontal Sinus; Bronchitis; Broncho-Pneumonia; Lobar Pneumonia; Pneumonia Unspecified; Pleurisy; Pulmonary Embolus; Asthma; Other Respiratory Diseases; Vincents Angina; Parotitis; Appendicitis; Intestinal Obstruction; Injury to Intestine; Yellow Atrophy of Liver; Gallstones; Acute Nephritis; Chronic Nephritis; Laceration Pelvic Floor; Abscess of Neck; Diseases of Joints; Congenital Heart Disease; Anaesthesia Poisoning; Drug Poisoning; Fracture Skull

* 54.6 percent of 639 Puerperal Deaths

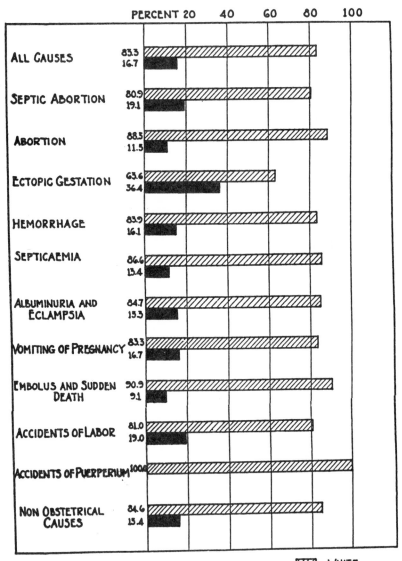

CHART 5

PERCENTAGE DISTRIBUTION OF DEATHS BY RACE AND CAUSE OF DEATH

| | PERCENT 20 | 40 | 60 | 80 | 100 |

ALL CAUSES — 83.3 / 16.7

SEPTIC ABORTION — 80.9 / 19.1

ABORTION — 88.5 / 11.5

ECTOPIC GESTATION — 63.6 / 36.4

HEMORRHAGE — 83.9 / 16.1

SEPTICAEMIA — 86.6 / 13.4

ALBUMINURIA AND ECLAMPSIA — 84.7 / 15.3

VOMITING OF PREGNANCY — 83.3 / 16.7

EMBOLUS AND SUDDEN DEATH — 90.9 / 9.1

ACCIDENTS OF LABOR — 81.0 / 19.0

ACCIDENTS OF PUERPERIUM — 100.0

NON OBSTETRICAL CAUSES — 84.6 / 15.4

WHITE

COLORED

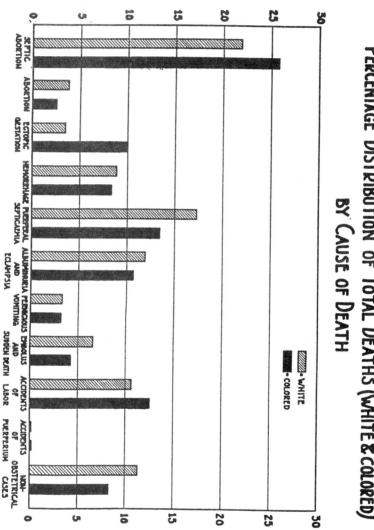

CHART 5a

PERCENTAGE DISTRIBUTION OF TOTAL DEATHS (WHITE & COLORED)
BY CAUSE OF DEATH

WHITE
COLORED

SEPTIC ABORTION
ABORTION
ECTOPIC GESTATION
HEMORRHAGE
PUERPERAL SEPTICAEMIA
ALBUMINURIA AND ECLAMPSIA
PERNICIOUS VOMITING
EMBOLUS AND SUDDEN DEATH
ACCIDENTS OF LABOR
ACCIDENTS OF PUERPERIUM
NON-OBSTETRICAL CASES

CHART 6

PERCENT DISTRIBUTION OF DEATHS BY NATIVITY AND CAUSE OF DEATH

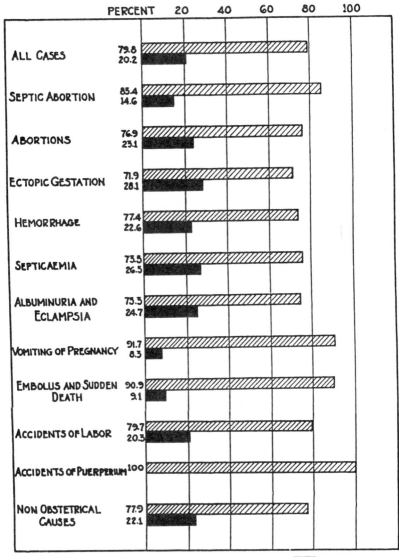

| | NATIVE BORN |
| FOREIGN BORN |

Other factors whose bearing on the problem may be more definitely evaluated are: age, parity, social status, prenatal care, place of delivery, character of attendant, the type and extent of operative intervention. The Committee has recognized the importance of these factors in its discussions and their influence will be discussed in the various correlations.

RACE AND NATIVITY AS FACTORS IN MATERNAL MORTALITY

The estimated population of Philadelphia during the three years of the survey averaged 1,978,879. During this survey a total of 99,579 births were recorded, of which 95,394 were born alive and 4,185 were stillborn. The distribution of these births may be seen in Table No. 15.

TABLE 15

TOTAL WHITE AND NEGRO BIRTHS* 1931-1932-1933

Year	Total	White Births			Negro Births		
		Total	Live Births	Still Births	Total	Live Births	Still Births
TOTAL	99,579	84,470	81,272	3,198	15,109	14,122	987
1931	35,284	30,028	28,860	1,168	5,256	4,913	343
1932	33,542	28,472	27,385	1,087	5,070	4,708	362
1933	30,753	25,970	25,027	943	4,783	4,501	282

*Source: Bureau of Vital Statistics, City of Philadelphia.

The maternal death rate as calculated by this survey gave 717 deaths to 99,579 total births or a maternal mortality rate of 7.09 per thousand total births. Eliminating the 78 non-obstetrical causes of death and calculating the rate on live births, we have a ratio of 639 deaths to 95,394 births or a puerperal death rate of 6.69 per thousand live births.

The nature of the admixture of negro and alien born residents lends interest to a survey of this nature. There are 235,383 negroes in Philadelphia. This is 11.8 percent of the population and it is a much greater proportion than any other large Northern city.

It has not been possible to determine the nativities of the mothers who gave birth during these three years, but figures of the negroes are available. The birth rate for the negro in Philadelphia was 21.3 per thousand negro population for the three years; 15.0 for the white population and 17.0 for the entire population.

During the survey there were 717 deaths, 639 puerperal and 78 non-obstetrical. Of the puerperal causes of death, 529 occurred in white women and 110 in negroes. Figuring in the manner of the local bureau of vital statistics on total births, we have for the three years a puerperal death rate of 6.1 in the white women (529 to 84,470), and a puerperal death rate of 7.2 in the negroes (110 to 15,109). The number and ratio of deaths to race from each of the puerperal causes and from the non-

TABLE 16

CAUSE AND PERCENTAGE DISTRIBUTION OF DEATH IN WHITE AND NEGROES

CAUSE OF DEATH	TOTAL		WHITE		COLORED	
	Number	Percent	Number	Percent	Number	Percent
TOTAL	717	100.0	597	100.0	120	100.0
Septic Abortion	162	22.6	131	21.9	31	25.9
Abortion	26	3.6	23	3.9	3	2.5
Ectopic Gestation	33	4.6	21	3.5	12	10.0
Hemorrhage	62	8.7	52	8.7	10	8.3
Septicæmia	119	16.6	103	17.3	16	13.3
Albuminuria and Eclampsia.	85	11.8	72	12.1	13	10.9
Vomiting of Pregnancy	24	3.4	20	3.3	4	3.3
Embolus and Sudden Death	44	6.1	40	6.7	4	3.3
Accidents of Labor	79	11.0	64	10.7	15	12.5
Accidents of Puerperium ...	5	.7	5	.8	..	....
Non-Obstetrical	78	10.9	66	11.1	12	10.0

obstetrical causes appears in Table No. 16 and Charts No. 5 and 5a. The figures of this survey are small, but are offered for comparison with the figures of other reports. The rates for the first two years of the survey were obtained for us by the Children's Bureau from the United States Bureau of the Census, and show that in 1931 there were 63 maternal deaths per 10,000 live births among white women and 59 among the colored; in 1932 there were 101 among the whites and 90 among the negroes.

Among the white women, the patient was considered responsible for 150 or 28.3 percent of the 529 puerperal deaths. Among negroes, the patient was considered responsible in 30 or 27.2 percent of the 110 puerperal deaths. Of the 529 white women who died, 49 or 9.2 percent were illegitimately pregnant; of the 110 deaths in negroes, 30 or 27.2 percent were illegitimate pregnancies. Prenatal care was adequate in 33 percent of the deaths in white women and in 14 percent of the negroes.

Of the 320 deaths following hospital deliveries, the white women had 198 planned deliveries (72.5 percent); 71 were emergencies (26 percent), and 4 cases were not recorded (1.5 percent). The negroes had 38 planned deliveries (80.8 percent) and 9 emergencies (19.2 percent).

The relation of nativity and puerperal causes of death is shown by percentage distribution in Table No. 16a and Chart No. 6. There were 565 native-born women who died during the survey and 143 foreign born, while in 9 deaths the birthplace was not recorded. The number of deaths of foreign-born women was largest among the Italians, being 34. There were 27 Russians and 19 Poles. The remaining 63 were distributed among 13 other foreign nativities.

TABLE 16a

CAUSE OF DEATH
BY NATIVITY

CAUSE OF DEATH	TOTAL		NATIVE BORN		FOREIGN BORN		NATIVITY NOT RECORDED	
	Number	Percent	Number	Percent	Number	Percent	Number	Percent
TOTAL	717	100.0	565	100.0	143	100.0	9	100.0
Septic Abortion	162	22.6	134	23.7	23	16.1	5	55.6
Abortion	26	3.6	20	3.5	6	4.2	.	....
Ectopic Gestation ...	33	4.6	23	4.1	9	6.3	1	11.1
Hemorrhage ..	62	8.7	48	8.5	14	9.8	.	....
Septicæmia	119	16.6	86	15.2	31	21.6	2	22.2
Albuminuria and Eclampsia ..	85	11.8	64	11.3	21	14.7	.	....
Vomiting of Pregnancy ..	24	3.4	22	3.9	2	1.4	.	....
Embolus and Sudden Death	44	6.1	40	7.1	4	2.8	.	....
Accidents of Labor	79	11.0	63	11.2	16	11.2	.	....
Accidents of Puerperium .	5	.7	5	.9	..	....	.	....
Non-Obstetrical	78	10.9	60	10.6	17	11.9	1	11.1

AGE

The relation of the age groups to the causes of death is shown in Table No. 17. In Table No. 18 the estimated deaths per 1,000 live births is shown by age groups. As shown in similar surveys, the most favorable time for childbirth is in the years from 21 to 25.

ILLEGITIMACY

During the period of the survey, 3,885 illegitimate births occurred among 99,579 total births, or almost 4 percent. Of these illegitimate births, 234 were stillbirths and 3,651 were live births. Six percent of the total stillbirths of the period were in illegitimate pregnancies, and 3.9 percent of the live births. In the same period 79 deaths occurred among the illegitimately pregnant women, a death rate of 20 per 1,000 births. These 79 illegitimate pregnancies were divided among 65 single women, 9 widows, 3 married women, and 2 divorcees. Thirty-three deaths occurred in patients under 21 years of age, 19 from 21 to 25 years, 14 from 26 to 30 years, 9 from 31 to 35 years, 2 from 36 to 40 years, and 2 in women over 40 years of age.

Of the 79 deaths occurring in illegitimate pregnancies, 40 were in white women and 39 in negroes. Seventy-two were native born and 7 foreign born. Fifty-nine of these deaths occurred in the 241 first preg-

TABLE 17

CAUSES OF DEATH
BY AGE GROUPS

CAUSES OF DEATH	AGE GROUPS						
	Total	Under 21	21-25	26-30	31-35	36-40	Over 40
TOTAL	717	72	146	169	154	135	41
Septic Abortion	162	22	43	43	34	15	5
Abortion Without Sepsis.	26	..	3	5	10	4	4
Ectopic Gestation	33	1	4	7	10	8	3
Hemorrhage	62	2	9	10	17	18	6
Puerperal Sepsis	119	14	19	35	22	26	3
Albuminuria and Convulsions	85	10	19	15	17	19	5
Vomiting of Pregnancy..	24	3	10	6	1	4	..
Embolus and Sudden Death	44	4	8	12	7	9	4
Accidents of Labor	79	9	17	19	17	12	5
Accidents of Puerperium.	5	1	2	..	1	1	..
Non-Obstetrical	78	6	12	17	18	19	6

TABLE 18

DEATHS PER 1,000 LIVE BIRTHS
BY AGE OF MOTHER

Age of Mother	Estimated Total Live Births*	Number of Maternal Deaths	Est. Deaths per 1,000 Live Births
TOTAL	95,298	717	7.5
UNDER 21	9,981	72	7.2
21-25	28,620	146	5.1
26-30	26,202	169	6.4
31-35	17,004	154	9.1
36-40	10,173	135	13.3
OVER 40	3,162	41	13.0
UNKNOWN	156	..	....

*As the classification by age of mothers for 1931 and 1933 was not available, the classification for 1932 was used. The estimate was obtained by trebling these figures as the deaths over the years 1931, 1932, 1933. The actual number of live births as reported by the Bureau of Vital Statistics for the three years was 94,780.

nancies of the series, 4 in the second, 7 in the third, and the remainder were scattered.

Fifty-three women were under 28 weeks pregnant and 26 over 28 weeks. Thirty-eight were less than three months pregnant. In 9 or the 26 women over 28 weeks pregnant, contributory causes of death were recorded, while in 3 others intercurrent diseases had been present but were not listed on the death certificates.

Of the 26 women over 28 weeks pregnant, only 2 had had adequate prenatal care, 23 had had none or inadequate care, and in one case nothing was known about the prenatal care.

Of the 53 women under 28 weeks pregnant, 15 had operative deliveries. Of the 26 women over 28 weeks, 10 were delivered spontaneously, 14 had operative deliveries, and 2 were delivered post mortem. These operations included 2 elective Cesarian sections, 10 forceps, 4 versions and 2 multiple operations.

Of the puerperal causes of death, 48 died of septic abortion, 1 from abortion with no mention of sepsis, 2 from ectopic gestation, 2 from post-partum hemorrhage, 5 from puerperal sepsis, 6 from eclampsia, 5 from embolus and sudden death, 5 from accidents of labor, and 1 from an accident of the puerperium. There were 4 non-obstetrical deaths in the illegitimate group. None of the women who died from eclampsia had had adequate prenatal care. All of the women who died from puerperal sepsis had been operated for delivery. Twenty stillbirths occurred among the 26 women over 28 weeks pregnant.

In the group of 49 abortion cases, 22 were criminally induced, 18 self-induced, and 9 recorded as having no interference.

The Analysis Committee decided that in 11 of the 79 deaths, the certificates were not correct as to the primary cause. The corrections made were largely in the group of septic abortions.

The Analysis Committee placed the responsibility for death on the patient in 51 instances or 63 percent of this group; upon the physician in 13 cases, and considered 15 of the deaths non-preventable. Included in the unavoidable deaths were four non-obstetrical cases.

In the 13 cases in which the responsibility was assigned to the physician, the avoidable factors were: error of judgment in 9 deaths and error of technique in four.

In the 51 cases in which the patient was considered responsible, the avoidable factor was ignorance. This was manifested by lack of knowledge of the consequences of induced abortion in 39 cases, failure to obtain prenatal care in 4, and disregard of symptoms in 8.

PRENATAL CARE

As previously mentioned in the section on preventability, the amount and degree of prenatal care must be assessed. In considering antenatal care as a factor in preventability, the Analysis Committee used as a standard the requisites outlined by the Children's Bureau of the United States Department of Labor in Publication No. 153, 1925, "Standards of Prenatal Care." These standards, as well as those used in the "Fifteen States Study,"[1] are considered more stringent than the requirements set forth by the British Departmental Committee on Maternal

---

[1] Maternal Mortality in Fifteen States. Children's Bureau, U. S. Department of Labor. Publication No. 223.

Mortality. Of necessity, a certain degree of latitude was allowed by the Analysis Committee in evaluating the type of prenatal care given certain individual cases. The classification of the "Fifteen States Study" by grades was abandoned for the more simple groupings of Adequate, Inadequate and None. Prenatal care was considered adequate if the standards were met; inadequate if they failed in frequency or quality; and none if no care was given in the antenatal period. The usage of the New York Academy of Medicine Study was closely followed in this survey. Their basis for prenatal care is quoted. "First visit to clinic or physician to be made at or before the fifth calendar month of gestation. A general physical examination, including an examination of the heart and lungs, at this time. Pelvic measurements at or before the seventh month. Urinalysis and systolic and diastolic blood pressure readings at the time of the first visit and at all subsequent visits. Visits to the physician or clinic monthly up to the ninth month and weekly thereafter. A careful personal history, including infectious diseases and past pregnancies. A history of the present pregnancy to elicit any symptoms bearing on possible abnormalities or a toxemia. Social service for clinic patients adequate to ensure the patient's co-operation with the clinic."

The relation of prenatal care to the causes of death has been shown in Table No. 19.

The result of the analysis of Maternal Mortality in Canada[2] is of interest in estimating the influence of prenatal care. A specific question was asked in connection with each of the 481 maternal deaths: "By what means might this death have been prevented?". The answer, "By having prenatal care," was given 276 times, in contrast to the varied answers for the other 205 deaths.

In recent years, health demonstrations and campaigns, often sponsored by benevolent trusts or funds, have been carried on in various parts of the country, in sections of cities or counties. The maternal health of the community is usually made a part of such work and the frequent consequent reduction in maternal mortality is pointed to as an indication of the enormous value of prenatal hygiene. The figures of such reports are not invariably comparable to the remainder of the city or state in question.

In evaluating the effect of prenatal care, four factors must be considered:[3] first, deaths in all periods of pregnancy must be included; second, the distribution of the pregnant women must be studied by nativity; third, they must be considered by age groups; and fourth, the attendant and place of delivery must be analyzed. The quality of judgment shown in indication for and selection of type and operation might be added.

The Analysis Committee considered all these factors in their decisions regarding the adequacy or lack of prenatal care. Accordingly, the grading of prenatal care in the 717 pregnancies was listed as follows: adequate

[2] Maternal Mortality in Canada. Department of Health of Canada. Ottawa, 1928
[3] "Prenatal Care in Relation to Mortality." American Public Health Association Year Book, 1931-32, p. 201.

TABLE 19

RELATION OF PRENATAL CARE TO CAUSES OF DEATH

(EXCLUSIVE OF ABORTIONS AND ECTOPICS)

	Total Deaths		Adequate		Inadequate		None		Unknown	
	Number	Per cent	Number	Per cent	Number	Per cent	Number	Per cent	Number	Per cent
TOTAL	496	100.0	207	100.0	188	100.0	93	100.0	8	100.0
Premature Separation of Placenta ...	12	2.4	6	2.9	2	1.1	4	4.3	0	...
Placenta Prævia	23	4.6	5	2.4	14	7.4	4	4.3	0	...
Postpartum Hemorrhage	27	5.4	11	5.3	13	6.9	3	3.2	0	...
Puerperal Sepsis	119	24.0	59	28.5	48	25.5	10	10.7	2	25.0
Albuminuria and Convulsions	85	17.1	34	16.4	29	15.4	21	22.6	1	12.5
Other Toxemias	24	4.9	10	4.8	4	2.1	9	9.7	1	12.5
Embolus and Sudden Death	44	8.9	18	8.7	17	9.1	9	9.7	0	...
Accidents of Labor	79	15.9	35	17.0	31	16.5	13	14.0	0	...
Accidents of Puerperium	5	1.0	2	1.0	3	1.6	0	...	0	...
Non-Obstetrical	78	15.8	27	13.0	27	14.4	20	21.5	4	50.0

in 216 cases, inadequate in 193, none in 297, and unknown in 11. The relation of prenatal care to various other factors appears in Tables Nos. 20, 21, 22, and 23. It must be realized that prenatal care cannot be defined in a satisfactory manner in cases under 28 weeks pregnant. Lack of prenatal care was mentioned specifically as the avoidable factor 28 times. In many instances, however, it was also the real agent expressed as error in judgment on the part of the physician or as lack of co-operation by the patient in failing to carry out instructions or advice.

TABLE 20

RELATION OF PRENATAL CARE TO PREVENTABILITY

PRENATAL CARE	TOTAL		PHYSICIAN'S RESPONSIBILITY		PATIENT'S RESPONSIBILITY		NON-PREVENTABLE	
	Number	Percent	Number	Percent	Number	Percent	Number	Percent
TOTAL	717	100.0	230	100.0	177	100.0	310	100.0
Adequate	216	30.1	95	41.3	6	3.4	115	37.0
Inadequate	193	27.0	85	36.9	17	9.6	91	29.4
None	297	41.4	48	20.9	152	85.9	97	31.3
Unknown	11	1.5	2	.9	2	1.1	7	2.3

TABLE 21

RELATION OF PRENATAL CARE TO PREVENTABILITY
(OVER 28 WEEKS PREGNANT)

PRENATAL CARE	TOTAL		PHYSICIAN'S RESPONSIBILITY		PATIENT'S RESPONSIBILITY		NON-PREVENTABLE	
	Number	Percent	Number	Percent	Number	Percent	Number	Percent
TOTAL	425	100.0	185	100.0	43	100.0	197	100.0
Adequate	183	43.1	88	47.6	4	9.3	91	46.2
Inadequate	176	41.4	78	42.2	15	34.9	83	42.1
None	61	14.3	17	9.2	24	55.8	20	10.2
Unknown	5	1.2	2	1.0	..	....	3	1.5

TABLE 22

NON-OBSTETRICAL CASES*

PRENATAL CARE	NUMBER	PERCENT
TOTAL	78	100.0
Adequate	27	34.6
Inadequate	27	34.6
None	20	25.7
Unknown	4	5.1

*Non-Obstetrical cases are also included in the preceding table.

TABLE 23

NON-OBSTETRICAL CASES*

(OVER 28 WEEKS)

PRENATAL CARE	NUMBER	PERCENT
TOTAL	51	100.0
Adequate	16	31.4
Inadequate	24	47.0
None	8	15.7
Unknown	3	5.9

*Non-Obstetrical cases are also included in the preceding table.

PARITY

The relationship of parity to death is shown in Tables Nos. 24 and 25 The majority of the deaths were among primiparas. There was a gradually diminishing numerical incidence of deaths in the succeding pregnancies. On a percentage distribution it was seen that the peaks were in the first pregnancy and in the very late ones. This fact has been demonstrated in other surveys. The relation of pregnancies to age groups is shown in Table No. 26. This table shows an additional factor of importance other than mere age or multiparity in the spacing of pregnancy. This factor of additional risk in too frequent pregnancies was

TABLE 25

DEATHS PER 1000 LIVE BIRTHS

BY GRAVIDITY

GRAVIDITY	ESTIMATED TOTAL LIVE BIRTHS*	NUMBER OF MATERNAL DEATHS	ESTIMATED DEATHS PER 1,000 LIVE BIRTHS
TOTAL	95,298	717	7.5
First	33,771	241	7.1
Second	22,761	115	5.1
Third	13,431	95	7.1
Fourth	8,361	67	8.0
Fifth	5,235	60	11.5
Sixth	3,756	28	7.5
Seventh	2,613	25	9.6
Eighth	1,722	25	14.5
Ninth	1,455	16	11.0
Tenth and Over	2,088	40	19.2
Unknown	105	5	...

*As the classification by age of mothers for 1931 and 1933 were not available, the classification for 1932 was used. The estimate was obtained by trebling these figures as the deaths over the years 1931, 1932, 1933. The actual number of live births as reported by the Bureau of Vital Statistics for the 3 years was 94,780.

TABLE 24

COMPARATIVE DANGER OF FIRST AND SUBSEQUENT PREGNANCIES BY CAUSE OF DEATH

Cause of Death	Total	Unknown	Number of Pregnancies											
			1	2	3	4	5	6	7	8	9	10	11	Over 11
TOTAL	717	5	241	115	95	67	60	28	25	25	16	19	10	11
Septic Abortion	162	1	57	24	23	25	12	4	6	:	2	5	1	2
Abortion	26	1	2	1	5	4	5	:	2	3	1	1	:	1
Ectopic Gestation	33	:	5	7	6	7	4	3	1	:	:	:	:	:
Hemorrhage	62	:	14	6	7	5	5	4	1	7	5	4	3	1
Puerperal Septicaemia ...	119	:	53	24	12	6	8	4	3	3	2	1	2	1
Albuminuria and Eclampsia	85	:	39	11	9	4	6	3	3	5	:	2	:	3
Pernicious Vomiting	24	:	12	5	5	:	:	1	1	:	:	:	:	:
Embolus and Sudden Death	44	:	13	10	5	4	4	1	1	1	1	2	1	1
Accidents of Labor	79	2	28	13	9	6	7	1	2	3	2	3	2	1
Accidents of Puerperium	5	:	2	1	1	1	:	:	:	:	:	:	:	:
Non-Obstetrical Cases	78	1	16	13	13	5	9	7	5	3	3	1	1	1

TABLE 26
RELATION OF AGE GROUPS TO PARITY

PARITY	Total	AGE GROUPS					
		Under 21 Years	21-25 Years	26-30 Years	31-35 Years	36-40 Years	Over 40 Years
TOTAL	717	72	146	169	154	135	41
Parity Not Reported	5	...	...	1	4	...	...
Primipara	241	57	81	54	34	15	...
Multipara	471	15	65	114	116	120	41
Second	115	12	30	43	9	15	6
Third	95	3	22	23	23	20	4
Fourth	67	...	8	21	17	17	4
Fifth	60	...	3	19	20	16	2
Sixth	28	...	1	3	11	12	1
Seventh	25	...	1	5	8	7	4
Eighth	25	...	...	...	8	11	6
Ninth	16	...	...	...	6	7	3
Tenth	19	...	...	...	8	8	3
Eleventh	10	...	...	...	5	3	2
Over Eleventh	11	...	...	...	1	4	6

commented upon in the Report of the British Departmental Committee. It is often difficult to induce tired mothers of large families to avail themselves of prenatal care or hospital facilities. Mudaliyar[4] summarizes this situation very concisely in his report on Maternal Mortality in Madras: "The question of the 'spacing of pregnancies' on which some emphasis has been laid, is a matter that requires attention, and undoubtedly mothers must be told of the added risk that they submit themselves to by frequent pregnancies at short intervals. What form of advice this should take, and whether it is at all justifiable or necessary in antenatal clinics to offer advice which will really be practicable, is a consideration that has got to be borne in mind."

PERIOD OF GESTATION

The relation of the duration of pregnancy to the various causes of death has been shown in Table No. 27.

SEPTIC ABORTION

One of the outstanding facts of this survey is that 22.5 percent or over one-fifth of the total deaths studied (162 of the total of 717), were caused by septic abortions. Of the 639 puerperal causes of death, over one-fourth came under this category.

[4] "Report on an Investigation Into the Causes of Maternal Mortality in the City of Madras." A. L. Mudaliyar. Government Press, Madras, 1933, p. 25.

TABLE 27

CAUSES OF DEATH BY MONTHS OF PREGNANCY

CAUSE OF DEATH	MONTHS PREGNANT								
	Total	Unknown	1-3	4	5	6	7	8	9
TOTAL	717	17	162	42	21	48	45	56	326
Septic Abortion	162	10	109	22	10	8	3	..	...
Abortion Without Sepsis	26	1	12	6	5	2	..	..	...
Ectopic Gestation ...	33	2	28	1	..	1	..	1	...
Placenta Prævia	23	..	...	..	..	1	2	5	15
Premature Separation of Placenta	12	..	...	..	..	2	..	3	7
Postpartum Hemorrhage	27	..	...	..	..	..	..	2	25
Puerperal Sepsis	119	..	...	..	..	..	6	7	106
Albuminuria and Convulsions	85	1	...	1	1	11	14	16	41
Vomiting of Pregnancy	24	..	9	6	2	2	2	1	2
Embolus and Sudden Death	44	1	1	..	..	2	3	2	35
Accidents of Labor ..	79	1	...	1	..	2	3	4	68
Accidents of Puerperium	5	..	...	..	..	1	..	1	3
Non-Obstetrical	78	1	3	5	3	16	12	14	24

In this study, the term abortion has been used to signify the expulsion of a non-viable fetus, that is, one of under 28 weeks. Of the 292 deaths in pregnancies under 28 weeks, 56 percent were cases of septic abortion. When contrasted with septic deaths following deliveries after the twenty-eighth week, there were 36 percent more deaths from septic abortion than from puerperal septicemia.

Of the 162 deaths from abortion, 56 cases were self-induced; 46 cases were induced by some one other than the patient, i. e., criminal abortions; 3 were therapeutic abortions; and in 57 cases interference was denied. Included in the 46 criminal abortions are 16 cases which the Bureau of Vital Statistics classified as homicides.

Among the 57 reputedly spontaneous abortions with septic infection, the inference was so strong in many cases that the abortion was either criminal or self-induced, that the figures in this group were not considered valid. Two-thirds of the entire abortion group admitted intra-uterine manipulations and undoubtedly many of the remainder had had interference in spite of their denials.

One hundred and fifty of the 162 abortion deaths occurred in hospitals and 12 at home. One hundred and fourteen or 70.3 percent of these deaths were in married women. Forty-eight of the whole group were illegitimately pregnant, including 42 single women, 4 widows and 2 divorcees. The deaths among the illegitimate pregnancies occurred in 37 white women and 11 negroes. One hundred and thirty-one of the septic abortion deaths occurred in white women, 31 in negroes; 134 were in native-born women, 23 in foreign-born, and for 5 the nativity was not given. One hundred and nineteen occurred in the first three months of pregnancy, 22 in the fourth month, 10 in the fifth, 8 in the sixth, and 3 just beyond the sixth month. Fifty-seven occurred in the first pregnancy, 25 each in the second, third and fourth pregnancies, 12 in the fifth, and the remaining 18 were distributed in the higher pregnancies up to the twelfth. Of the 57 septic abortions in the first pregnancies, 39 were illegitimate and 30 of these were in white women.

In 6 of the multiparas there had been complications in 11 previous pregnancies, with operative deliveries. There were 37 cases with contributing causes of death given on the certificate; 29 had other complications not mentioned on the certificates; and 18 had intercurrent diseases as shown by the histories.

Fifty-one of these cases had operations, 5 were not recorded, and 106 had no operation. In 38 operated cases, the procedure was given as curettage. Eleven patients who were afebrile at operation developed sepsis later. Curettage or evacuation was done on 27 women, even though they were running varying degrees of fever at the time.

The Analysis Committee considered that such curettements were performed in the face of evident or potential sepsis, as shown by the fever. The stated indications for operation in these cases were as follows: excessive hemorrhage in two, placental tissue protruding from the cervix in three, in another therapeutic abortion for pyelitis, the patient dying forty-eight hours later, and in seventeen the indication for the operation was not stated, except for the diagnosis of incomplete abortion with fever. In one case the only indication was associated pelvic abscess. Statements found in hospital records accounted for the following three operations performed in the presence of fever: *First*, Diagnosis: septic abortion with peritonitis. General condition was poor and, as abortion was incomplete, dilation and evacuation was done. A small amount of necrotic tissue was obtained and patient died five days later. *Second*, Diagnosis: Puerperal sepsis following septic abortion. Peritonitis was present. As Fowler position and transfusion were of no avail dilatation and evacuation was done. Death occurred on the following day. *Third*, Diagnosis: Septic abortion, incomplete, with pelvic abscess. On the day after admission, under morphine and hyocine narcosis, a dilatation and curettage was done and a small amount of gangrenous placental tissue was obtained. Death followed in four days. The futility of surgery in these three cases needs no comment.

In each of the following three cases of therapeutic abortion, death resulted from sepsis following the operation. One was performed on a woman six weeks pregnant, for a true chronic nephritis with a blood pressure of 248/100. Another was done at six months for continued vomiting of pregnancy and bilateral pyelitis. The patient died on the twenty-fifth day after the abortion and the cause of death was certified as chronic colon bacillus septicemia. Autopsy of the kidneys showed no changes in the parenchyma or pelvis. Blood culture was sterile; urine cultures showed colon bacillus. The third case was operated because of pyelitis. The patient was acutely ill and died in two days.

The interval between abortion and death and operation and death varied widely, ranging from a few days to prolonged illnesses of several weeks or even months in cases of long-drawn-out pyemias with ultimate toxic exhaustion. The majority of the deaths, however, occurred within the second week. Operation other than intrauterine manipulation was performed in two cases of septic abortion. In one, a laparotomy was performed for drainage of a spreading peritonitis. In the other, an abscess in the stump of a previous salpingectomy was excised. Later, in this same case, a colpotomy was performed to drain a pelvic abscess.

Autopsies were obtained in 95 of these 162 deaths. Many of them were performed by coroner's physicians and showed little of scientific interest other than to disclose the spread of the infection.

In studying the death certificates of these cases of septic abortion, the Analysis Committee decided the cause was not correctly stated in 25 or 15.5 percent. This percentage of error approximates that obtained for septic conditions in other similar surveys, even before the last revision of the International List of the Cause of Death divided puerperal septicemia into classes: septic abortion and puerperal septicemia. The certificates changed by the Analysis Committee contained many indefinite causes of death, such as: curettage and evacuation of the uterus; self-induced abortion in a few cases; terms denoting evidence of terminal sepsis as toxic nephritis, bronco or lobarpneumonia or abscess of lung, or finally, such general terms as toxemia, endocarditis or pelvic inflammatory disease, often with no mention of the true cause except in a few instances where "abortion" was listed as a contributing cause.

In regard to preventability, the Analysis Committee considered 39 deaths as non-preventable and 123 as preventable. Of the preventable abortion deaths, the responsibility was ascribed to the physicion in 15 cases or 12.3%, and to the patient in the remaining 108 cases or 87.8%. The patient was responsible for 66.6% of the total septic abortion deaths.

The avoidable factors in the preventable deaths assigned to the physician were errors in judgment in 60% of the cases and errors in technic in 40%. In the cases ascribed to the patient, the performance of abortion either personally or by connivance with a second party, was considered the avoidable factor in the entire group or 100%.

The Analysis Committee regarded the following case as an example of error in technic on the part of the physician: A woman a little over two months pregnant had an apparently spontaneous abortion at home and was referred to the hospital because of bleeding. Pieces of placenta were removed from the cervix digitally and the vagina was packed. The following day dilatation and currettage was done. Within two days a febrile reaction occurred, becoming septic in type. A right sided mass developed. Repeated transfusions were given as well as other supportive measures, but death followed in a few weeks.

The Analysis Committee selected the next case to illustrate error in judgment on the part of the physician. A woman had repeated hemorrhage during the third month of pregnancy. The vagina was packed on admission to the hopital. Two days later a dilatation and evacuation was attempted but was unsuccessful as the cervix was hard to dilate, but the history stated the uterus was packed. On the third day a dilatation and evacuation was done and a transfusion was given for hemorrhage. The patient developed a septic temperature and died on the eleventh day after the final operation. This case was one of a number where the uterine cavity was entered more than once.

In placing the responsibility upon the patient, the Analysis Committee attributed such deaths as the following to ignorance of the probable results of the induction of abortion. A thirty-four year old patient, gravida five, second month, inserted a piece of wood into the cervix. After a week of intermittent bleeding, an abortion occurred. Fever had been present, but now became septic in type. Death occurred eighteen days after the induction.

The Analysis Committee considered the following case typical of a non-preventable death in septic abortion. A thirty-three year old woman, having had ten pregnancies and with seven living children, aborted spontaneously at the second month. After bleeding for two weeks she called a physician, who prescribed rest and medication. Even with the help of her unemployed husband, the nursing care of her small children prevented her from following directions. A phlebitis developed, accompanied by chills, sweats and vomiting. The patient finally entered the hospital on the twenty-fourth day and died six hours after admission.

Comment on Septic Abortion.

Septic abortion was responsible for over one-fifth of all the maternal deaths reviewed. One hundred and two of these 162 deaths followed illegal induction. The laity has not been educated sufficiently to realize the dire consequences of illegally induced abortion. Nor is the seriousness of the criminal act recognized. This is shown by the fact that, during the three years of the survey, no conviction was obtained for this crime in Philadelphia.[*] If this group of 102 cases could have been eliminated, the deaths would have been reduced fourteen percent. The death rate from sepsis was far greater in the cases under twenty-eight weeks pregnancy than in those over twenty-eight weeks.

Of the 162 deaths following septic abortion, 114 were in married women, and 48 were in illegitimate pregnancies. This ratio of almost three to one indicates clearly that the cause of self-induced or criminal abortion is not, as has been commonly believed, the result of illegitimate pregnancies, but, in far greater measure, is a direct corollary of economic and social conditions.

---

[*] Personal Communication from the District Attorney of the County of Philadelphia.

The Committee feels that a dictum should be laid down in regard to treatment of these cases. In septic or potentially infected abortions, the uterus should not be invaded further than to remove material from the cervix for better drainage of the uterine cavity or for the control of hemorrhage.

ABORTION, WITH NO MENTION OF SEPSIS

In this survey of 717 maternal deaths during three years there were 26 deaths, 3.6 percent under 28 weeks pregnancy, due to abortion which was not associated with septic infections. These deaths were classified under Title Number 141, International List of the Causes of Death. In this survey every fetus under 28 weeks of gestation is considered as non-viable and its premature expulsion is classified as an abortion.

Three and six-tenths percent of the whole series and eight and two-tenths percent of the 292 deaths under twenty-eight weeks come under this title. There were two cases of non-septic abortion to every thirteen cases of septic abortion.

Twenty-two of these abortions were spontaneous in origin, two were criminal, one self-induced, and one therapeutic. Twenty-four of the women died in a hospital and two at home. Twenty-three of the women were white and three were negroes. Twenty were native-born and six foreign-born. In a study of the age groups, it was found that over half were past the third decade. In regard to parity, over half were in the third, fourth and fifth pregnancies, while only two were primiparas.

Ten multiparas had had complications in previous pregnancies; four had had previous operative deliveries. Ten had intercurrent diseases in the present pregnancies. One woman in this group was illegitimately pregnant.

In this group of twenty-six abortions, the causes of death were: hemorrhage in fifteen; toxemia and complicating broncho-pneumonia, pneumonia, type unspecified, or influenza in six; complications of renal or cardio-renal disease in three; pulmonary embolus in one, who died undelivered; and shock, possibly perforated uterus, in one. The one therapeutic abortion in the group was done in a case of chronic renal disease, accompanied and followed by profuse vaginal bleeding.

In this group of deaths an operation other than to deliver the fetus was performed in three cases. In one an exploratory laparotomy was done to ascertain if there was an intraperitoneal hemorrhage. In the second an exploratory laparotomy was done to remove an ovarian cyst. The mass was found to be an enlarged uterus and the abdomen was closed. Two days later the woman died from hemorrhage incident to the removal of a hydatid mole. The third operation was a supravaginal hysterectomy performed to check a persistent profuse hemorrhage in connection with a five months' miscarriage.

The causes of death were changed to abortion with no mention of sepsis, by the Analysis Committee, on three certificates. One had been certified as "pregnancy," one as "extra uterine pregnancy," and was changed to pulmonary embolus, to account for sudden death following an exploratory laparotomy, one was changed from broncho-pneumonia to abortion, under the rules of the Manual of the Joint Causes of Death.

The Analysis Committee considered these deaths as non-preventable in thirteen cases, and assigned the responsibility to a physician in six, and to the patient in seven instances. In the latter class the avoidability was called ignorance and lack of co-operation of the patient and her family in six, and lack of prenatal care in one. In the physicians' group, all were decided as being due to errors of judgment.

The Analysis Committee ascribed to a physician under error of judgment the death of a woman between five and six months pregnant who was subjected to laparotomy, on the diagnosis of extrauterine pregnancy, for an attack of abdominal pain. A normal intrauterine pregnancy was found. The woman died on the operating table evidently from pulmonary embolus.

The same avoidable factor was assigned to a physician who retained at home a woman spontaneously aborting in the third month. The resulting hemorrhages persisted and when hospitalization occurred, two weeks later, the hemoglobin was below thirty percent and the erythrocyte count well below two million. Transfusions and other supportive measures failed to prevent death.

The avoidable factor of ignorance of significance of symptoms on the part of the patient was assigned by the Analysis Committee in the case of a woman para x, who bled for a month following a two months abortion. Medical advice was not sought because of the family's financial condition. Finally a severe hemorrhage necessitated hospitalization seven weeks after the abortion. Transfusions and infusions were of no avail. The patient died twelve hours after admission.

The Analysis Committee considered as non-preventable practically all the medical complications of early pregnancy, complicating abortion or associated with abortion.

Comment on Abortion with no Mention of Sepsis.

The outstanding feature of this section is the predominance of hemorrhage as a cause of death. Early recognition and prompt treatment of this condition should be borne in mind. Ignorance of the patient and lack of co-operation on her part signifies again the need for earlier and more instructive prenatal care.

THERAPEUTIC ABORTION

In the deaths studied during this survey there were sixteen deaths following abortion performed for therapeutic reasons. The indications for these operations may be summarized as follows: in eight cases, vomiting of pregnancy; in one, pyelitis; in four, chronic renal disease; one each of toxemia, bleeding and multiple neuritis, all of which are classed under Title 147. All of these deaths occurred in hospitals. The causes of death may be summarized as follows: septic infection in three cases, two of which developed in hospital; abortion without septic infection in one case, with hemorrhage in a nephritic; pernicious vomiting of pregnancy in eight cases; toxemia in one; and three cases in which the causes were non-obstetrical.

The interval between operation and death was less than twenty-four hours in eight instances, or 50 percent of the deaths; it was between one and three days in three; and between three and six days in two, and over seven days in three.

Thirteen of the deaths occurred in native-born women, three in foreign-born; eleven in white women, five in negroes. All of the deaths occurred in married women. A study of the age groups showed no fact of value; four deaths occurred in women between 26 and 30 years of age, and four in women between 36 and 40 years. As to the gravidities represented, three were in primiparas and thirteen in multiparas. Of the multiparas, eight were in the second and third pregnancies, the remainder were scattered up to the eighth pregnancy. All were under twenty-eight weeks pregnant, eleven were under four months, while one case in the sixth month gave birth to a living fetus.

In five instances where sufficient information was available it was considered by the Analysis Committee that prenatal care had been adequate. The time element and quality of supervision were the deciding factors in determining that nine women had had no care.

In eight previous pregnancies of the multiparas of this group there had been complications. In the present pregnancies of the entire group, intercurrent disease had complicated eight, three of whom had pyelitis.

The Analysis Committee felt that the certificate of death had not been correctly filed in three; the Committee in evaluating the conditional elements which might have averted the fatal outcome considered thirteen deaths as non-preventable. In all instances where religion was the reason for non-interference, the death was termed non-preventable. In one instance the physician was considered responsible through error in technic, and in two deaths the patient was held responsible through lack of co-operation.

Autopsies were performed in five of these cases. The clinical diagnosis was not altered as a result of any of these examinations, except that the diagnosis of acute yellow atrophy was not sustained in two cases of vomiting of pregnancy.

ECTOPIC GESTATION

During the period of this survey, 33 women died from causes connected with ectopic gestation. This is 4.6 percent of the total number of deaths studied, 717; and 11 percent of the 292 cases under 28 weeks pregnant. The hospitals of the city reported having treated 703 cases in that same time. As one patient died at home, the hospital mortality for this condition was 4.55 percent for the three years. Over half the cases, 18, occurred in the fourth decade of life. As to gravidity, the cases were almost equally divided between primigravida and multigravida. Two cases occurred in illegitimate pregnancies. Twenty-one occurred in white women and twelve in negroes. Twenty-eight were native-born, five foreign-born. Twenty-nine cases were under three months pregnant, one was four months, and one over seven months pregnant, and in two the duration of the pregnancy was unreported.

Twenty-six patients were operated upon and seven died without operation. Eight of the women operated upon, approximately one-third, developed sepsis; ten of the twenty-six had procedures other than the removal of the affected tube. These additional operations, which included three appendectomies and three hysterectomies, ranged from diagnostic dilatation and curettage to a rather formidable list in one case of dilatation and curettage, amputation of the cervix, perineorrhaphy, suspension of the uterus and salpingo-oophorectomy. Laparotomy for intestinal obstruction preceded one death in a case where the tubal pregnancy had been successfully removed by a bilateral salpingo-oophorectomy, supravaginal hysterectomy and incidental appendectomy.

The duration of the symptoms before operation ranged from a few hours to three and four weeks in a number of cases. In the majority the symptoms were present for five days. Only three of the operations were recorded as elective and in two of them the ectopic gestation was not diagnosed prior to operation. In ten of the twenty-three operations, recorded as emergencies, the patient was in the hospital from over one day to eight days before operation. In the two cases that were in the hospital for eight days, the patients had already been operated on (perineoorhaphy and other plastic procedures in one and dilatation and curettage in the other), several days previously, although the symptoms of amenorrhea, lower abdominal pain and bleeding were present. Blood transfusions were given in eleven cases.

Autopsies were performed in eleven cases. In three of these no operation had been done and the autopsy disclosed the true cause of death.

The causes of death were decided by the Analysis Committee to have been incorrectly certified in ten cases. Corrections were made to include six with septic conditions specified; four, ruptured ectopic gestation; and one operative shock.

The causes of death for the group were decided to have been hemorrhage in twenty-one cases, septic infection in eight, and operative shock in four. Death occurred within six hours in seven of these, and within twenty-four hours in three others of the twenty-six operated cases; septic infection caused death after several days in the majority of the remaining cases.

In the discussion of preventability, the Analysis Committee ascribed the responsibility to the physician in sixteen cases, to the patient in six, and regarded eleven as non-preventable. In regard to the responsibility of the physician, the avoidable factor, error in judgment, consisted of faulty diagnosis, delay in operation, too much operating in some cases, particularly an unnecessary appendectomy in a blood filled abdomen, and the omission of transfusion as a supportive measure. In regard to the patient, ignorance as shown in refusal of hospitalization and lack of prenatal care furnished the avoidable factors. In eleven cases no avoidable factors were discernable.

As an example of preventability due to failure in diagnosis may be cited the case of a woman who was referred to the hospital with a diagnosis of "probable extrauterine pregnancy." She had had three months amenorrhea, severe pain in the abdomen, nausea and vomiting and intermittent slight flow for two weeks. The abdomen was tender; an irregular semi-solid mass was present in the region of the left tube. On the fifth day in the hospital the woman died without operation. Autopsy disclosed a left tubal pregnancy of three months, with perforation of the tube.

In another case the preventability was ascribed to error in judgment. A woman who gave typical symptoms of ectopic gestation had a preoperative diagnosis, among other items, of bilateral ectopic pregnancy. She was submitted first to a plastic operation and removal of hemorrhoids. The abdomen when opened showed the peritoneal cavity filled with blood. In addition to removing the affected tube, the other tube and ovary were removed and an operation performed on the uterus. The woman gradually developed a toxic condition and died on the third day postoperative. Here the Analysis Committee felt that too much surgery had been performed.

Under the responsibility of the patient as to prevention of such deaths may be mentioned the record of a woman who, after two months amenorrhea, was seized with abdominal pain and had bleeding from the vagina. The diagnosis of ruptured ectopic pregnancy was made, but hospitalization was refused until twelve hours later. An emergency laparotomy, with infusion, was followed by death an hour later.

A typical non-preventable death was that of a luetic woman in whom the condition was diagnosed soon after her symptoms began. Prompt hospitalization was followed by an immediate operation and subsequent transfusion. On the ninth day of a satisfactory convalescence the woman expired suddenly on sitting up in bed. The contributory cause of death was given as postoperative pulmonary embolism.

Comment on Ectopic Gestation.

The outstanding fact developed in this section was failure in diagnosis of the condition. Ignorance of the significance of symptoms demands more instruction of the laity. That one-fifth of the cases were not operated upon reflects upon both physician and patient. This could be eliminated in part by early examination of women with amenorrhea during the reproductive period. That gratuitous surgery added its burden is shown in the finding that almost half the cases discussed here had had coincident operative manipulations other than the removal of the affected tube. It was noteworthy that one-fourth of this group of deaths was caused by septic infection after operation.

PUERPERAL HEMORRHAGE

During the period of the survey there were 77 deaths from hemorrhages, or nine percent of the total deaths. Sixty-two hemorrhages were primary causes of death and fifteen were secondary or contributory causes. Placenta previa occurred twenty-five times, in two it was contributory to a sepsis which developed at delivery. Accidental or premature separation of the placenta occurred nineteen times, in seven of which it was listed as a secondary cause. Postpartum hemorrhage occurred thirty-three times, in six it was a contributory cause of death.

PLACENTA PREVIA

The 25 cases of placenta previa, two of which died of sepsis, were all hospital cases. During the period of the survey the hospitals of the city reported a total of 342 cases of placenta previa, giving a death rate of 7.31 percent. There is no information available as to how many women with placenta previa were delivered safely at home, consequently, the calculations on birth numbers may not be valid. Evidently the average for the three years for the hospitals is one placenta previa to every 201 deliveries.

A study of the age group shows five deaths occurred in women under 31 years; eight occurred in the age group from 31 to 35 years; eleven in the group from 36 to 40; and one in the group over 40 years. On the other hand, a study of the relationship to the gravidity shows four cases in the fourth pregnancy as the largest number in any one pregnancy. There was one case in the sixth month, two in the seventh, the others were seven in the eighth and fifteen in the ninth month. There were twenty-two white women and three negroes in this group, seventeen native-born and eight foreign-born. All the women were married.

Prenatal care was inadequate or none had been given in twenty cases, in five it had been adequate. Eleven of the previous pregnancies of these women had been complicated. Five had been previously delivered by operation. Two had intercurrent diseases. The symptom of painless hemorrhage was recorded in eighteen cases as to its duration before delivery; in one case it had lasted eleven weeks; another, eight weeks; in four cases, four weeks; in a seventh, three weeks; in the eighth, two weeks; in the ninth, six days; in the tenth and eleventh, five days; and in seven, one day or less.

Labor was spontaneous in nine cases, induced in four, unknown in one, and none in eleven. The duration of labor was over twenty-four hours in two, under twenty-four hours in eleven, unknown in one, and none in eleven. Twenty-two women were delivered while alive, three died undelivered, in one of these a postmortem delivery was accomplished. One woman was delivered spontaneously, twenty-one by operation. The operations included surgical induction in four, Cesarean in five, forceps in five, version in twelve. There were three multiple operations in this group. The placenta was removed manually in eight cases. Postpartum hemorrhage occurred in twelve cases. Six women died within one hour after delivery, eight others within twelve hours, and two within twenty-four hours. Three women died undelivered. There were no multiple pregnancies. Transfusions were used in only five of these cases.

The Analysis Committee felt that the cause of death was not accurately filed in four cases. The changes were made from postpartum hemorrhage, uterine hemorrhage of pregnancy, dilatation of the heart and slow cortical hemorrhage.

The Analysis Committee considered fourteen of these deaths as preventable and eleven as non-preventable. In the preventable group a physician was held responsible in nine cases and the patient in five. Avoidable factors were error in judgment in eight, error in technic in one, and ignorance of the patient in five.

As examples of preventability, the Analysis Committee regarded the physician responsible under error in judgment in cases similar to the following: A multipara in the eighth month had a moderate hemorrhage, for which she was packed. The packing was removed the following day, but repacking was necessary two days later. At this time the patient was transferred to a hospital. The packing was removed and the woman kept in bed. The child was viable, the woman in good condition. On the fifth day a severe hemorrhage occurred. Manual dilatation of the cervix and internal podalic version were performed with a central placenta previa. The woman died six hours later in shock, although transfused twice in the interval.

The Analysis Committee regarded error in technic with question as to judgment in the performance of Cesarean section in a para iii, with a marginal placenta previa. One vaginal examination had been made. Sepsis developed on the third day and autopsy after death on the sixth day showed purulent peritonitis.

The Analysis Committee regarded ignorance in lack of co-operation on the part of the patient as the avoidable factor in the following case: A patient had had slight bleeding, irregularly, for six weeks. The day before her admission to the hospital, when she was eight and a half months pregnant, she had a profuse hemorrhage, but refused hospitalization. A second profuse hemorrhage on the day of admission caused her to go into shock. On admission a bag was inserted in the cervix and the shock treated, but death occurred before labor began.

As a non-preventable death, the following example was regarded as typical by the Analysis Committee: A para x, with no prenatal care, called a physician for moderate vaginal bleeding at the eighth month. She was hospitalized at once, and found to be in labor, half dilated with a partial placenta previa. Braxton-Hicks version was performed and delivery followed two hours later. A massive hemorrhage followed delivery and death occurred within six hours, although the patient was actively treated. Autopsy revealed intense anemia of all organs and no rupture of the uterus.

Comment on Placenta Previa.

Frequently the diagnosis of placenta previa was not made until a serious or at times fatal hemorrhage had occurred. The improper management of such a case, however, presented a more serious problem than the failure in diagnosis.

The choice of means to control the hemorrhage was often questionable. The application of the method of delivery was unskillful and the lack of asepsis was shown in the proportion of septic infections incurred. Induction of labor in placenta previa is a debatable question. Failure to properly pack the uterus after delivery in these cases and the omission of transfusions shows evidence of lack of preparedness for emergencies. When placenta previa is diagnosed a method of delivery for the particular case should be selected and properly performed and the necessary adjuvant measures should be carried out promptly.

PREMATURE SEPARATION OF THE PLACENTA

During the period of the survey 19 women died of premature separation of the placenta. In 12 cases it was the primary cause, and in 7 cases it contributed to the death. This group forms 30 percent of the hemorrhage deaths. One in every 43 deaths of the entire series of 717 occurred from this cause. All of these women died in the hospital. One died undelivered.

Eighteen were white women, one a negro. Fifteen were native-born, four foreign-born. All were married women. A study of the age groups shows 10 of the 19 were 36 years or older. A study of the number of the pregnancies showed nothing of value. Three cases were in pregnancies under 28 weeks. Six had had complications in previous pregnancies; three had had previous operative deliveries; and twelve had complications in the present pregnancy. Six had albuminuria, four had hypertension, five had edema, two had had pernicious vomiting in the present pregnancy. There was a history of scarlet fever in three, and of abnormal kidneys in four cases. There had been bleeding in early pregnancy in ten of these patients.

The prenatal care was regarded as inadequate or none in eleven, and adequate in eight. Only three of the sixteen cases over 28 weeks pregnant had planned to have hospital delivery.

Symptoms of the final illness began in the majority of instances within twenty-four hours of admission to the hospital; in four they had been present over a week. There was but one case of concealed hemorrhage. Fifteen women over 28 weeks pregnant were delivered alive and one died undelivered. Of the three cases under 28 weeks pregnant, two were delivered by operation and one spontaneously.

Labor was induced in three cases. Nine Cesarean sections were done, and all were recorded as emergency operations. Three forceps and four versions were done, one had a multiple operation. The third stage was completed by manual removal in eleven cases, and postpartum hemorrhage occurred five times. The attendant was a physician except in two instances where an interne was in charge. Death followed quickly in most of these cases. In two death occurred on the delivery table, four died in less than an hour, and five others within the first twelve hours. Four living over seven days, died of sepsis. There were two autopsies in the group. Transfusion of blood was practiced three times in the nineteen cases. There were two live births in these cases.

The Analysis Committee regarded eleven of the deaths as nonpreventable and eight as preventable. In the latter group the responsibility was assigned to the physician in six, and to the patient in two. In the group in which the physician was regarded responsible, the avoidable factor of error in judgment operated in five and error in technic in one case. The ignorance of the patient was the avoidable factor in the other two preventable deaths.

In the group in which a physician was responsible under error of judgment, the Analysis Committee considered the following example as a typical case: A multipara was admitted to the hospital with a history of bleeding for two days. A medical induction was tried. Slow labor ensued, with slight to moderate vaginal bleeding and passage of clots of blood. No mention was made of blood count or pulse rate during the labor. Delivery was spontaneous after eighteen hours of labor, under rectal analgesia. Following delivery the placenta was expressed and was covered with firm clotted blood. The uterus did not contract well and bleeding continued. Not until an hour after delivery was packing inserted. The bleeding continued and the patient died four hours after delivery.

As an example of error in technic, the Analysis Committee gave the following: A Cesarean section was performed on a woman who had bleeding at term, associated with abdominal pain, without any preliminary vaginal examination. The woman died of peritonitis on the tenth day. No condition predisposing to infection was noted on the history.

Ignorance of a patient was regarded by the Analysis Committee as a deciding factor in the following case: A multipara, with a history of previous toxemia, had no prenatal care. She had abdominal pain for two days, and on the second day bleeding began moderately. This was disregarded until it became excessive during the night. She was admitted to the hospital, where intravenous glucose was given during an emergency version, followed by manual removal of a partially separated placenta and by packing. Notwithstanding a blood transfusion after delivery, death occurred fifteen hours later. There was no autopsy.

As an example of a non-preventable death, the Analysis Committee regarded the following case as typical: A primipara with good prenatal care, in the ninth month had abdominal pain but no bleeding. This led to hospitalization. Within two hours after consultation, a Cesarean section was performed and a dead fetus and a two-thirds separated placenta were removed. The patient died suddenly a few hours later.

Comment on Premature Separation of the Placenta.

The most important conclusion to be drawn from this section is that the women who died of premature separation with other complications of pregnancy, whether toxic or otherwise, all showed preliminary symptoms, so that there was sufficient time for more prompt treatment. The error in judgment on the physician's part was often poorly selected time of operation. All cases of premature separation delivered by the vaginal route should be packed immediately after delivery, and blood volume should be restored by blood transfusion or by the intravenous injection of other fluids.

POSTPARTUM HEMORRHAGE

During the period of this survey there were 33 deaths in which postpartum hemorrhage was the primary cause of death in 27 and the contributory cause in 6. In other words, one death in every 22 of the 717 of the series resulted from postpartum hemorrhage. In addition there were 62 deaths in which the records stated there had been severe or more than usual postpartum blood loss.

Twenty-three of these deaths were in white women, ten in negroes. Twenty-six were native-born, six foreign-born, one not recorded. A study of the age groups and number of pregnancies showed the majority of these deaths in the years and gravidities which held the largest number of pregnancies. Five deaths occurred after deliveries in the eighth month, the remainder during the ninth month and at term.

There had been adequate prenatal care in eleven cases or one-third; in the other two-thirds it had been either inadequate or none had been given. There had been complications in nine previous pregnancies, with previous operations to deliver in the nineteen multiparas of the group. During the present pregnancy, there were complications or intercurrent diseases in sixteen cases, some of which given as contributory causes of death appear in Table No. 14. Eight women had had albuminuria, two convulsions, seven high blood pressure, and eight edema.

Labor was induced before five deaths and was spontaneous in the remainder. Twelve of the women were in labor over twenty-four hours, eight over forty-eight hours, and four over seventy-two hours. Two fetuses presented by the breech, two were transverse, one position was unknown, and the remainder, or twenty-eight, were vertex presentations. There were no multiple pregnancies in this group.

The attendant at origin of the case was a physician in twenty-one instances, interne in nine, and midwife in three. The delivery was spontaneous in ten cases. In the other twenty-three it was operative. No woman is recorded as having bled to death following a Cesarean section. There were sixteen forceps deliveries, version occurred in six of these cases, and twice version followed attempted forceps in this hemorrhage group.

The third stage varied in duration from a few minutes to ten hours. The placenta was removed manually in nine cases. The time following delivery of the child varied from a few minutes to a number of hours. The indication for the manual removal was uniformly not stated upon the hospital records. In nineteen of these thirty-three postpartum hemorrhages the uterus was packed, in three instances the uterus was packed twice before death. Fifteen of the cases received intravenous injections of saline or glucose solution. One case, only, was transfused. There were recorded three tears of the cervix, in one no attempt to suture to control hemorrhage was mentioned. The perineum was lacerated in varying degrees eighteen times. In three cases hysterectomy was performed in an attempt to check the bleeding.

There were twenty-eight hospital deliveries and five home deliveries. Three of the home deliveries died in the hospital later. Of the twenty-eight hospital deliveries, twenty-five were planned admissions. Postpartum hemorrhage was given as a contributory cause in one septic death, in four deaths from accidents of labor (rupture of uterus), and in one death from placenta previa.

In five instances the Analysis Committee decided the true cause of death had not been certified and made appropriate changes from the following certified causes: hemophilia, childbirth and myocarditis, interstitial nephritis and fibroid uterus, uremia, and acute dilatation of heart in childbed.

The Analysis Committee decided that in these thirty-three cases of postpartum hemorrhage there were fifteen non-preventable deaths and eighteen preventable. Of the eighteen preventable deaths, sixteen were decided to have been the responsibility of a physician and two of a patient. In the latter, lack of prenatal care was considered the avoidable factor. In the group assigned to a physician, the avoidable factors were considered as error in judgment in fourteen cases and error in technic in two.

The Analysis Committee regarded the following case as typical of error in judgment: A woman was admitted to a hospital in inactive labor. On the following day a surgical induction was done, by means of rectal tubes inserted into the cervix, under gas anesthesia. With full dilatation an elective version and extraction were done. The third stage was normal but the vagina was packed. Bleeding was moderate when the patient left the delivery room. Two hours later a cervical tear with a torn artery was discovered. The patient was exsanguinated before the sutures could be completed. All the operative procedures were done by an interne. No mention was made on the record as to supervision.

The Analysis Committee considered as typical of error in technic the following case. A multipara was admitted in labor. After two days of ineffectual labor with occiput posterior, and after failure of forceps delivery, a version was performed to deliver a stillborn child. The placenta was removed manually and the vagina packed. Bleeding occurred through the packing, which was removed. The uterus was found distended to the umbilicus and filled with blood clots. It was emptied and packed but no transfusion was given. The patient died six hours later. There was no autopsy.

Ignorance and lack of co-operation on the part of the patient in refusing hospitalization was considered the avoidable factor by the Analysis Committee in the following case: A para ix registering late in pregnancy, had a hypertension and albuminuria. Hospitalization was refused for three weeks. Labor was induced and after spontaneous delivery, postpartum hemorrhage occurred which could not be checked by intrauterine packing and stimulants. The patient died before hysterectomy could be arranged. No transfusion was available. There was no autopsy.

The Analysis Committee regarded as non-preventable deaths in postpartum hemorrhage cases similar to the following: A multipara iv was delivered spontaneously after twelve hours in labor. The placenta delivered spontaneously. About five minutes later profuse bleeding occurred. The uterus was packed. Intravenous saline and glucose were given. A hysterectomy was performed for continued bleeding one hour after delivery. Several small intramural fibroids were found. Transfusion was given. The patient died six hours later. There was no autopsy.

Comment on Postpartum Hemorrhage.

This section shows that postpartum hemorrhage was twice as common in deaths following operative delivery as in those after spontaneous delivery. The cases of operative delivery, however, were difficult and postpartum hemorrhage was necessarily more liable to occur.

In twenty-four of these cases labor had continued for more than twenty-four hours. The relation of labor to non-contractility of the uterus seems to have been overlooked. The technic of packing the uterus must be questioned when it is shown that nineteen of these cases died in spite of uterine tamponade. An outstanding suggestion is that vaginal packing be discarded for full intrauterine packing. That but one case received a blood transfusion is a shocking admission of lack of preparedness for such emergencies, provided it was not due to error in judgment in the handling of the case. The relation of manual removal of the placenta to postpartum hemorrhage was high, and the need for the operation was not explained sufficiently in the records. It appears incredible that a woman should bleed to death from a torn cervix with no attempt at repair.

PUERPERAL SEPTICEMIA, NOT SPECIFIED AS DUE TO ABORTION

During the three years of the survey 119 women died of puerperal sepsis. This term, Title No. 145, does not include septic abortions or septic infections following ectopic gestation. The group of 119 is 16.6 percent of all the cases studied, 18 percent of the puerperal causes of death, and accounts for 28 percent of the deaths in women over 28 weeks pregnant. Contrasted with the births in Philadelphia during the three years a septic death occurred once for every 35 stillbirths, once to every 800 live births, and once to every 838 total births.

Hospital delivery preceded 98 deaths from puerperal sepsis and home delivery 21. Twelve of the women delivered at home were later transferred to the hospital. These 98 deaths represent 30.6 percent of the 320 deaths following hospital delivery in women over 28 weeks pregnant. Of the 98 hospital deliveries followed by septic death, 77 records showed that the sepsis developed in the hospital. Sixty-five of this number were deliveries planned to occur in the hospital. In 21 cases the sepsis was recorded as originating before admission, although delivery occurred in the hospital. There were also 21 septic deaths following home deliveries in pregnancies of over 28 weeks duration in which the sepsis originated in the home. The incidence of hospital delivery sepsis is 77 to 65,626 live births in hospitals or a rate of 1.17 septic deaths per thousand live births. The incidence of home delivery sepsis (21 cases) plus sepsis originating outside of the hospital (21 cases), is 42 to 29,154 live births in homes, or a rate of 1.44 septic deaths per thousand live births.

One hundred and fourteen women were married, the pregnancy was illegitimate in five. One hundred and three were white women, sixteen were negroes. Eighty-six were native-born, thirty-one were foreign-born, and the nativity of two women was not recorded. In the various age groups there were 14 under 21 years; 19 were 21 to 25 years; 35 were 26 to 30 years; 22 were 31 to 35 years; 26 were 36 to 40 years; and 3 were women of 40 years or over. See Chart No. 7. In regard to the present pregnancy of these women, 53 septic deaths occurred in the 241 first pregnancies, 24 in the 115 second pregnancies; 12 in the 95 third pregnancies; 6 in the 67 fourth pregnancies; 8 in the 60 fifth pregnancies; 4 in the 28 sixth pregnancies; and 12 scattered by one and two through the remaining gravidities. See Chart No. 8.

Prenatal care was considered adequate in 59 cases, and inadequate, none or not recorded in 60. Pelvic measurements were given as abnormal in 20 cases, normal in 80, and unrecorded or unknown in 19.

In addition to the complicating conditions mentioned on the death certificates as contributing causes, Table No. 14, there were 16 cases who had had intercurrent diseases during the present pregnancy. Eighteen women had had complications in previous pregnancies and 19 had had previous operative delivery.

There were 94 live births; 28 stillbirths, or one in every four cases. Three deaths were in multiple pregnancies with live births. The onset of labor was induced artificially in 12 cases, or approximately 10 percent. Labor was less than 24 hours in 89 cases where labor occurred or was recorded. No labor occurred in the elective Cesareans. While it is acknowledged that internal pelvic examinations during labor bear some relation to the development of infection, the figures on vaginal and rectal examination would be invalid unless closely controlled. No figures on this factor have been compiled. There were 18 cases in which no internal examination whatever was made, and 19 in each of which but one rectal examination was made. Rubber gloves were used in 92 cases, while they were either not used or no mention made of their use in 27 cases.

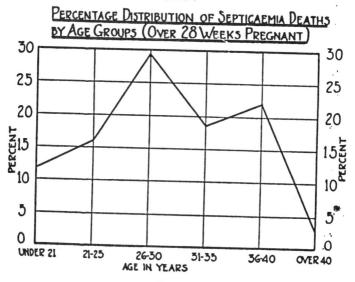

CHART 7

PERCENTAGE DISTRIBUTION OF SEPTICAEMIA DEATHS BY AGE GROUPS (OVER 28 WEEKS PREGNANT)

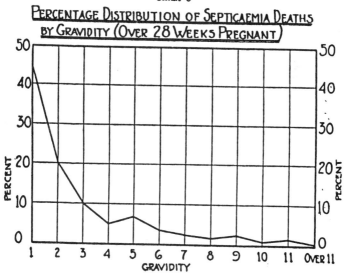

CHART 8

PERCENTAGE DISTRIBUTION OF SEPTICAEMIA DEATHS BY GRAVIDITY (OVER 28 WEEKS PREGNANT)

The attendant at the origin of the case was a physician in 96 cases, an interne in 15, a student in 2, and a midwife contact in 2. There were non-medical attendants in 4 cases, 1 of whom was a Faith Healer.

The presentation of the fetus was recorded as vertex 108 times out of the 358 head presentations, including 3 multiple pregnancies; as breech 8 times of the 37 breech presentations; as transverse 4 times of the 14 transverse lies; as face once of the 3 face presentations, and the presentation in one case was unknown.

The delivery was spontaneous in 39 of this group of 119, 32.8 percent. In 80 cases the delivery was accomplished by operative measures, 67.2 percent. Of these, either the attempted method or the final procedure was forceps in 29 instances; version in 13; breech extraction in 4; and Cesarean section in 45. One destructive operation and one hysterectomy were recorded. In eleven cases multiple operations of various combinations had been done. Cesarean section was performed in hospitals 92 times on women over 28 weeks pregnant. Forty-five of these women or 48.8 percent died of puerperal sepsis. Of the 1,775 Cesarean sections reported in the hospitals for the three years, 47 or 2.64 percent died of puerperal sepsis, and 49 or 2.7 percent died of all other causes. Version was performed in hospitals on 63 women in pregnancies of over 28 weeks duration who died. Of these, 13 or 2.06 per cent died of puerperal sepsis. Of the 1,050 versions reported in hospitals during the three years, 13 or 1.23 percent of the women died of puerperal sepsis and 50 or 4.76 percent died of all other causes.

One hundred and three women over 28 weeks pregnant who died had had forceps operations performed in hospitals. Twenty-four of these or 23.3 percent died of puerperal sepsis. Of the 14,292 forceps operations reported in hospitals during the three years, 24 or 0.0167 percent died of puerperal sepsis and 79 or 0.055 percent died of all other causes.

There were 36 lacerations of the perineum and 7 tears of the cervix. Postpartum hemorrhage of varying degrees, but of sufficient severity to be recorded, occurred in 18 cases.

The interval of death after delivery was longer than seven days in 83 or 70 percent of the cases. Eleven or 10 percent died in three days or less. Autopsies were performed in 36 cases. In no instance did the autopsy seem necessary for diagnosis. Death was preceded by operation, other than that for delivery, in 14 of the 119 patients who died of sepsis. These operations consisted of explorations, under various terms, of the uterine cavity, and five abdominal operations, including removal of the uterus in two cases and a resection of gangrenous intestine in one. The remaining four operations were for drainage of pelvic or other abscesses.

The specific etiological organism was sought for by blood culture in 36 of the 119 cases. In 18 no growth was recorded. One was recorded as contaminated, two showed staphylococcus aureus, five staphylococcus albus, which were questionable findings, one showed a non-hemolytic streptococcus, and nine showed hemolytic streptococcus. There was no mention of anaerobic organisms.

Two pelvic abscesses were cultured, one showed streptococcus viridans. One throat culture was done and showed non-hemolytic streptococcus. The one urine culture recorded showed streptococcus. The one peritoneal fluid culture recorded showed non-hemolytic streptococcus. One infected Cesarean incision was cultured and showed staphylococcus aureus.

Of the five illegitimately pregnant women who died of sepsis, four were negroes of 16 and 17 years of age. Two had high forceps deliveries of stillborn children. In the third, a blind imbecilic epileptic, a Cesarean section with sterilization was done. One woman, a syphilitic, was delivered spontaneously of a seven months stillborn fetus, and later had a curettage. None of these cases had had prenatal care and all were emergency admissions. The fifth, a white woman, had a profound nephritic toxemia with a blood urea nitrogen of 85. She had had no prenatal care and was an emergency admission. Sepsis followed a surgical, rectal tube, induction of labor. A bilateral pyelonephritis and a broad ligament abscess developed before death.

In 42 or 28 percent of the 119 death certificates filed for this group the Analysis Committee made a change to list the case under puerperal septicemia. The original causes of death as stated may be included in groups: three were stated as pregnancy; five as Cesarean sections; eleven as various cardiac lesions, dilatation, myocarditis and failure; seven as some form of toxemia or renal lesion; four as pulmonary disease or embolus; three as lesion of gastrointestinal tract; three as hemorrhage; and a scattered number of synonyms of terminal pathological lesions in the remaining ten deaths.

The Analysis Committee decided, in regard to preventability, that 99 or 83 percent of these 119 septic deaths could have been avoided. This fact is regarded as one of the most outstanding developed from this survey. To the physician was ascribed the responsibility in 97 cases; to the patient in 2; 20 deaths were regarded as non-preventable.

In the 97 cases in which the physician was held responsible for the death, the avoidable factor, error in judgment, was decided by the Analysis Committee to be operative in 38, and error in technic in 59 cases.

In both instances in which the responsibility was assigned to the patient the avoidable factor was considered as ignorance and lack of co-operation.

The Analysis Committee regarded as preventable such cases as the following, which was attributed to an error in judgment. A woman who had received adequate prenatal care, as far as the number of visits was concerned, but who had a flat pelvis, was admitted to the hospital after twenty-four hours in labor. The membranes had ruptured and frequent vaginal examinations had been made. Delivery was completed by a destructive operation after forceps and version had failed. The patient died on the ninth day of a stormy puerperium. Autopsy revealed a widespread septic infection of the pelvic tissues.

The Analysis Committee regarded error in technic as the avoidable factor in cases of which the following is an example: A woman, admitted to a hospital at term with a contracted pelvis, was given a test of eighteen hours in labor, during which no vaginal examinations were made. At the end of this time a low cervical section was performed and a living baby delivered. On the third day, temperature rose to 104 degrees, following a chill. The patient died on the seventh day of a septic puerperium.

In the two cases in which the Analysis Committee ascribed the preventability to the patient under the avoidable factor of ignorance, one was delivered by a religious healer and died of sepsis a week later. Few details of the conduct of the delivery could be obtained. In the other case the women left one hospital on the ninth day after a normal delivery and convalescence. Within a few days she was admitted to another hospital with lower abdominal pain, foul lochia and fever. The diagnosis on admission to the second hospital was pelvic peritonitis and cellulitis. She died six weeks later, being constantly septic. No autopsy was permitted.

The Analysis Committee regarded as non-preventable such deaths as the following: A para ii, having had adequate prenatal care and having planned for a hospital delivery, was admitted in labor with membranes ruptured. After a short labor, with only one rectal and no vaginal examinations, she delivered a live baby spontaneously. The third stage was normal and there were no lacerations. Three days postpartum, the lochia became offensive, and on the fifth day the temperature rose and became septic. Death followed on the sixteenth day. Blood cultures showed no growth and transfusions were done repeatedly. No autopsy was permitted.

Comment on Puerperal Sepsis.

The Committee believes that deaths from puerperal sepsis could be reduced materially, and that they are essentially a medical responsibility. This section demands very careful consideration. Rather than make definite comments, the Analysis Committee urges that the reader study these facts and draw his own conclusions.

ALBUMINURIA AND ECLAMPSIA

Of all the deaths studied during the survey, 114 had albuminuria and eclampsia. This was the primary cause of death in 85 cases or 13 percent of the 639 puerperal deaths. In the remaining 29 cases, albuminuria and eclampsia was classed as a secondary factor according to the rules of preference in the joint causes of death. This group of 114 is 15.8 percent of all the maternal deaths (717) and 26.8 percent of those over 28 weeks pregnant (425).

Twenty-two of the 114 patients or 19.2 percent, died undelivered, and five had postmortem deliveries. Seven of the women died at home and 107 in the hospital. Of the 52 cases over 28 weeks pregnant, in which albuminuria and eclampsia was the primary cause, 31 had planned hospital deliveries and 21 had emergency admissions.

Fifty-nine of these women, or a little over half, had entirely inadequate or no prenatal care. The remaining 55 received at least the minimum amount of supervision required for adequate prenatal.

Among the patients who had inadequate or no care, there were three times as many white as colored women, and three times as many native as foreign-born women. In the entire group of 114 there were 97 white women and 17 colored; 85 native-born women and 29 foreign-born.

As to age, the groups were as follows: under 21 years, 14; 21 to 25 years, 23; 26 to 30 years, 23; 31 to 35 years, 21; 36 to 40 years, 26; and over 40 years, 7. Fifty-one or almost half of these deaths occurred in the 241 first pregnancies of the entire series; 16 in the 115 second pregnancies; 10 in the 95 third pregnancies; 7 in the 67 fourth pregnancies; 8 in the 60 fifth pregnancies; 4 each in the 28 sixth and 25 seventh pregnancies; 8 in the 25 eighth; and the other 6 in the 57 remaining pregnancies of higher parities.

Four cases occurred in the fourth month, 2 in the fifth, 14 in the sixth; 15 in the seventh; 19 in the eighth; and 60 in the last month and at term. It is probable that the cases of albuminuria and eclampsia occurring in the fourth and fifth months of pregnancy may have been uremic manifestations of chronic kidney disease, but in at least two of these six cases autopsy findings showed hepatic damage of eclamptic type.

Complications had occurred in past pregnancies in 20 women. Nine had had albuminuria and convulsions previously. Other obstetrical complications, such as operative deliveries, were noted in 15 cases. There was a history of disease of the kidneys in 25 cases or 21.9 percent, of heart disease in 11, and of scarlet fever in 10. Four of the women had pernicious vomiting during the early weeks of pregnancy.

Table No. 14 shows the complicating factors recorded as contributory causes when albuminuria and convulsions was the primary cause. Twenty-nine cases had intercurrent diseases not mentioned on the death certificate. Three patients had vaginal bleeding during the present pregnancy, and 8 had postpartum hemorrhage following operative vaginal delivery.

The onset of symptoms has not been calculated, but 52 of the 78 cases over 28 weeks pregnant entered the hospital before delivery.

Convulsions occurred in 45 cases, albuminuria in 55, edema in 58, and high blood pressure in 70. Persistent headache was recorded in only 24 case histories.

In 23 cases labor was induced surgically. Forty-nine women with eclampsia were delivered by operation; 43 had spontaneous deliveries, and 22 died undelivered, of which five had post mortem deliveries. The operative deliveries included 16 Cesareans, of which 12 were recorded as emergencies and 4 as elective; 21 forceps operations; 8 versions and 4 breech decompositions and extractions. Four cases had multiple operative procedures. In the group of 92 women who were delivered before death, the operative incidence was over 50 percent, and in the cases over 28 weeks pregnant the operative incidence was 60 percent.

The anesthesia employed was mainly ether or gas-ether, but three cases had chloroform and three had spinal anæsthesia. Two of the spinal group were actively convulsive. In the first patient, low spinal anæsthesia was used for forceps delivery; death occurred within an hour from respiratory failure. The second patient had had but one convulsion; death followed immediately after the anæsthetic agent was injected. Cyanosis and respiratory failure were recorded. The third case was first seen at eight months, when her blood pressure was 222/156. She was given hospital treatment, but her blood pressure rose and a Cesarean section was performed under spinal anæsthesia. Four hours later she went into shock and died six hours after delivery.

One-half of the babies or 57 were stillborn. Four stillborn babies resulted from postmortem deliveries in the 22 women who died undelivered. Thirty-six viable fetuses were delivered alive. From a sociological angle it is of interest to note that the deaths of 90 woman in this group left 170 orphaned children. The importance of this problem has been discussed in a separate section.

The greatest number of the eclamptic patients died within twelve hours after admission or delivery. Autopsies were held in 28 cases and showed in the great majority typical parenchymatous changes in the liver, kidneys and heart muscle. In two cases massive cerebral hemorrhage was demonstrated at necropsy.

The Analysis Committee decided that in 21 of the 114 death certificates the cause was stated incorrectly. The 85 cases in which albuminuria and convulsions was considered the primary cause of death include eight cases incorrectly certified as follows: 1, fractured skull; 2, acute hemorrhagic nephritis with thrombosis; 3, multiple hemorrhages; 4, Cesarean section; 5, acute yellow atrophy of liver (no autopsy); 6, cardiac dilatation; 7, pregnancy; 8, coronary thrombus (no autopsy). In each of these cases the certificate was changed to albuminuria and convulsions, as this was indicated clearly by the histories.

The 29 cases in which albuminuria and convulsions was a contributing cause include 13 that were certified incorrectly and the causes of death recorded were as bizarre as those just mentioned. Thirteen of these 29 women died of sepsis, 8 developing the infection in the hospital. When septicemia and toxemia coexist as causes of death, septicemia takes preference under the rules of the Manual for Joint Causes of Death.

The Analysis Committee regarded 63 of the 114 cases in this group as preventable and 51 as non-preventable. In the entire group of 114 deaths, the responsibility was credited to the physician in 32 cases, to the patient in 31, and 51 were considered non-preventable. Included in the unavoidable group were 14 fulminant cases, of which 6 were hepatic in type.

In regard to the 32 cases assigned to the physician the avoidable factor was error in judgment in 25 deaths: error of technic, 1; and lack of proper prenatal care, 6.

Lack of prenatal care was considered the fault of the patient in 16 instances, while in 14 her own ignorance and lack of co-operation, or the refusal of her family to allow hospitalization, were given as the avoidable factors.

In the group of 85 primary eclampsias, the responsibility was assigned to the patient in 29 cases and to the physician in 19, while 37 were regarded as non-preventable.

The Analysis Committee considered the physician responsible for death in some cases of primary eclampsia in which the patient had failed to obtain prenatal care. For example, a patient, thirty-six years of age, made infrequent visits to her physician. At the sixth month she had a blood pressure of 145-85 and abdominal pain, and was warned of the danger of increased blood pressure. At her next visit, two months later, her pressure was 185-100. Urinalysis had not been made, although specimens had been requested repeatedly. One month later, convulsions began. The physician was called and twelve hours afterward referred her to the hospital. A Cesarean was performed immediately, with the patient in coma. Death occurred in an hour. While the outlook in this case was bad, the abrupt surgical measure for delivery prejudiced the patient's only chance. The Analysis Committee felt the physician's judgment was faulty.

Another of the primary eclampsias was assigned to the physician because of error in judgment, as he failed to recognize the significance of elevated blood pressure and albuminuria. This patient made semi-monthly visits to her physician. Her urine showed four plus albumin constantly. Her blood pressure rose in six weeks from 155 systolic to 180-100. She was then sent to the hospital. Labor was induced, but death occurred in convulsions before delivery.

The following case, in which eclampsia was a contributory cause of death, was assigned to the physician: The patient was referred from clinic for admission because of pressure of 188-96 and albumin and casts. On the second day and again on the fourth a rectal tube was inserted into the cervix to induce labor. Twenty-four hours after the second induction, a full term stillbirth was delivered. The placenta was removed manually. The following day the temperature rose to 103, and on the eighth day the patient died of sepsis. The avoidable factor was considered error in technic.

The cases in which the Analysis Committee ascribed the responsibility to the patient were uniform in that they had all failed to seek medical aid until marked toxemic symptoms developed.

The Analysis Committee considered these two cases as typical of many non-preventable deaths.

In the first case, a multipara had had eclampsia in her first two pregnancies, and her third had resulted in a miscarriage. She consulted her physician every two weeks until the middle of the sixth month. Because of rising blood pressure, at the twenty-sixth week she was hospitalized. In spite of the well-considered, conservative treatment she received, convulsions ensued. A live baby was delivered spontaneously, but death followed three days later. As in all cases of this nature, religious belief was considered as excepting the general rule.

In the second, the woman had adequate prenatal care. Within a period of five days after normal findings were registered, a fulminant toxemia developed. Treatment was instituted and no attempt made at delivery. The patient died in two days.

Comment on Albuminuria.

The third largest cause of death in this survey was albuminuria and eclampsia. As half of these women received at least the minimum amount of supervision necessary for adequate prenatal care, one must be skeptical as to the exact quality of such care. Every pregnant woman should be regarded as a potential eclamptic. More thorough study in early pregnancy is necessary to determine possible functional inabilities. Earlier hospitalization is essential for mild degrees of toxemia. Prompt termination of pregnancy is imperative in toxic cases failing to respond to treatment. Emergency surgery showed to no advantage in the treatment. Of the 57% of cases regarded as preventable, the patient was considered responsible in 61%. The avoidable factors were failure to obtain suitable prenatal care and lack of co-operation on the part of the patient.

VOMITING OF PREGNANCY

"Other toxemias of Pregnancy," or Title No. 147 of the International List, comprises mostly cases of pernicious vomiting of pregnancy. For this reason, "Vomiting of Pregnancy" is used as the heading for this section, including thirty deaths from this cause. It was the primary cause in twenty-four cases and contributory in six according to the rules of the Manual of Joint Causes. The causes of death in these latter six cases were two septic abortions, one premature separation of the placenta, two puerperal sepsis (delivery at seventh month), and one lobar pneumonia. The ratio of deaths from vomiting of pregnancy to the whole series was 4.1 percent and to the cases under 28 weeks pregnant, 10.3 percent.

There were twenty-four white women and six negroes in the group; twenty-seven native-born and three foreign-born. All of the women were married. Seventeen deaths occurred in the first pregnancy; ten in the second and third, and the other three in higher pregnancies. There were two sets of twins in the groups.

Antenatal supervision in the ordinary sense could not be calculated for this group; however, the Analysis Committee felt that thirteen women had received adequate care. Physical examinations were made on seventeen of the patients. Five multiparas had had complications in previous pregnancies, including one with pernicious vomiting. Twenty-five of the thirty patients had complications in the present pregnancy and ten had intercurrent diseases.

In eighteen cases the vomiting was regarded as pernicious on admission to hospital.

Pregnancy was less than seven months in twenty-one cases, including nine under three months, six in the fourth month, and three each in the fifth and sixth month. Nine pregnancies were in the seventh month, of which four had stillbirths. Of the twenty-one patients under twenty-eight weeks gestation, ten died undelivered or had stillborn babies.

Abortion occurred in fifteen patients or half of the vomiting of pregnancy group. It was spontaneous in five and therapeutic in ten. One of the latter cases died of sepsis. Six of the therapeutic abortions died within twenty-four hours of the operation, one in four days, and one in nine days.

The duration of symptoms prior to the attendance of the physician could not be obtained in every case, but sixteen were recorded as follows: one week or less in eight; two weeks in two; three weeks in three; and one, two and three months for the remaining three cases. The condition of the patient at time of hospitalization was recorded in half the histories. It was bad in ten cases and fair in five. One patient in bad condition was discharged on release and died at home later. The duration of symptoms prior to interference in the ten patients having therapeutic abortions was as follows: six days, one case; two weeks, two; three weeks, three; one month, one; three months or more, three.

In two cases, acute yellow atrophy of the liver was given as either primary or contributory cause of death. There was no autopsy in either of these cases to confirm the diagnosis. Four autopsies were performed in the whole group of thirty cases.

The Analysis Committee decided that seven certificates failed to state the correct cause of death. These included acute myocarditis; acute nephritis; general toxemia; acute yellow atrophy; influenzal toxemia; chronic interstitial nephritis and angina pectoris. The true cause in each of these cases was hyperemesis gravidarum.

The Analysis Committee decided that twenty-two of these deaths were non-preventable and eight avoidable. The responsibility was credited to the physician in three cases and to the patient in five. The avoidable factors in the latter group were uniformly stated as ignorance or lack of co-operation of the patient or her family. In this study, cases in which religion was given as a reason for refusal of operation, were regarded as non-preventable. Error of judgment was the avoidable factor in the three cases assigned to the physician.

Typical case histories of the vomiting of pregnancy deaths show two outstanding factors among the preventable cases: first, treatment continued too long before hospitalization for operation; and second, refusal by the patient of permission for operation.

Comment on Vomiting of Pregnancy.

The majority of the cases of pernicious vomiting occurred in primiparous women, who failed to seek medical assistance early. Sixty-six percent of the hospitalized patients were in only fair condition on admission. The number of deaths occurring soon after therapeutic abortion would seem to show that the operation had been postponed beyond a reasonable time for expectancy of recovery. There was a high incidence of other puerperal complications or intercurrent diseases to further lower the resistance of these women.

EMBOLUS AND SUDDEN DEATH

During the period of the survey 44 deaths, 6.12 percent of the 717 deaths studied, were certified to have occurred from phlegmasia alba dolens, embolus or sudden death. These cases are listed under Title No. 148 of the International List of Causes of Death. The cases were divided into 14 pulmonary embolus, 5 cerebral embolus, 2 cardiac embolus, 2 embolus not otherwise specified, 1 venous thrombosis, 1 coronary thrombosis, and 19 cases of sudden death from shock after delivery. In 13 of the certificates of death the Analysis Committee decided the stated cause was not correct, and made appropriate change to include the cause of death in this category.

There were 39 white and 5 negroes in this group. Five of the group were under, and 39 over 28 weeks pregnant. A study of the age groups showed the largest number proportionately occurred in the more advanced years. A study of the gravidities showed no fact of value. Fourteen of these deaths occurred in home cases and 30 in the hospital. Twenty-six had inadequate or no prenatal care.

Thirteen of the 39 cases over 28 weeks pregnant were delivered spontaneously. The 20 operative deliveries included: forceps 13, version 4, Cesarean section 7, and breech extraction 1. In four multiple methods were used. Six women pregnant over 28 weeks died undelivered.

The time of death after delivery for this group was studied with especial care, as most instances of emboli occurring late in the puerperium are regarded as manifestations of a septic process. Of those delivered, 4 died within a hour, 12 within 12 hours, and 5 within 24 hours after delivery. There were 11 women who died after the seventh day of the puerperium. In this group of 11 there was no sepsis noted. In the cases in which the symptoms were observed prior to death, there were present classical respiratory distress with sudden onset, cyanosis and rapid pulse. Not all the deaths were observed, however, as several of the women were found dead in bed or on the floor of their rooms.

The Analysis Committee regarded 32 of this group as non-preventable deaths and 12 preventable. In this latter group a physician was considered responsible for the death in ten cases and the patient in two. The avoidable factor in the entire first group was decided by the Analysis Committee to have been error in judgment; in the latter, ignorance of the patient.

There were four autopsies performed after these forty-four deaths. Two were made by a coroner's physician and it cannot be said that anything definite was learned from these autopsies. The others, made in a hospital, were equally inconclusive in establishing a more exact cause of death than that clinically certified as "Sudden Death."

Comment on Embolus and Sudden Death.

In this connection a paragraph may be quoted from Kerr: "There is little doubt that a considerable number of deaths are attributed to pulmonary embolism which should really be relegated to trauma or shock or both. The diagnosis of embolus is a simple explanation and salves the conscience of the person in attendance." The Registrar-General (England) refers to this very point in the 1930 *Statistical Review:* "In 1928 in only 14 percent of the deaths assigned to this cause (embolus) was the condition verified by post-mortem examination, and in the absence of such verification, this form of return is not above suspicion."

ACCIDENTS OF LABOR

Title No. 149 of the International List of the Causes of Death, Accidents of Labor, includes as a subtitle Cesarean Section and Other Operations to Deliver. Included also in the subtitles are such traumatic conditions as rupture and inversion of the uterus and other injuries, abnormal positions of the fetus, shock and various conditions which are synonyms for dystocia. It has been rather difficult at times to separate "sudden death from shock after delivery," which pertains to Title No. 148, from "shock of birth" or "post-puerperal shock." ·

During the period of the survey 79 deaths occurred from accidents of labor. Two deaths included in this group were pregnancies just under 28 weeks. Eleven of the deliveries in pregnancies over 28 weeks were spontaneous, 9 deaths were recorded during labor and before birth occurred. The remaining 59 deaths, in women over 28 weeks pregnant, were in connection with operative deliveries. There were 76 operations attempted or completed. In 12 instances the operations were multiple, in one instance there were 5 operations performed before delivery was accomplished. Cesarean section was done 18 times, forceps used 29 times, versions tried in 22, and breech extraction in 2. There was one hysterectomy and one abdominal section. Seven deaths occurred at home, 72 in the hospital.

The history of previous pregnancies in the multiparous women showed complications had occurred in 15, while 17 records showed previous operative deliveries. There had been puerperal complications in 32 pregnancies represented in this group, and intercurrent diseases had occurred in 24. A study of the age groups and gravidities showed that over half of the deaths were in the first, second and third pregnancies.

The presentation was vertex in 63, face in 2 (this presentation occurred but 3 times in the whole series), transverse in 5 (fourteen in the whole series), unknown in 1.

Labor began spontaneously or there was none in 58 instances. Labor was induced in 21 cases. The duration of labor was over 24 hours in 32, under that in 33. The placenta was removed manually in 36 cases, exclusive of the Cesarean sections.

Nine women died undelivered and over half the deaths associated with delivery occurred within 12 hours. There were 32 stillbirths in the 79 cases. The attendant during labor was a physician in 65 deaths, interne in 9, student in 1, midwife in 2, and no attendant in 2. Prenatal care was considered to have been adequate in 35, inadequate or none in 44 instances. The delivery was planned to occur in a hospital in 51 cases, in 27 the admissions were emergencies, and 1 case was unknown.

The causes of death in this category may be divided into seven groups: shock, 12 cases; rupture of the uterus, 20 cases; inversion of the uterus, 6 cases; respiratory complications, 12 cases; cardiac complications, 22 cases; spinal anesthesia, 2 cases, and a miscellaneous group in which there were 5 cases.

The Analysis Committee regarded 23 certificates of death as not expressing the true cause. The two largest groups added under this category were ten under rupture of the uterus and seven under shock as the primary cause. Autopsies were performed after nineteen deaths.

The Analysis Committee felt that 37 of these deaths were non-preventable. Forty-two were considered preventable and a physician was held responsible in 37, the patient in 5. Ignorance and lack of co-operation in four and lack of prenatal care in one made up the avoidable factors in the patient group. Error in technic in 3, lack of prenatal care in 1, error in judgment in 33, comprised the avoidable factors in the group listed under physician's responsibility. Of the 35 cases which had had adequate prenatal care, error in judgment on the part of the physician was the avoidable factor in 15. In the 51 cases where hospital deliveries were planned, error in judgment was the avoidable factor 22 times.

In 12 of the 29 cases where prenatal care was adequate error in judgment was the avoidable factor. In 9 of the 27 cases where the hospital admission was an emergency, error in judgment was the avoidable factor.

OPERATIONS TO DELIVER

In routine obstetric practice, operative delivery, in certain instances, becomes absolutely necessary. When seriously regarded as a major surgical procedure and technically performed in accordance with major surgical practice, the measure, irrespective of its type, will prove a life saving recourse for both the mother and her child.

Delivery by operative means, be it by forceps or any other method, unless instituted for compelling indications and performed according to sound surgical tenets, must inevitably lead to grave danger and frequently it may lead to disaster, either for the mother, the baby or both.

Surveys made regarding the obstetrical death rate throughout the world, but more especially in our own country, disclose that delivery effected by operative means, manual or instrumental, without good indications and in unskilled hands, is a mortality factor of disquieting proportions. Plass, in his White House Conference report, stated: "The most striking change in obstetric practice in the past decade and a half has been the great increase in operative deliveries. A certain few have raised their voice on every occasion against the tide of radicalism, but apparently without stemming the rise."[6]

Reference to Table No. 8 will show that the operative incidence in some hospitals in Philadelphia is indisputably high. On Chart No. 3 the hospital data are expressed graphically. The mortality rate is the total gross uncorrected puerperal and non-obstetrical rate for each hospital. It was difficult for the Analysis Committee in reviewing the answers to the hospital questionnaire received each year, to believe that 18 Cesarean sections were even relatively indicated in a one year delivery service of 142 births. For a period of six months during the survey the figures on operations in one general hospital maternity service with a practically open staff showed an operative incidence of 50 percent in the private floor service and 4 percent in the ward service. The comment of the Resident Obstetrician of this hospital was that either the ward patients were being neglected, which did not seem to be true, in view of the results obtained, or that some of the forceps applications on private patients were unnecessary. To what extent obligatory consultation before operative obstetric procedures would serve to reduce the number of unnecessary operations, is problematic, but such consultation might be a salutary measure. The inevitable risk of injury to the baby in operative delivery is well recognized. What the increase in artificial delivery has meant in Philadelphia is shown by the figures on birth injury deaths by the Bureau of the Census. In 1920 the rate of death of infants from birth injuries in Philadelphia was 2.9, in 1929 it was 4.7 per thousand live births, an increase of 62 percent in a decade.[7]

There were 68,733 hospital deliveries in the three years. This number was computed from the answers to the hospital questionnaire. The Bureau of Vital Statistics, City Hall, stated that 65,626 live births were recorded in the hospitals during the survey. There were 19,237 operative deliveries and 49,496 spontaneous deliveries. The total operative incidence was 27.9 percent. There were 1,775 Cesarean sections in hospitals, an incidence of 2.58 percent. If the ratio of type of operation of the 1931 survey of Cesarean section, by the Obstetrical Society, had held good throughout the three years of the survey, there would have been 1,423 classical Cesarean sections or 80.2 percent, and 320 cervical or extraperitoneal Cesarean sections or 18 percent, and 32 Porro or celiohysterectomy Cesarean sections or 1.8 percent.

---

[6] Forceps and Cesarean Section by E. D. Plass. Fetal, Newborn and Maternal Morbidity and Mortality. D. Appleton-Century Co., New York, 1933.
[7] "The Challenge of the Falling Birth Rate." J. C. Litzenberg, Am. J. Obst. and Gyn., 1934, xxvii, 317.

There were 14,292 forceps deliveries, an incidence of 20.7 percent. According to the percentages of types of forceps reported on the hospital questionnaire for the third year of the survey, there would have been 485 high forceps or 3.4 percent of the total forceps operations, 3,174 midpelvis forceps or 22.2 percent, and 10,633 low or outlet forceps, 74.4 percent of all the hospital forceps operations in the three years. Plass stated (l. c.): "When the use of forceps is limited to the actual need, instrumental delivery is uncommon and probably represents not more than 5 percent in any given series. Any great increase over this figure savors of meddlesome midwifery."

There were 1,050 versions performed in the hospitals during the survey; no information was available as to the number in this group which were elective. There was an incidence of 1.52 percent versions performed in 68,733 hospital deliveries.

There were 18 craniotomies performed in the 68,733 hospital deliveries. There were 2,039 breech extractions or breech decomposition and extractions performed among the 68,733 hospital deliveries—an incidence of 2.96 percent.

The relation of the type of delivery to cause of death appears in Table No. 28, while the relation of the method used in 245 operative deliveries to the cause of death appears in Table No. 29. It may be noted that the majority of deaths from sepsis and accidents of labor followed operative deliveries, and it can hardly be felt that operation added anything to the chance for recovery in the group of eclampsias.

TABLE 28

TYPE OF DELIVERY BY CAUSE OF DEATH

(Pregnancies of 28 Weeks and Over)

Cause of Death	Total Deaths	Died Under-livered	Delivered While Alive		
			Total	Spontaneous	Operative
TOTAL	425	50	375	132*	245*
Ectopic Gestation	1	1	...	...	...
Premature Separation of Placenta	10	1	9	1	8
Placenta Prævia	22	3	19	1	18
Postpartum Hemorrhage..	27	..	27	9	18
Sepsis	119	..	119	39*	81*
Albuminuria and Eclampsia	69	14	55	25*	31*
Other Toxemias	5	..	5	2	3
Embolus and Sudden Death	39	5	34	12	22
Accidents of Labor	77	9	68	11	57
Accidents of Puerperium..	5	..	5	5	...
Non-Obstetrical	51	17	34	27	7

* Twin Pregnancies.

TABLE 29

RELATION OF METHOD OF DELIVERY (ATTEMPTED OR SUCCESSFUL)
TO CAUSE OF DEATH IN 245 OPERATIVE DELIVERIES

TYPE OF DELIVERY

CAUSE OF DEATH	TOTAL OPERATIVE DELIVERIES	MULTIPLE METHODS	CESAREAN SECTION	FORCEPS	VERSION	CRANIOTOMY	BREECH	ABDOMINAL SECTION	HYSTERECTOMY
TOTAL	245	34	93	107	64	4	13	1	2
Premature Separation of Placenta	8	...	4	1	3	...	...	...	...
Placenta Prævia	18	3	3	5	12	...	...	...	...
Postpartum Hemorrhage	18	2	...	13	5	...	2	...	...
Sepsis	81	11	45	29	13	1	4	...	1
Albuminuria and Eclampsia	31	2	11	15	4	...	2	...	...
Other Toxemias	3	...	...	1	...	...	2	...	...
Embolus and Sudden Death	22	4	7	13	4	...	1	...	...
Accidents of Labor	57	12	18	22	22	3	2	1	1
Non-Obstetrical	7	...	5	1	1	...	...	...	...

It is a striking fact that almost half of the deaths following Cesarean section were caused by sepsis, and that death from accidents of labor was recorded in one-third of the version deaths. Practically two-thirds of the deaths following forceps deliveries resulted from sepsis and accidents of labor, both regarded as largely preventable causes of death.

CESAREAN SECTION

During the period of the survey there were 98 deaths following Cesarean sections performed while the patients were alive. Eleven other sections were done post-mortem in an effort to obtain live babies. In this same period the hospitals of the city reported 1,775 Cesareans, Table No. 8. The incidence of deaths following Cesarean section was 13.6 percent or 98 out of a total of 719. Many weeks after the tabulations had been completed, two "lost" Cesarean deaths were discovered by chance and are included in this section, although they do not appear in general tables. Both cases were septic and the cause of death was so incorrectly certified, with no mention of the associated puerperal state, that it was impossible for the local Bureau of Vital Statistics to classify them as puerperal deaths. The addition of these cases makes a true total of 719 deaths. The incidence of deaths following Cesarean section to the total reported Cesarean sections was 5.52 percent. The incidence of deaths following Cesarean sections to all hospital deliveries with live births was 0.103 percent. There was an incidence of 2.58 percent Cesarean sections to all hospital deliveries and 1.78 percent to all births in the city for the three years. Forty-four of the 98 Cesarean section deaths or 45 percent, were in primiparas, and 54 or 55 percent in multiparas. All of these deaths occurred in hospitals. The 91 operations in this group which were performed after the seventh month form 34.4 percent of the 264 operative deliveries in the cases over 28 weeks.

The indications, Chart No. 9, as stated on the histories were: contracted pelvis, 26, 14 of which were elective sections; disproportion, 20, 7 of which were elective sections; heart disease, 14, 9 of which were elective sections; toxemia, 11, 1 of which was an elective section; placenta previa, 8; premature separation of the placenta, 7; obstructed labor, 3; transverse position, 2; and 1 case each of the remainder—brow position, previous elective section, Bandl's ring, psoas abscess, meningitis, purely elective and myomata.

By age groups, Cesarean sections were done 9 times in women under 21 years; 20 times from 21 to 25 years; 27 times from 26 to 30 years; 17 times from 31 to 35 years; 21 times from 36 to 40 years; and 4 times in women over 40 years. Two Cesareans were done on illegitimately pregnant women. Of these 98 women, 73 were native-born and 25 foreign-born; 88 were white and 10 were negroes.

Forty-four of these patients were primiparas and 54 were multiparas. Among the multipara, 22 were in their second pregnancies, 8 in the third, 6 in the fourth, 5 in the fifth, 6 in the sixth, 1 each in the eighth, ninth and tenth, 3 in the eleventh, and 1 over the eleventh.

CHART 9

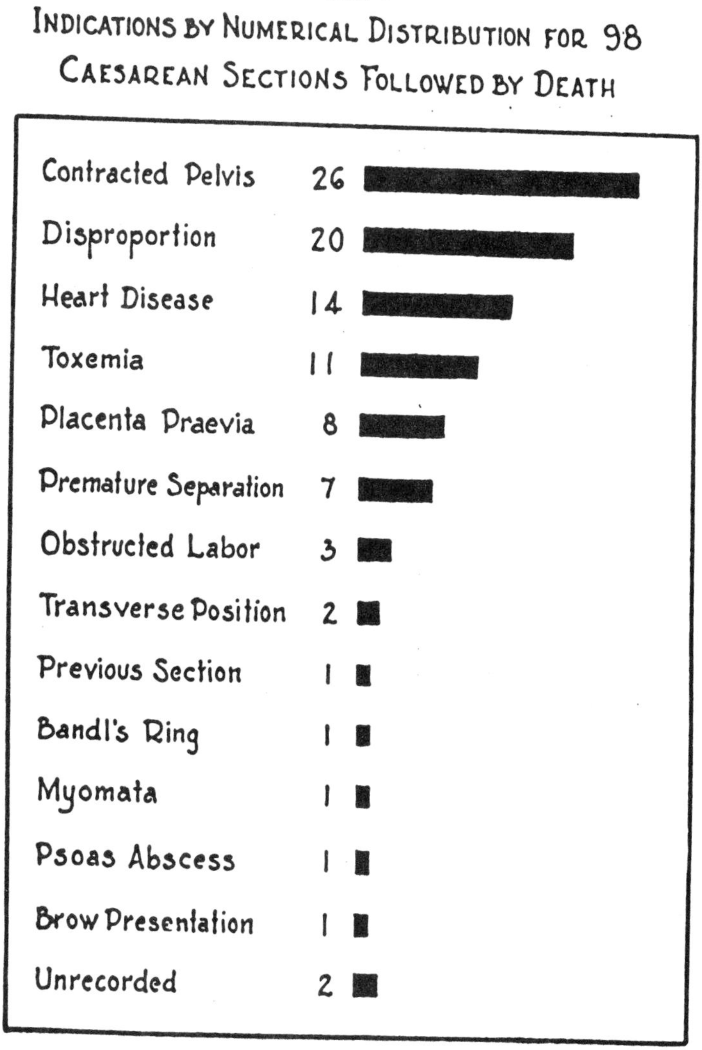

INDICATIONS BY NUMERICAL DISTRIBUTION FOR 98 CAESAREAN SECTIONS FOLLOWED BY DEATH

Contracted Pelvis	26
Disproportion	20
Heart Disease	14
Toxemia	11
Placenta Praevia	8
Premature Separation	7
Obstructed Labor	3
Transverse Position	2
Previous Section	1
Bandl's Ring	1
Myomata	1
Psoas Abscess	1
Brow Presentation	1
Unrecorded	2

Two of the operations were done in women just under 28 weeks pregnant; 5 were in the seventh month; 12 in the eighth month; and the remaining 79 were in the ninth month or at term.

As to prenatal care, 61 women had had adequate supervision, 28 inadequate, while in 9 the care was not given or not recorded. Pelvic measurements were not taken in 12 of these cases and in 4 there was no record. In 28 the measurements were recorded as abnormal and in 54 as normal.

Of the 54 multiparas, 25 had complications in previous pregnancies. Twenty multiparas had required previous operative interference. Six women had had previous Cesarean sections, repeated in two cases; 9 had had forceps deliveries, 2 high forceps, 1 extraction, 1 embryotomy, and 1 operative delivery the nature of which was not recorded.

Sixty-one of these 98 women had complications in their present pregnancies. Thirty-nine had albuminuria, 5 had convulsions, 18 high blood pressure, 33 marked edema, 16 bleeding from vagina, and 7 had persistent headaches. In addition, 24 of the Cesarean group had intercurrent diseases. The heart was recorded as abnormal 24 times, the lungs as abnormal 6 times. The fetus was born alive 73 times and stillborn 25 times in these 98 cases. In three cases there were multiple pregnancies. The presentation of the fetus was recorded in 94 cases—it was vertex in 79 cases, breech in 11, and transverse in 4.

The admission to the hospital was planned in 67 cases, emergency in 27, and unknown in 4. Cesarean section was elective in 33 cases and emergency in 65. The type of operation is shown in Tables Nos. 30 and 31. Of the 67 planned admissions to the hospital, the Cesarean section was recorded as an emergency operation in 34 instances. There had been previous attempts to deliver vaginally in five cases; forceps in one, high forceps in one, forceps and craniotomy in one, and version in two. All these cases died of septic infection. In many cases there were other operative procedures beside the Cesarean section. Thirteen cases, exclusive of the Porro operations, were sterilized, and four others had myomectomies. All of this latter group died of septic infection.

TABLE 30

DEATHS FOLLOWING CESAREAN SECTION BY ELECTIVE AND EMERGENCY OPERATIONS AND TYPE OF OPERATION

	TOTAL		CLASSICAL OR INTRA-PERITONEAL		LOW OR EXTRA PERITONEAL		PORRO OR CELIOHYS-TERECTOMY		TYPE UNKNOWN	
	Number	Per-cent	Number	Per-cent	Number	Per-cent	Number	Per-cent	Number	Per-cent
TOTAL	98	100.0	73	100.0	14	100.0	5	100.0	6	100.0
Elective	33	33.7	30	41.1	2	14.3	1	20.0	...	.....
Emergency	65	66.3	43	58.9	12	85.7	4	80.0	6	100.0

TABLE 31

TYPE OF OPERATION IN 98 DEATHS FOLLOWING
CESAREAN SECTIONS
AND
TYPE OF OPERATION IN 1931 SURVEY OF
CESAREAN SECTIONS*

| | MATERNAL MORTALITY SURVEY | | 1931 SURVEY | |
	Number	Percent	Number	Percent
TOTAL	98	100.0	571	100.0
Type Unknown	6	6.1	...	...
Classical or Intra-Peritoneal	73	74.5	458	80.2
Low or Extra-Peritoneal	14	14.3	103	18.0
Porro or Celiohysterectomy	5	5.1	10	1.8

*A Survey of Cesarean Sections Performed in Philadelphia During 1931. C. B. Lull, Amer. Jour. Obst. and Gyn., 1933, XXV, 426.

In 33 cases the duration of labor was over 24 hours; 24 of these died of septicemia. In 14 the labor was under 24 hours; 7 of these died of septic infection. In 47 cases there was no labor and 15 died of sepsis. These included elective, toxemic, cardiac and hemorrhage cases. In 4 cases the duration of labor was not recorded. Labor was induced surgically in 7 cases, of which 3 died of septic infection. In 53 cases the membranes had ruptured previous to the Cesarean section; 28 of these died of septic infection. In 42 instances the membranes had not ruptured prior to the operation; 16 of these died of septic infection. In 3 cases the condition of the membranes was not noted; 1 of these died of septic infection.

Vaginal examinations had been made during labor in 49 patients, 26 of whom died of septic infection. No vaginal examinations were made in 48 patients, 17 of whom died of septic infection. In one case there was no record of vaginal examination. Control data are not available and these figures are offered merely as a statement of fact. Rectal examinations alone were made in 21 cases, 11 of which died of septic infection. Neither vaginal nor rectal examinations were made in 24 cases, and 8 of these died of septic infection.

The interval between childbirth and death was less than an hour in 5 mothers, between 5 and 12 hours in 12, between 12 and 24 hours in 7, from 1 to 3 days in 14, from 3 to 6 days in 29, and over six days in 28, while three patients died during delivery. The majority of deaths in the last two groups, that is, after the third day, were due to septic infection.

The causes of death, Chart No. 10, in these 98 Cesareans were as follows: septic infection, 47, almost 50 percent; accidents of labor, 18; toxemia, 12; embolus and sudden death, 7; non-obstetrical causes, 6; premature separation of placenta, 5; placenta previa, 3. Of the 47

CHART 10

INCIDENCE BY NUMERICAL DISTRIBUTION OF CAUSES OF DEATH IN 98 CAESAREAN SECTIONS

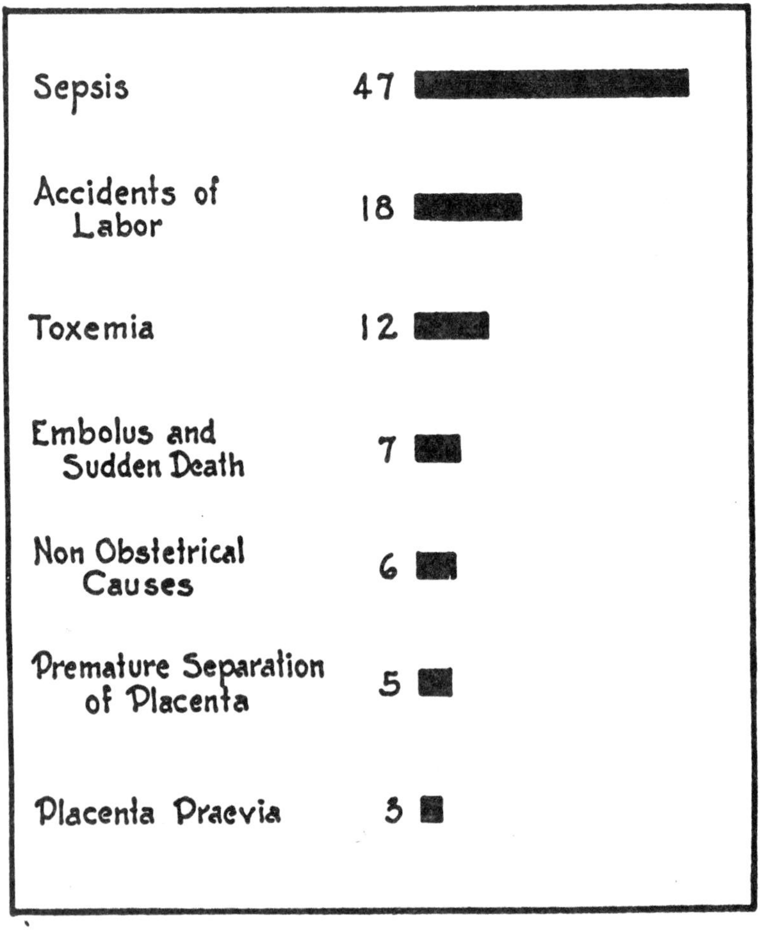

Sepsis	47
Accidents of Labor	18
Toxemia	12
Embolus and Sudden Death	7
Non Obstetrical Causes	6
Premature Separation of Placenta	5
Placenta Praevia	3

deaths from septic infection, 29 had had emergency operations and 18 elective. The Analysis Committee considered that 31 of the Cesarean death certificates were incorrect and changed 22 of them to septic infection.

The Analysis Committee regarded 61 of these deaths as preventable, and 37 as unavoidable disasters (Table No. 32). Among the prevent-

TABLE 32

PREVENTABILITY AND RESPONSIBILITY IN CESAREAN
SECTION DEATHS

	Number	Percent
TOTAL CÆSAREAN DEATHS	98	100.0
Not Preventable	37	37.8
Preventable	61	62.2
ASCRIBED TO PHYSICIAN	57	100.0
Error in Judgment	29	50.8
Error in Technique	26	45.6
Lack of Prenatal Care	1	1.8
Combination of Factors	1	1.8
ASCRIBED TO PATIENT	4	100.0
Ignorance of Patient	3	75.0
Lack of Prenatal Care	1	25.0

able deaths, the patient was considered responsible in four cases. Three of these were due to lack of co-operation and the fourth to lack of prenatal care. In the remaining 57 cases a physician was considered accountable. Error in judgment was the determining element in 29, error in technic in 26, lack of proper prenatal care in 1, and a combination of several responsible factors in 1.

Post-mortem Cesarean sections were performed 12 times. The causes of death in this group were: cardiac failure, 3; toxemia, 3; hemorrhage and shock from ruptured uterus, 2; spinal anesthesia, 2; suppurative appendicitis, 1; and intestinal obstruction 1. Nine of these patients had no labor, and in one the duration was 15 hours. One patient was in labor two days and an attempt had been made to deliver the child by forceps from a ruptured uterus. Another patient was in labor three days and delivery had been attempted twice by forceps and once by version. Among the post-mortem Cesareans there were two deaths from respiratory failure following the administration of 150 mgm. neocain for spinal anesthesia. In neither chart was it recorded that the requirements for spinal anesthesia had been estimated. In two of the twelve post-mortem deliveries the child was born alive.

The Analysis Committee concluded that four of these deaths were unavoidable and eight might have been prevented. The responsibility rested with the patient in two cases because of lack of prenatal care; the physician was accountable for six through error in judgment or technic.

The Analysis Committee selected the following case as typical of the proper use of Cesarean section in convulsive toxemia of pregnancy: A primipara, having had no prenatal care, was admitted to the hospital as an emergency case. She was at term and had had four convulsions before admission. She was treated conservatively for two days, but, as the convulsions recurred, and as other objective symptoms of a severe nature persisted, delivery was decided upon. A long, narrow cervix with no dilatation favored Cesarean section as the best method of delivery. After operation, the toxemia did not regress and death followed in 24 hours. The responsibility of this case was assigned to the patient because of failure to obtain prenatal care.

In another death, the Analysis Committee concluded that Cesarean section had not favored the possible recovery of a woman with eclampsia. A multipara, in labor at term, had one convulsion at home. She was admitted in coma. An immediate Cesarean section was performed and the patient died on the operating table.

From a similar viewpoint the Analysis Committee considered the use of Cesarean section in placenta previa. In the following case, Cesarean section was performed for central placenta previa: A primipara, at the thirty-sixth week, was admitted after a single, large, painless hemorrhage. One vaginal examination was made after aseptic precautions and after vaginal instillation of mercurochrome. A classical Cesarean section was followed by transfusion. The patient developed a low grade fever and on the ninth day died very suddenly, evidently from embolus. Although the embolus was possibly of septic origin, the death was regarded as non-preventable.

Cesarean was used in the following case of marginal placenta previa: A multipara, para iv, in her eighth month, was admitted to the hospital as an emergency. She had had two small hemorrhages in the twenty-four hours before admission. After five days in the hospital, an alarming hemorrhage occurred and an emergency Cesarean section was performed. Death occurred on the operating table from shock. The Analysis Committee regarded this as a preventable death and the avoidable feature as error in judgment.

In premature separation of the placenta, the Analysis Committee considered Cesarean as a debatable procedure in the following case: A multipara at the eighth month of pregnancy, with albuminuria and moderately elevated blood pressure, had uterine contractions associated with vaginal bleeding. On admission to the hospital, she was in labor and her condition was fair. The diagnosis of premature separation of the placenta was followed by immediate Cesarean section. Sterilization was done on account of an underlying nephritis which had been recognized in clinic. Death followed from septic infection.

The Analysis Committee regarded the termination of the following case of premature separation of the placenta as unavoidable. A primipara at term was in the hospital under treatment for nephritic toxemia of pregnancy. Signs of an abruptio placenta, without external hemorrhage, led to an immediate section under local anesthesia. The diagnosis was confirmed at operation, the placenta being almost entirely separated. The baby was dead. Following delivery, a blood transfusion was given. Death followed in two days from progressive toxemia and coma.

All heart patients who had been carefully studied and who died from cardiac lesions, following elective Cesareans, were classified as unavoidable by the Analysis Committee. If patients with decompensation or acute cardiac failure were subjected to immediate Cesarean section, without preliminary treatment, the Analysis Committee considered the procedure as inadvisable and prejudicial to the recovery of compensation. Such deaths were regarded as due to errors in judgment.

In many emergency cases where Cesarean section was performed for contracted pelvis and disproportion, the Analysis Committee felt that a possible source of infection was the frequency of previous vaginal examinations associated with maternal exhaustion.

In elective Cesarean sections, performed for contracted pelvis and disproportion, in which death resulted from septic infection, the Analysis Committee considered the sepsis due to some unnoticed break in technic.

FORCEPS

During the period of the survey there were 112 deaths associated with either attempted or successful forceps deliveries. This group represents 15.6 percent of the 717 deaths studied, and 42.4 percent of the 264 operative deliveries of women over twenty-eight weeks pregnant. One hundred and three of the forceps deliveries occurred in hospitals and nine at home. Of the nine home cases three were later sent to hospitals for further treatment.

During the survey there were 14,292 forceps deliveries in all the hospitals of Philadelphia. The group of women who died, following hospital forceps deliveries, forms .0783 percent of hospital forceps deliveries and .0163 percent of all hospital deliveries. Comparison cannot be made with forceps deliveries in home practice, as figures for such study are not available. As 33 cases or nearly 30 percent of the 112 forceps cases were emergency admissions to hospitals, such a comparison might be considered unfair.

In this group of 112 cases there were 90 white women and 22 negroes; 97 native-born and 15 foreign-born. Thirteen of the women were illegitimately pregnant, 12 single and 1 widow. A study of the age groups showed 16 under 21 years; 29 between 21 and 25 years; 22 between 26 and 30 years; 23 between 31 and 35 years; 19 between 36 and 40 years; and 3 women over 40 years of age. As to gravidity, 65 were primiparas, 47 multiparas. Of the multiparas, 18 were in the second pregnancy; 8 in the third; 4 in the fourth; 5 in the fifth; 2 in the sixth;

3 in the seventh; 2 in the eighth; 2 in the tenth; and 3 in pregnancies over eleven.

Prenatal care was adequate for 53 cases (47.3%), inadequate for 35 (31.2%), none for 11 (9.8%), and unknown for 13 (11.6%). In the physical examinations recorded the heart was abnormal in 13 patients but it was the indication for the operation in only four. The pelvis was abnormal in twelve cases, yet this complication indicated interference only six times. The hospital admissions were planned in 76 instances, emergency in 33, and unknown in 3. Fifteen of these 112 women had had complications in previous pregnancies, while operations to deliver had been necessary in 17 previous labors in the multiparas. In the present pregnancy there were complications in 52 patients, including albuminuria in 28, edema in 27, high blood pressure in 17, and convulsions in 13. Toxemia was the indication for the use of forceps in 17 cases. In nine cases there was antepartum bleeding. The indications are shown in Chart No. 11.

A physician performed 98 of the 112 operations, an interne the remaining 14. Three cases arose in the practice of a midwife. As to type, the operations were divided into high 27, mid 17, low 50, and unknown 28. Of the low forceps, 15 were recorded as elective or prophylactic, of which 5 or one-third died of septicemia. The indications for the use of forceps as stated in the hospital records or as obtained by a personal interview by the Recorder, are shown graphically as to percentage distribution.

The operation of forceps was associated with that of version 15 times, with Cesarean section 4 times, and with craniotomy once. In 27 instances or 24.1% there were other multiple operations associated with the 112 forceps deliveries. In 14 cases in which forceps failed version was used to complete delivery; in one case a Cesarean and in one a craniotomy completed a failure to deliver by version after attempted forceps. The cause of death in the cases where multiple operations were used for delivery was divided almost equally between sepsis and shock. The Analysis Committee judged them largely preventable.

The presentation was vertex in all but two instances: there was one face and one brow presentation. Only seven errors of rotation of the vertex were stated as indications for operative delivery.

In 92 cases, labor began spontaneously, in 11 it was induced, and in 9 the type of onset was not known. The duration of labor was under 24 hours in 50 patients, over 24 hours in 45, and unknown in 17. The cervix was manually dilated before the application of forceps in 10 cases. The causes of death in these 10 patients were: septic infection, 3; shock, 2; eclampsia, 2; and 1 each of ruptured uterus, postpartum hemorrhage and rheumatic fever.

Of the 120 babies, which included 8 sets of twins, 42 or 35 percent were stillborn. The placenta was manually removed in 26 cases or 21.6 percent of the 112 forceps deliveries. Four of this group died of sepsis and 9 of postpartum hemorrhage. Nine cases of rupture of the uterus

CHART 11

PERCENTAGE DISTRIBUTION OF INDICATIONS FOR FORCEPS DELIVERIES IN 112 DEATHS

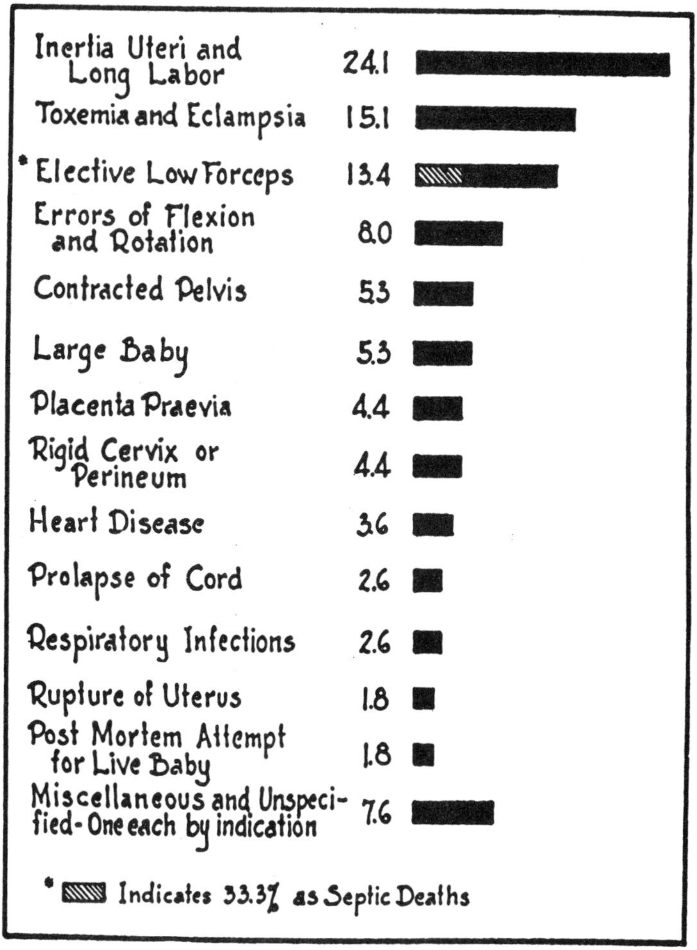

Inertia Uteri and Long Labor	24.1	
Toxemia and Eclampsia	15.1	
* Elective Low Forceps	13.4	
Errors of Flexion and Rotation	8.0	
Contracted Pelvis	5.3	
Large Baby	5.3	
Placenta Praevia	4.4	
Rigid Cervix or Perineum	4.4	
Heart Disease	3.6	
Prolapse of Cord	2.6	
Respiratory Infections	2.6	
Rupture of Uterus	1.8	
Post Mortem Attempt for Live Baby	1.8	
Miscellaneous and Unspecified- One each by indication	7.6	

* Indicates 33.3% as Septic Deaths

were associated with forceps delivery. In five instances the Analysis Committee felt that the rupture resulted from poorly performed operations, or that there was clearly an error in judgment in the choice of forceps for such cases. In the remaining four cases the forceps deliveries had no part in producing the rupture. Postpartum hemorrhage occurred after thirty-six of the 112 forceps deliveries, but it was actually the cause of death in 13 cases or 11 percent of this group.

The interval between birth and death was less than an hour in 12 cases; between one and twelve hours in 32; and between twelve and twenty-four hours in 8. Twenty-two other deaths occurred from the first to the seventh day after delivery, and 30 women died more than seven days following delivery.

The causes of death are given in Chart No. 12.

In eight cases delivery was effected by forceps after the death of the woman, but in only one case was the delivery truly a post-mortem attempt to obtain a live baby. In the other seven cases delivery by forceps had been attempted before death and the patients died on the delivery table. The indications for using forceps in these eight deliveries were maternal exhaustion or long labor in three; eclampsia in one; rupture of uterus in one; fetal distress in one; and attempt to obtain a live baby in two. The causes of death in this group were: shock, four; eclampsia, one; rupture of the uterus, one; cerebral syphilis, one; and embolus, one.

Twenty autopsies were performed after these 112 deaths. The diagnosis was not changed in any instance, nor did the Analysis Committee make any corrections after reading the autopsy protocols. There were, however, 31 other certificates of death regarded by the Analysis Committee as incorrect. Nine of these were changed to sepsis as the primary cause of death. The Analysis Committee concluded that the origin of the sepsis had been in the hospital in 20 cases and outside prior to admission in 12 cases.

In studying the avoidability in this group of deaths following forceps deliveries, the Analysis Committee regarded 40 as unavoidable disasters and 72 as possibly preventable. Of this latter group, the responsibility was assigned to the physician in 60 cases and to the patient in 12. The responsible factors in the 60 physicians' cases were error in judgment in 40 and probable error in technic in 20 cases. Among the 12 cases assigned to the patient, the avoidable element was lack of co-operation in seven instances and failure to obtain prenatal care in five.

The Analysis Committee selected the following case to illustrate a preventable death following delivery by forceps in which the avoidable factor was error in judgment: A primipara two weeks over term was in labor for twelve hours. The vertex was presenting with the occiput posterior and the head floating. It was a dry labor. The cervix was manually dilated and axis traction forceps applied. The attempt at delivery was unsuccessful. A few hours later, a consultant was called and found the patient in poor condition with the head in mid pelvis.

CHART 12

PERCENTAGE DISTRIBUTION OF CAUSES OF DEATH AFTER 112 FORCEPS DELIVERIES

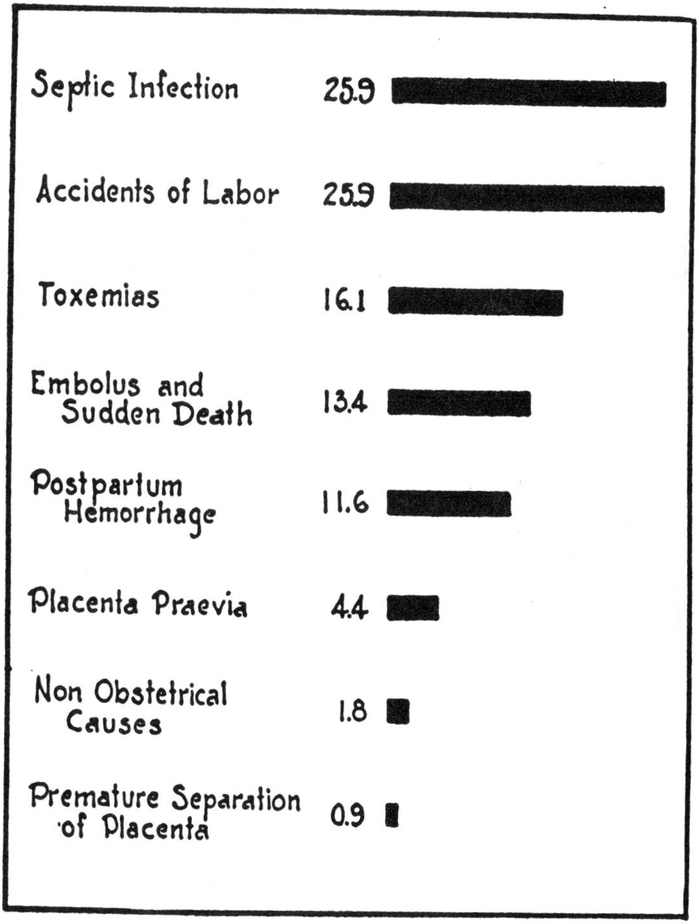

Septic Infection	25.9	
Accidents of Labor	25.9	
Toxemias	16.1	
Embolus and Sudden Death	13.4	
Postpartum Hemorrhage	11.6	
Placenta Praevia	4.4	
Non Obstetrical Causes	1.8	
Premature Separation of Placenta	0.9	

Delivery was effected by forceps. After delivery the placenta was removed manually and repairs were made. The patient became shocked and died two hours postpartum. Autopsy disclosed a rent in the lower uterine segment extending into the broad ligament. The certificate of death attributed the demise to embolus.

To illustrate a preventable death resulting from some unseen break in technic, the Analysis Committee cites the following case: A young primipara at term was in labor for nineteen hours. With the head on the perineum for one hour an elective low forceps was performed. A first degree tear was repaired. The placenta was spontaneously delivered. Three days later chills and high fever developed and the blood culture was positive for hemolytic streptococcus. Metastic foci developed in various portions of the body. Death occurred on the twenty-first day after delivery.

The Analysis Committee regarded the following case as an example of an unavoidable disaster associated with forceps delivery: A primipara with a negative past history and negative physical examination, had a dry labor at term. There was a spontaneous rotation of a posterior occiput presentation after twenty-four hours. The head was on the pelvic floor, the cervix fully dilated for three hours; delivery was easily effected by low forceps. The placental stage was unassisted and there was no hemorrhage. Sixteen hours after delivery the patient developed cyanosis, air hunger and other signs of respiratory distress, and died suddenly.

VERSION

During the period of the survey, 65 deaths followed attempted or successful deliveries by internal podalic version. This constitutes 9 percent of the 717 deaths studied or 25 percent of the 264 deaths following operative deliveries in women over 28 weeks pregnant. Sixty-three of these cases were delivered in hospitals and died in hospitals; two patients were delivered at home and died at home—one of embolus, the other of shock. The incidence of version in Philadelphia hospitals to total hospital births for this period, was 1.52 percent. The 63 deaths following hospital version deliveries represents 6 percent of the 1,050 versions reported by all of the hospitals for the three years.

In the total of 65 fatal versions, 51 were white women and 14 negroes; 48 were native-born and 17 foreign-born. Four of the women were illegitimately pregnant. A study of the age groups showed 35, or over half, between the ages of 31 and 40 years; 9 between 21 and 30 years; and 21 under 21 years. Fifteen women were primiparas and 50 multiparas. The multiparas showed eight each in the second and third pregnancies; five in the fourth; nine in the fifth, and the remaining twenty almost equally divided in the higher parities. The position of the fetus was transverse in five, face in three, and vertex in the remainder.

Prenatal care had been adequate in only one-third of the cases. Ten women in the group had had no prenatal care. The heart was found to be abnormal ten times. The pelvis was contracted in five patients, while in fourteen the measurements were recorded as not taken or unknown. The percentage of rupture of the uterus was divided almost equally among the three groups of cases, namely: those with normal pelves, those with abnormal pelves, and those in which measurements were not recorded.

Of the 63 hospital versions, 42 women had planned admissions and 21 had emergency admissions. There were 9 cases of ruptured uterus among the 40 planned admissions and 3 among the 21 emergencies.

Among the 50 multiparas, 13 previous pregnancies had been complicated. There had been previous operative deliveries in 12 instances, which included one Cesarean and eleven forceps, four of which had been high forceps operations. Intercurrent diseases had been present in eight of the present pregnancies, while 33 had had other complications, including 11 antepartum hemorrhages, 18 albuminurias, 12 cases of high blood pressure, and 2 convulsive toxemias.

The indications, Chart No. 13, for which versions were attempted or performed in these 65 cases, were: placenta previa, 13; prolonged labor, 11; premature separation of placenta, 7; contracted pelvis, 4; disproportion, 3; errors in rotation or flexion of the head, 4; transverse position of the fetus, 3; Bandl's ring or tetanic contraction of the uterus, 3; elective version, 3; rigid birth canal, 2; attempt for live baby in dying woman, 2; heart disease, 3; influenza, 1; toxemia, 2; and 1 each for partial embryotomy by the mother; traction on scar of old suspension operation; prolapsed cord; and polyhydramnios.

The histories showed that labor was induced in fourteen of the cases, resulting in delivery by version. Four of these cases died of rupture of the uterus. Where the duration of the labor was recorded on the hospital charts, it was under 24 hours in 21 cases, over 24 hours in 23 cases, unknown in 2 and none in 8.

It was interesting to study the line of attack and the indications for version in the eight cases having no labor. Three were in lateral placenta previa, in two of which the cervix was dilated manually and immediate version and extraction performed. Two were for central placenta previa, one of which had manual dilatation; both of these versions were followed by immediate extractions. Three versions were for premature separation of the placenta, all of which were preceded by manual dilatation of the cervix. In other words, six of these cases without labor were virtually accouchement forcè.

The attendant at delivery in this group of versions was a physician in fifty-nine cases and an interne in six. One case originated in the practice of a midwife. After this patient had been in labor twenty-four hours, two physicians were called and each made an unsuccessful attempt at forceps delivery. The patient was then transferred to a hospital, where another attempt at forceps delivery failed. Delivery was then accomplished by version, but the patient died a few hours later of hemorrhage and shock. The child was stillborn.

CHART 13

PERCENTAGE DISTRIBUTION OF INDICATIONS FOR 65 VERSIONS FOLLOWED BY DEATH

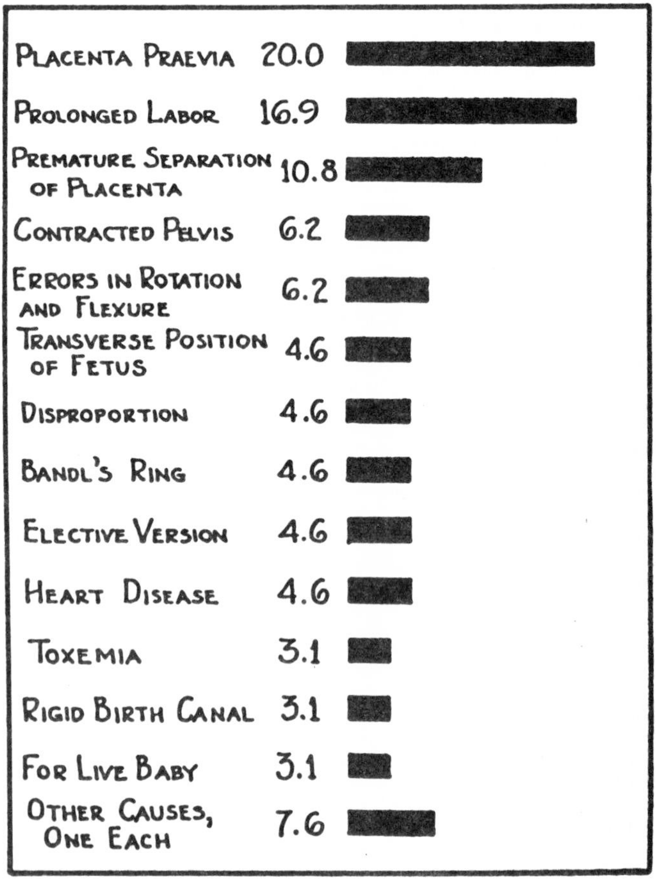

Indication	Percentage
PLACENTA PRAEVIA	20.0
PROLONGED LABOR	16.9
PREMATURE SEPARATION OF PLACENTA	10.8
CONTRACTED PELVIS	6.2
ERRORS IN ROTATION AND FLEXURE	6.2
TRANSVERSE POSITION OF FETUS	4.6
DISPROPORTION	4.6
BANDL'S RING	4.6
ELECTIVE VERSION	4.6
HEART DISEASE	4.6
TOXEMIA	3.1
RIGID BIRTH CANAL	3.1
FOR LIVE BABY	3.1
OTHER CAUSES, ONE EACH	7.6

Seven of the pregnancies were multiple. In the first instance, version was used to deliver a twin presenting by the chest with a prolapsed cord. The woman died of sepsis. In the second instance, a second twin was delivered by version because of a face presentation. The patient died of operative shock. In the third, a version was used on a second twin because of a rigid perineum. The woman died of postpartum hemorrhage. The fourth version was done on a second twin to obtain a live baby, as the woman had died of embolus. In the fifth, twins were delivered by forceps and version after a four-day labor with full dilatation for two and a half days. The woman died of sepsis. In the sixth, the first twin was delivered precipitately, a version was done on the second twin to deliver it, after due preparation. The woman died of sepsis. In the seventh, the twins were delivered by breech extraction and version to relieve strain on a damaged heart. The woman died on the fifth day of an embolus.

The cervix was manually dilated before the version in fifteen of the sixty-five deliveries considered here. Eighteen versions were preceded by other operations. One version failed and was followed successfully by forceps delivery. In these eighteen versions, four had craniotomy after the version and one had craniotomy before the version; two were followed by Cesarean section and one by hysterectomy.

The interval between birth and death was less than an hour in 12 women; from 1 to 12 hours in 23; from 12 to 24 hours in 8; 1 to 3 days in 7; 3 to 6 days in 3; over 6 days in 8, and in the remaining 4 cases the patients died during delivery. In 3 of these last 4 cases, version followed attempted forceps, and in the other a Cesarean was being performed after unsuccessful version when the patient died.

Thirty-four babies were stillborn—over 50 percent of the 65 version deaths. Operations, other than to deliver, preceded death in three cases: one drainage of abscess of right broad ligament, one supravaginal hysterectomy and one secondary repair.

The causes of death (Chart No. 14) as decided by the Analysis Committee, were as follows: Shock and rupture of the uterus, 22; sepsis, 13; placenta previa, 12; embolus and sudden death, 5; postpartum hemorrhage, 5; toxemia, 4; premature separation, 3; and non-obstetrical cause, 1. The Analysis Committee considered that the cause of death had not been certified correctly in 22 cases or 33 percent of the 65 deaths associated with version. Eight certificates were changed to shock, six to ruptured uterus, five to sepsis, and three to puerperal hemorrhage.

The Analysis Committee decided that 15 deaths were unavoidable disasters and that 50 might have been averted. Of the 50 preventable deaths, the responsibility was assigned to the physician in 43 cases and to the patient in 7. The avoidable factor in the physician's group, was error in judgment in 36 instances, and error of technic in 7. Where the responsibility was assigned to a patient, the determining element in each instance was thought to be ignorance and lack of co-operation.

Illustrative cases in which version acted as an influence in maternal mortality have been described in other sections, and will not be repeated here.

CHART 14

PERCENTAGE DISTRIBUTION OF CAUSES OF DEATH IN 65 VERSIONS

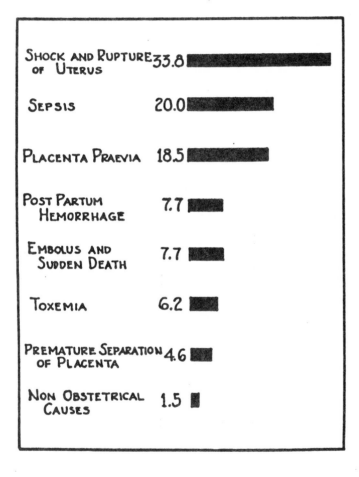

BREECH EXTRACTION OR DECOMPOSITION AND EXTRACTION AND BREECH PRESENTATIONS

During the period of the survey there was reported a total of 2,039 breech extractions or decompositions and extractions which were performed in the hospitals. This group represents an incidence of 2.9 percent of the 68,733 hospital deliveries. There were 37 deaths associated with breech presentations, 5.1 percent of the 717 cases studied. Thirteen deaths in this group of 37 cases followed breech extraction or decomposition and extraction. The causes of death in the breech presentation cases were septic abortion in one; abortion without sepsis in one; placenta previa in one; postpartum hemorrhage in two; puerperal septicemia in eight; albuminuria and eclampsia in 6; vomiting of pregnancy in two; embolus and sudden death in five; accidents of labor in eight; and non-obstetrical causes in three deaths. The causes of death in the cases where extractions were done were two deaths each from postpartum hemorrhage; albuminuria and eclampsia; vomiting of pregnancy; embolus and sudden death and accidents of labor. The remaining three of this group of thirteen died of puerperal sepsis. In eight of the thirty-seven deaths the Analysis Committee considered the death certificate incorrect as to the cause of death.

Thirty-six of the breech presentation cases died in the hospital, and one at home, all of the extraction cases died in hospitals. Thirty of the breech case deaths and eleven of the extraction case deaths were in white women. There were seven breech presentation deaths and two extraction deaths in negroes. A study of the age groups showed an almost equal division in the four age groups from 21 to 40 years. Nineteen of the deaths were in multiparas, 18 in primiparas. The deaths in this group were associated with multiple pregnancies, twins, six times. In three of these multiple pregnancies breech extractions were performed.

Three of the deaths were in illegitimately pregnant women. Twenty of the 43 children in deaths associated with breech presentation were stillborn, 9 children in the 13 breech extraction cases were stillborn. In the pregnancies of the 37 deaths discussed here prenatal care was considered adequate in 20, inadequate in 11, and was unknown in 1. There was no prenatal care in 5 cases. In the 13 cases in which extractions were done, prenatal care had been adequate in 7 and inadequate in 6. Measurements of the pelvis were normal in 18 of the 37 presentation cases and in 10 of the extraction cases. The pelvis was abnormal or deformed in 8 breech presentation cases and in one of the extraction cases. In the remaining 13, 11 cases were unknown and 2 not done.

Ten of the 13 breech extractions which were followed by death were performed by a physician and three by an interne. The 37 breech presentation cases were attended by a physician in 27 instances, by an interne in 9, and a student in 1.

The length of labor was recorded in nine histories of the breech extraction cases. In five of these labor was under 24 hours, in two over 24 hours, in one the duration of labor was recorded as unknown, and in one as none. In three histories it was recorded that labor had been induced before the breech extraction occurred. The placenta was delivered manually 5 times after the 30 breech presentation deliveries by the vaginal route in pregnancies over 28 weeks duration.

Thirty women of this group were delivered alive in pregnancies of over 28 weeks duration, and one woman died undelivered. There were six cases under 28 weeks pregnant. Of the 30 women delivered alive in pregnancies of over 28 weeks duration, 7 delivered spontaneously, 10 had Cesarean sections performed, and 13 had breech extractions. The indications for the Cesarean sections were four cases of contracted pelvis, four cases of toxemia, one case of endocarditis with decompensation, and one case of inertia uteri. The indications for the 13 breech extractions were: toxemia in 7 cases, which was associated in 1 case each of a frank breech, a monster and a twin pregnancy; cardiac disease in 2 cases; and 1 case each of a large baby, frank breech, delay in labor and dystocia.

In the 9 septic deaths in the 37 breech presentation cases, 8 were considered to have had the infection originate in the hospital, 2 of these being among the 13 breech extractions.

The Analysis Committee regarded 19 of the deaths associated with breech presentations as non-preventable, and 18 as preventable. Six of the deaths following breech extraction were regarded as non-preventable and 7 as preventable. Of the 18 preventable deaths, the responsibility was assigned to a physician in 14, and to the patient in 4. In the 7 preventable deaths following breech extraction, the responsibility was assigned to a physician in 5, and to the patient in 2.

MANUAL REMOVAL OF PLACENTA

It was disclosed in this survey that the placenta had been removed manually from the uterus forty-three times or in fifteen percent of the 286 women over twenty-eight weeks pregnant and delivered by vagina while alive. This procedure was used after twenty-four versions, seven forceps, one breech decomposition and extraction, two combined forceps and versions in two sets of twins, one craniotomy, and after eight spontaneous deliveries. Cesarean section was not included in this group.

The causes of death following the combined versions and manual removal of the placenta were: placenta previa, 8; shock, 8; postpartum hemorrhage, 2; sepsis, 2; premature separation of placenta, pneumonia, tuberculosis and toxemia, one each.

After the combined forceps and manual removal of the placenta the causes of death were: shock, 4; postpartum hemorrhage, 2; and toxemia, 1. After the multiple pregnancies, operations with added removal of the placenta, one woman died of shock and one of sepsis. The craniotomy and manual removal combination had a ruptured uterus as the cause of death. The breech extraction and manual removal case died of a postpartum hemorrhage.

Of greater interest was the group of eight deaths where the delivery was spontaneous and the placenta removed manually. All but one of these women were multiparas, all but two were over thirty years of age. The indication for the removal or extraction in six of these cases was adherent placenta, in one retained placenta, and in the remaining case no indication was given. The time interval for removal of placenta after birth varied greatly. In four it was less than an hour, in two the interval was three hours, in one seven hours, and in the last case ten hours. Death occurred in from three hours to thirteen days after delivery. In the two cases dying in three hours, one woman died from shock and the other case the one in which no indication was given for the extraction of the placenta after a thirty minute interval from birth, the death resulted from postpartum hemorrhage. Three others died of septic infection. One died of toxemia, one of secondary postpartum hemorrhage, and one of tuberculosis.

OTHER OPERATIONS TO DELIVER

CRANIOTOMY

Beside the operative deliveries just described, several others, either attempted or successful, were recorded in the obstetrical histories. Among these were four craniotomies. Prenatal care had been inadequate in all of them. In only one case was the pelvis deformed. Three patients had emergency admissions to hospitals, while the one woman who had planned an admission, failed to register until the ninth month. Her history showed she had had forceps deliveries in three of her four previous labors. All four cases having craniotomies had other operations associated with them, some of which have been discussed in other sections. Two cases had rupture of the uterus, in the third this condition was considered probable, while in the fourth, rupture of the uterus was ruled out by internal examination.

The hospital questionnaire revealed that eighteen craniotomies were done during the three years of the survey. In this particular group of four cases, one of the women died of sepsis and the others of operative shock. The Analysis Committee considered all of these four deaths preventable and the responsibility was assigned to a phyician in each instance; the determining factor being error in judgment.

LAPAROTOMY

In this series of deaths, laparotomy was performed only once and that to deliver a fetus from the abdominal cavity after rupture of the uterus. The uterus was removed. The woman, a para viii, was overdue and had had no prenatal care. Hospitalization was delayed by refusal of the patient. The Analysis Committee assigned the responsibility to the patient.

HYSTEROTOMY

Hysterotomy was performed three times; twice for nephritis and once for vomiting of pregnancy. The nephritis was regarded as influencing the onset of uremia and both of these cases were considered non-preventable.

In the vomiting of pregnancy, the determining factor was refusal of permission for operation.

MULTIPLE METHODS OF OPERATIVE DELIVERY

Multiple methods of operative delivery were used in thirty-six cases, all over twenty-eight weeks pregnant. All of the final operations were performed in hospitals and nineteen resulted in stillbirths. The pelvic measurements were recorded as normal in twenty-four of these cases, abnormal in five, unknown in four, and not taken in three.

Cesarean section was associated with other operative procedures to deliver in six deaths; forceps in twenty-seven; version in twenty-six; and craniotomy in four.

By cause of death, the three largest groups were: sepsis, eleven; operative shock, rupture of the uterus or other accidents of labor, twelve; and embolus or sudden death, five.

The Analysis Committee decided twenty-nine of these cases were preventable and seven were non-preventable. The responsibility was assigned to the physician in twenty-six of these twenty-nine cases, and to the patient in three.

RUPTURE OF THE UTERUS

During the survey, twenty-eight deaths followed rupture or perforation of the uterus. Twenty-four occurred in pregnancies over twenty-eight weeks, three under four months, and one was at the sixth month. In the three cases under four months pregnant, rupture of the uterus was due to trauma caused by the instrument used to produce abortion. The rupture occurring at six months was in a patient who had convulsions. The membranes were ruptured artificially to induce labor. Delivery was spontaneous. The patient died in shock five hours later. Autopsy showed a laceration of the cervix extending into the lower uterine segment.

In the twenty-four cases over twenty-eight weeks pregnant, there were twenty-three white women and one negro. There were six primiparas, seventeen multiparas, and the gravidity in one case was not recorded. Three of these deaths occurred in the second and third pregnancies, four in the fifth, and the remainder were distributed among higher pregnancies up to the eleventh. Only one woman was illegitimately pregnant.

Of the seventeen multiparas, seven gave a history of complications in previous pregnancies, six had a record of one or more operative deliveries, including two Cesarean sections, and the remainder showed negative histories.

Certain facts were noted in the group of twenty-four patients over twenty-eight weeks pregnant. All died in hospitals. Prenatal care was adequate in nine and inadequate or none in the other fifteen. Fifteen had planned for hospital deliveries, while nine had emergency admissions. Labor was induced in six of the cases. The length of labor was less than twenty-four hours in thirteen and over twenty-four hours in eleven. The actual time in these eleven cases was recorded as follows: under thirty hours in two; thirty-six hours in three; forty-five hours in one; fifty-four hours in one; ninety-three hours in one; one hundred and four hours in two; and one hundred and eighty hours in one. There had been no labor in one death in which rupture occurred spontaneously in late pregnancy. Only two women in this group had abnormal pelves, according to their histories; in fourteen the pelves were recorded as normal; while in the remaining eight cases no measurements were recorded. Pituitrin was used four times in this group, twice in small doses to induce labor, once in a dose of three minims in the first stage, and once in a dose of ten minims in the second stage. In this last case delivery was finally accomplished by a difficult high forceps operation. History of previous pelvic operation was recorded in only one case. This patient had had an ophorectomy and uterine suspension a year prior to the delivery.

In this group of twenty-four patients, three died undelivered and twenty-one had operative deliveries. This represents 7.9 percent of the total or 264 operative deliveries in patients over twenty-eight weeks pregnant. Of the twenty-one babies, sixteen were stillborn and five born alive.

The operations performed on these twenty-one patients for delivery included an emergency Porro-Cesarean section; nine forceps applications; twelve versions; one breech decomposition and extraction; one craniotomy; a hysterectomy and an abdominal section. As will be noted by the figures, various types of operations were combined in many cases.

The presentation of the fetus in the twenty-four women over twenty-eight weeks pregnant was face in one; breech in two; transverse in four, and vertex in the remaining seventeen. Fifteen deaths occurred within the first twenty-four hours from shock, and six in the interval between the third and seventh day, from sepsis. The infection in two of the septic cases was considered as originating in the hospital.

Operations other than for delivery were performed in three cases. In two, hysterectomy was done, but in each case death followed within three days. In the third, an exploratory laparotomy was performed and a rent in the uterus was closed. Death occurred two hours later.

Autopsies were done in seven of the twenty-four deaths of women with ruptured uteri over twenty-eight weeks pregnant. It was possible to establish a correct final diagnosis in each of these cases. In all four cases under twenty-eight weeks, autopsies were performed by coroner's physicians and the correct diagnosis made.

The Analysis Committee felt that the cause of death had been certified incorrectly in eleven cases. Three had been recorded as postpartum hemorrhage; five as various indefinite cardiac lesions such as acute myocarditis, heart failure and coronary occlusion; and the other three as *"hyperstatic"* pneumonia, intestinal paresis, and difficult labor. The clinical notes or autopsy findings were sufficient to establish the correct diagnosis of ruptured uterus.

The Analysis Committee regarded the deaths of the four cases under twenty-eight weeks as preventable and ascribed the responsibility to the patient. The avoidable factor was ignorance of the patient either in induction of abortion or in failing to obtain prenatal care.

In the twenty-four deaths over twenty-eight weeks pregnant the Analysis Committee regarded only one as non-preventable (Table No. 33),

TABLE 33

PREVENTABILITY AND RESPONSIBILITY FOR DEATHS FOLLOWING RUPTURED UTERUS

	TOTAL DEATHS*	DEATHS FOLLOWING RUPTURED UTERUS	
		Number	Percent of Total Deaths
TOTAL	425	24	5.6
Not Preventable	196	1	.5
Preventable	229	23	10.0
Responsibility Ascribed			
Physician	186	21	11.3
Patient	43	2	4.7

* Pregnancies of 28 weeks and over.

and 23 as preventable. The responsibility was assigned to the physician in twenty-one cases and to the patient in two. Concerning the physician's responsibility, error in judgment was considered the avoidable factor in eighteen cases and error in technic in three.

The following case was selected by the Analysis Committee as an example of a preventable death: A woman had had a Cesarean section in her first pregnancy for a flat pelvis with disproportion. In her second pregnancy she fell in labor at term. On admission to the hospital, she had severe, continuous abdominal pains out of proportion to the uterine contractions. The vertex was presenting and unengaged. After six hours' labor the pain became more intense; the pulse rate rose rapidly and became imperceptible; the presenting part was no longer palpable. Shock treatment was of no avail. The patient died undelivered. Autopsy revealed rupture of the uterine scar. The avoidable factor was considered error in judgment.

In another avoidable death, labor was induced at term for no stated indication. After thirty hours dilatation was complete and forceps delivery was attempted unsuccessfully on a high head. Six hours later the patient was delivered by internal podalic version. She was badly shocked and the uterus was packed. Death followed in an hour. A partial autopsy revealed a rent in the bladder and vaginal vault and a rupture of the lower uterine segment extending into the broad ligament, which was distended by an enormous hematoma.

The Analysis Committee regarded this next death as non-preventable: A multipara had had a forceps delivery in her first pregnancy. Her second delivery was spontaneous. With the present or third pregnancy, after an eight hour labor, the head reached the pelvic floor. Before prophylactic low forceps could be used the patient fainted. Delivery was accomplished, immediately following which a tear was found in the lower uterine segment on the left side. The woman died before preparation could be made for a hysterectomy. This was considered as a spontaneous rupture occurring during labor.

The Analysis Committee assigned the responsibility to the patient in the following avoidable death: A woman, illegitimately pregnant, attempted a dismemberment of the fetus with scissors at the seventh month. The resulting traumatic injury to the cervix and uterus caused her death. A rent was found as high as the fundus on the right side.

INVERSION OF UTERUS

Included in the category, "Accidents of Labor," was a small group of six cases in which death resulted from inversion of the uterus. All these deaths occurred in young native-born, white, married primiparas, at term. In one case eclamptic convulsions occurred intrapartum. In four, the delivery was accomplished by forceps, for which the indications were uterine inertia in two and prophylactic in two. The third stage was spontaneous in two cases. In four, the placenta was removed manually. The placenta was still attached to the uterine wall after inversion in two of these cases, but in the other two there was no indication on the records for manual removal.

In two cases the condition was not recognized for three hours or longer after delivery, despite the fact that hemorrhage and shock were present. Replacement of the inversion was possible four times. In one case, where inversion occurred twice in the same patient, it was not possible to replace it the second time.

Three of the women were transfused. All but one had intravenous therapy. The interval between birth of the child and death varied from three hours in three cases to nineteen hours as the longest.

In two deaths such an outstanding accident did not appear as a cause of death, either primary or contributing, on the certificates of death. The Analysis Committee regarded three of these deaths to have been preventable and three non-preventable. All the preventable deaths were decided to have been due to errors in judgment or technic on the part of a physician.

As an example of a preventable death, the Analysis Committee regarded the following case as typical: A woman was delivered by forceps by an interne, without supervision. One-half hour after delivery fundal pressure and traction on the cord precipitated an inversion. The placenta was separated about an hour later by an attending obstetrician, the inversion replaced, the uterus packed and supportive treatment continued. The death occurred three hours after delivery.

The following case was considered as an example of a non-preventable death: Following delivery by prophylactic low forceps, the uterus inverted during suture of an episiotomy. The adherent placenta and membranes were stripped off, the uterus was reinverted and packed. Intravenous saline and stimulants failed to prevent death, which occurred three hours after delivery.

The Analysis Committee regarded as a preventable death the one instance where the first and partial inversion was replaced immediately after delivery without packing the uterus. When recurrence of inversion followed, replacement was not possible and death followed in a few hours.

ACCIDENTS OF THE PUERPERIUM

Under this title there are included five deaths from puerperal psychosis or the toxemia from exhaustion consequent to it. These deaths all occurred in hospitals. The interval between birth and death ranged from fourteen days to five months. They were all considered by the Analysis Committee to have been non-preventable.

In two there was definite history of previous mental disease, one gave a history of manic depressive insanity, one recurrent amnesia. Four were native-born, white, married multipara; one was a native-born single, negro primipara. All gave birth spontaneously to living children. One only had adequate prenatal care. As factors in the previous medical history one had chronic nephritis, one chronic endocarditis, and one was syphilitic.

NON-OBSTETRICAL CAUSES OF DEATH

During the three years of the survey there were 78 maternal deaths with non-obstetrical conditions as the primary cause of death. This group formed 10.9 percent of the entire series of 717 deaths. The number of non-obstetrical conditions which were certified as contributing causes, with a puerperal primary cause of death, are shown in Table No. 14.

The largest single group of this class was pneumonia, which included 23 deaths, 16 from lobar pneumonia and 7 from bronchopneumonia. The second largest group was cardiac disease, from which 16 deaths were certified. These 16 deaths and the deaths in which cardiac disease was given as a contributory cause, have been discussed in a separate section. The next largest group was tuberculosis of the lungs, from which there were 16 deaths. This was also a contributory cause in 7 puerperal cause deaths. As a large proportion of the deaths from tuberculosis occurred either at home or in the Philadelphia General Hospital, an inquiry was made as to the admission of tuberculous pregnant women to various maternity hospitals or wards. The Philadelphia Health Council and Tuberculosis Committee supplied the information that the lack of isolation rooms in most hospitals prevents them from accepting tuberculous women for care and treatment during pregnancy. Such cases are admitted to the wards of the Philadelphia General Hospital if the tuberculosis is active and the patient is indigent. The chest department of one of the teaching hospitals is apparently the only other institution accepting such cases.

There were only four deaths in which chronic nephritis was finally considered as the primary cause of death. There were twenty-eight deaths in which chronic nephritis was certified as a contributing cause. Of these, fifteen occurred in the group of albuminuria and eclampsia deaths. After a full study of the histories in these deaths, the Analysis Committee felt that the nephritis was but an underlying factor. In other instances the nephritis was made a secondary cause through the rules of the Manual of Joint Causes of Death.

The various causes remaining in this group were medical and surgical conditions, such as one might expect to obtain in a large group of women in the reproductive period. It was difficult to assess other than obstetrical values upon these case histories. They have not, therefore, been decided upon as preventable or unavoidable, nor was the avoidable factor so clearly determined in reviewing these deaths. Prenatal care was lacking in efficiency or amount in the majority of cases where the pregnancy had reached twenty-eight weeks. The Analysis Committee often felt that the influence of the pregnancy upon disease or upon certain procedures had not been estimated sufficiently.

OPERATIONS IN NON-OBSTETRICAL GROUP

Among the cases grouped in the non-obstetrical causes of death were seven women on whom operations had been performed. Two were appendectomies, one a choledochostomy, one a rib resection, one a cauterization of the cervix, and one debridement of gangrene of lower extremity.

NON-OBSTETRICAL CAUSES OF DEATH

Title No.	Name of Disease	Number of cases
11	Influenza with respiratory complications specified.	2
11b	Influenza without respiratory complications specified.	1
17	Lethargic or epidemic encephalitis.	1
18	Epidemic cerebrospinal meningitis.	
23	Tuberculosis of respiratory system.	14
35	Gonococcus infection and other venereal diseases.	1
48	Cancer and other malignant tumors of the uterus.	1
55e	Tumors of other organs (nature unspecified).	1
55d	Tumors of brain (nature unspecified).	1
56	Acute rheumatic fever.	1
59	Diabetes mellitus.	1
82b	Cerebral embolism and thrombosis.	1
87	Other diseases of nervous system.	1

Title No.	Name of Disease	Number of cases
90	Pericarditis.	1
91	Acute endocarditis.	1
92	Chronic endocarditis, valvular diseases.	10
93	Diseases of the myocardium.	4
107	Bronchopneumonia.	7
108	Lobar pneumonia.	16
110	Pleurisy.	1
112	Asthma.	1
121	Appendicitis.	2
122b	Intestinal obstruction.	3
125	Other diseases of liver.	1
131	Chronic nephritis.	4

Total non-obstetrical deaths 78

CARDIAC DISEASE

During this survey there were 69 maternal deaths in which heart disease was a factor. In 16, heart disease was the primary cause of death, and in 53 it was secondary. This corresponds closely to the state-

CHART 15

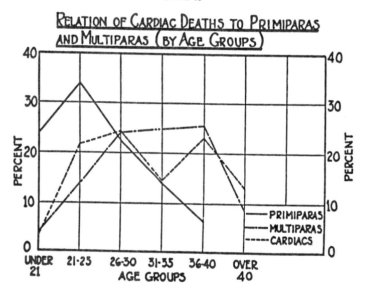

RELATION OF CARDIAC DEATHS TO PRIMIPARAS AND MULTIPARAS (BY AGE GROUPS)

CHART 16

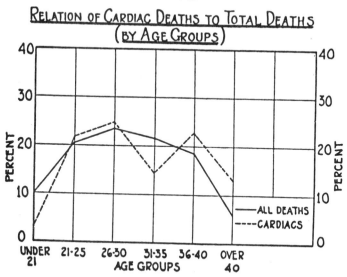

RELATION OF CARDIAC DEATHS TO TOTAL DEATHS
(BY AGE GROUPS)

ment by Herrick,[a] that one percent of all pregnancies are complicated by cardiac disease, and that six percent of these die. One percent of all the deliveries in Philadelphia, 99,579, is 995; six percent of this number is 60. This was nine percent of the total deaths in the series. The ratio of the primary cause cardiac deaths to the total non-obstetrical causes was twenty percent. The 69 cases in this survey equalled 0.4 percent of the total 15,702 deaths from heart disease in Philadelphia in the same period.

Sixty-one of the deaths occurred in white women, eight in negroes. Fifty-eight women were native-born, eleven were foreign-born. Three deaths were in illegitimate pregnancies. Two deaths occurred in women under 21 years; 15 in women from 21 to 25 years; 17 in women from 26 to 30 years; 10 in women from 31 to 35 years; 16 in women from 36 to 40 years; and 9 in women over 40 years. Charts Nos. 15 and 16. The period of gestation in relation to cardiac deaths is shown in Chart No. 17.

Forty of these women had had complications in previous pregnancies. In the present pregnancy, 10 had hypertension, 26 had edema, and 4 intercurrent diseases. The histories were noted in seven of the sixteen primary cause deaths and 14 of the 53 secondary cause deaths. The

[a] "Heart Disease in Pregnancy." W. W. Herrick, M.D. Fetal, Newborn and Maternal Morbidity and Mortality. D. Appleton-Century Co., 1933.

CHART 17

CARDIAC DEATH DISTRIBUTION (PRIMARY AND CONTRIBUTORY) BY PERIOD OF GESTATION

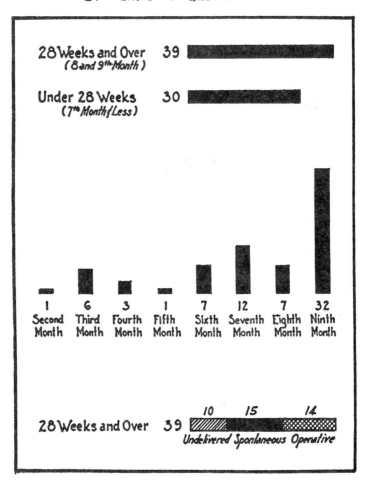

total of 21 was 30 percent of the cardiac group. Four women **gave** a history of chorea. Two women of the group in which cardiac disease was a primary cause, and 19 of the women in the group in which it was a secondary cause, had a positive diagnosis of mitral stenosis, again 30 percent of the entire cardiac group. Many of the histories were incomplete as to such details. It may be remarked in passing that in not one chart reviewed by the Analysis Committee was there recorded a classification of the cardiac lesion according to the system of the American Heart Association.

Heart disease was noted in two ways: in the history and from a physical examination. In 94 of the 717 histories the heart was recorded as abnormal. Forty-six of these cases were in the group of deaths from cardiac disease. Seventy-three women of the whole group, 717, studied in this survey, were recorded as having abnormal hearts on physical examination. Thirty-four of the heart disease deaths fell in this group. In forty-six case histories the heart was noted in both history and physical examination as being abnormal. Twenty-eight of the cardiac deaths fell in this latter group.

Prenatal care was considered adequate in 15 of the 69 cases; in 18 it was inadequate; 18 received no prenatal care; and in 18 cases there was no record.

Ten women died undelivered, 5 over and 5 under 28 weeks gestation. Thirty-four women were delivered while alive, 29 were over 28 weeks pregnant and 5 under. There were three postmortem deliveries. Thirty children were born alive, 29 were stillborn or undelivered. Labor was under 24 hours in 19, over 24 hours in 10. There was no labor in 29 cases, which included the undelivered women. There was no record in 11. Internes delivered seven women in this group. Physicians delivered 37. Thirteen of the deaths were in homes and 56 in hospitals. Fifteen were delivered spontaneously. Seventeen were delivered by Cesarean section, eight of which were elective and nine emergency operations. Four each were delivered by forceps and version and extraction. Nineteen of the 34 women delivered alive died within 24 hours of delivery.

The Analysis Committee considered 15 death certificates in the 53 contributory cause deaths as incorrect and made appropriate changes.

Four of the deaths in the group in which cardiac disease was the primary cause were thought by the Analysis Committee to have been avoidable. Responsibility was equally divided between physician and patient. In the first two deaths error in judgment, and in the last two deaths lack of co-operation were ascribed as the avoidable factor. In the group where heart disease was a contributory cause of death, 22 deaths were regarded as avoidable. In fifteen, the responsibility was assigned to a physician and in seven to the patient. In 43 cases of both groups the deaths were considered non-preventable. In 16 deaths the heart disease, by ruling of the Manual of Joint Causes of Death, became the primary cause, and assigned those deaths to the group of non-obstetrical causes.

Heart disease was a contributory cause of death in 6 septic abortions; 1 non-septic abortion; 2 ectopic pregnancies; 2 placenta previas; 6 cases of puerperal septicemia, exclusive of the septic endo- and myocarditis so frequently given as the cause of death in that condition; 10 eclampsias; 8 cases of embolus and sudden death; 16 accidents of labor, and 2 accidents of the puerperium.

The Analysis Committee regarded the following case typical of a non-preventable death: A woman with a history of rheumatic fever in childhood passed through a first pregnancy uneventfully. Because of a known heart lesion the labor was terminated with forceps. In the second pregnancy decompensation occurred in the sixth month. She was carried to term by constant rest in bed. A Cesarean section was done under local anesthesia, and a living baby obtained. Acute postoperative cardiac failure, twelve hours later, caused death.

Comment on Cardiac Disease.

Every cardiac patient should receive careful supervision during pregnancy, in order to assure the best possible health at the time of labor and puerperium. This necessitates a careful physical examination, repeated attempts at evaluation of cardiac reserve and close co-operation between obstetrician and cardiologist. A pregnant patient who goes into heart failure is a victim of neglect. "Every pregnant patient who, upon examination,[a] gives: (1) a positive etiologic history, such as acute rheumatic fever or chorea; (2) symptoms of heart disease, such as dyspnea, palpitation, edema, night starts, sighing, nose-bleeds; or (3) signs of heart disease, such as tachycardia, enlargement of the heart, venous pulsation, murmurs, whether basal or apical, systolic or diastolic, gallop rhythm or third sounds, should be referred to a cardiologist for complete diagnosis and recommendation for definite treatment."

SHOCK FOLLOWING DELIVERY

In the group of deaths classified under accidents of labor were twelve certified as due to shock of delivery. In some instances it has been difficult to ascertain whether or not certain deaths ascribed to embolus might not have been more properly included in this group. In a number of the graver traumatic puerperal injuries the associated or contributory cause of death is given as shock.

In one only of these deaths was the delivery spontaneous. In the eleven operative deliveries two only were emergency hospital admissions, the other nine were planned. Of these nine planned admissions, five only had had adequate prenatal care. The successful operative measures in eleven such cases were: forceps in three; versions in four; and Cesarean sections in four. In five cases multiple attempts were made. In one instance four separate operations were used. The indications

---

[a] "Reduction of Maternal Deaths from Heart Disease in Pregnancy." George C. Griffith, M.D. Weekly Roster and Medical Digest, August 19, 1933.

for the forceps and versions were usually exhaustion and long labor, protracted in one instance to five days. The indications for the four Cesarean sections were contracted pelvis and disproportion. In two the operation was done electively, in one after 54 hours, and in the fourth after 96 hours. In both of the latter cases classical Cesarean sections were performed.

In two instances death occurred intrapartum, the majority of deaths occurred within three hours after delivery, one woman remained alive for eighteen hours after delivery.

According to the records, hemorrhage played no part in these deaths. Eight cases were infused with saline or glucose solutions and one was transfused, along with other supportive or stimulative measures.

There were practically no complicating organic lesions or intercurrent diseases recorded in this group. One had a systolic mitral murmur on physical examination on admission and one gave a history of bronchitis in the seventh month.

Two patients in the group had no labor, two were in labor under twelve hours, three others under twenty-four hours, five over twenty-four hours. These figures may be contrasted with the indications for the various operations performed. While ether anesthesia in one and spinal anesthesia in another case may have contributed largely to the fatal termination, in the majority of instances vasomotor collapse, precipitated by trauma, and accelerated by acidosis in a few, seemed to be the cause of death. There were five multiparas in the group; of these, four had had previous operations to deliver. There were seven primiparas. Six live and six stillborn children resulted from deliveries in this group.

In four instances the Analysis Committee decided the certified cause of death did not express the true or correct cause of death. Changes were made in certificates reading "acute myocarditis" twice; "labor" and "acute cardiac failure" once.

The Analysis Committee considered that three deaths were nonpreventable, and that of the nine preventable deaths one was due to the lack of co-operation of the patient. Of the eight which were assigned to physician's responsibility, the avoidable factor in every instance was an error in judgment in the management of the case.

As an example of non-preventability in this group, the Analysis Committee regarded the following case: A primipara in good health and with a history and physical examination which were negative, had received excellent prenatal care. She entered the hospital in labor at term. After eighteen hours delivery of a live child occurred. The third stage was normal, slight perineal laceration was repaired and no hemorrhage noted. Within an hour the patient developed a rapid pulse, drop in blood pressure and weakness and pallor. Stimulative measures with intravenous therapy were of no avail and patient died four hours after delivery. Partial autopsy revealed no pelvic pathology. The absence of respiratory distress and cyanosis ruled out embolus in the opinion of the Analysis Committee.

The Analysis Committee_regarded as an example of a preventable death with error in judgment as the avoidable factor the following case: A primipara with adequate prenatal care entered a hospital in labor at term. Pelvic measurements indicated possibility of Cesarean section. After twenty-four hours in labor, with the membranes ruptured, the cervix was dilated manually. The head was noted as being engaged. Forceps were applied, but failed. Version was attempted, but failed. Craniotomy was performed, but after the head was made smaller the shoulders were found locked in the bony pelvic obstruction. A classical Cesarean section was then performed. Death occurred shortly afterward.

Another example of a preventable death was that of a woman with a contracted flat pelvis who had been in labor at term for twenty-four hours. Manual dilatation of the cervix and the membranes ruptured. The head was not engaged. Version was attempted but failed. The head was fixed in the inlet by pressure while axis traction forceps were applied. A stillborn child was delivered with difficulty. Death occurred within two hours of delivery with symptoms of shock. There was no autopsy.

There was only one death in which the patient was held responsible for prevention. This was the case of a woman who had not seen a physician before her admission to the hospital after having been twenty-four hours in labor. After being examined she signed her release and went home. On readmission she was found to have a transverse position, for which she permitted a version to be performed. She died in shock one hour after delivery. An autopsy was not permitted, but examination revealed no rupture of uterus.

SYPHILIS

The histories reviewed during this survey showed that twenty of the 717 cases were syphilitic, a much smaller percentage than might have been expected, in view of the number of deaths in negroes. There were nine white women and eleven negroes in this group. Eight were illegitimately pregnant. Six were in their first pregnancy and fourteen were multiparas. Of the latter, nine had from one to five living children. Fourteen were over and six under twenty-eight weeks pregnant. Four of the former group had stillborn infants.

The causes of death in this group were puerperal in fourteen cases; six deaths were from septic infection; two from hemorrhages; one from toxemia; five from other puerperal accidents; and six from non-obstetrical causes; two from arsphenamin shock; two from cerebral syphilis; one from cerebral embolus, and one from tuberculosis.

Prenatal care had been inadequate in all of these cases. In seven the diagnosis of syphilis was made clinically, in one skin lesions were present. In thirteen the Wassermann reaction ranged from weakly positive to four plus. Treatment had been instituted in but five of the fourteen women over twenty-eight weeks pregnant at the time of their deaths. In one, one injection of neoarsphenamin had been given a few days before a macerated fetus and placenta were expelled. This was followed by death from postpartum hemorrhage. In four deaths the fatal outcome appeared to have more than a casual connection with the treatment. In one instance a multipara had a weakly positive reaction found on routine admission examination at clinic. She gave a history of four living children born spontaneously. She had a moderately elevated blood pressure and slight albuminuria and a systolic murmur at the apex. One month after registering she received 0.45 neoarsphenamin, after which she felt nauseated and dizzy. One week later she received 0.6 neoarsphenamin. The following night she was admitted with a history of persistent headache and vomiting. Icterus was present. Spinal tap reduced pressure from 44 to 20 mgm. Further supportive and eliminative measures were carried out during the next day and a stillborn infant was delivered. Gradual coma developed and was followed by death forty-eight hours after the second injection of neoarsphenamin.

In a second instance, a multipara who had given birth to three living children had a faintly positive Wassermann reaction in her sixth month. She received two injections of neoarsphenamin, 0.3 and 0.6, a week apart. Two days after the second injection she was admitted mentally disoriented. Convulsions followed during the ensuing labor. A live baby was delivered by low forceps as the woman died. Autopsy disclosed a syphilitic encephalitis and gumma of the brain. The cause of death in one of the other two treated cases was considered arsphenamin shock and the other as cerebral thrombosis with hemiplegia. One woman had positive reactions and was being treated with injections of neoarsphenamin.

Comment on Syphilis.

Syphilis (per se) plays little part in maternal mortality. Its influence, however, may be a decided factor in producing other and more immediate hazards. A routine Wassermann test should be made at one of the early prenatal examinations. If the syphilitic patient is properly treated early enough in her pregnancy, she will usually give birth to a non-infected child. The treatment of syphilis in the pregnancy necessitates a fine sense of discrimination as to choice of method. This depends largely on the duration of pregnancy, the stage of the disease, and the physical condition of the patient. No definite rules can be advocated for the treatment of syphilis in pregnancy.

PYELITIS AND PYELONEPHRITIS

The Title Number 146, Puerperal Albuminuria and Eclampsia, of the International List of Causes of Death, includes pyelitis of pregnancy and pyelonephritis of pregnancy. In some respects this inclusion appears as a misnomer, since the toxemias are generally regarded as degenerative or toxic manifestations, while pyelitis is considered as a bacterial infection with different symptomatology. During the period of the survey pyelitis or pyelonephritis was recorded as a primary or contributing cause of death or an intercurrent disease in twenty-one deaths.

Eight of these deaths occurred in primiparas, thirteen in multiparas. Sixteen of the women were white and five negroes. The age group study proved irrelevant. Prenatal care had been adequate in two, inadequate in twelve, none in six, and unknown in one case. There were other complications in eleven of these cases. Fourteen women were over twenty-eight weeks pregnant, four of whom had stillbirths, and seven women were under twenty-eight weeks pregnant. Nineteen of the women died in the hospital, two at home. In one of the cases in which the woman died at home, the pyelitis was regarded as the focus of origin of a fatal septicemia. In the other case the woman died undelivered. She had been in the hospital under treatment for pyelitis for seventeen days, she signed a release, went home and died two days later.

The primary causes of death in which pyelitis was present were as follows: Puerperal sepsis, 10; septic abortion, 4; vomiting of pregnancy, 2; and one each of puerperal albuminuria and eclampsia, embolus and sudden death, accidents of labor, bronchopneumonia and lobar pneumonia. Of the fourteen women with pyelitis who were delivered alive and over twenty-eight weeks pregnant, ten had spontaneous deliveries and four operative deliveries. Of the seven cases under twenty-eight weeks pregnant, three aborted spontaneously, three had therapeutic abortions for this or other indications, and one woman died undelivered.

In the medical histories of these cases, it was recorded in the past history that the kidneys were normal in sixteen, abnormal in four, and unknown in one. The urine was studied by culture in but five of these twenty-one cases. The results obtained were as follows: B. Coli, 2; streptococcus viridans, 2; no growth, 1. In eight cases cultures were made from the blood with the following results: S. albus and B. diptheroid, 2; hemolytic streplococci, 1; hemolytic S. albus, 1; S. aureus, 1; pneumococcus, 1; and no growth, 2.

The onset of these renal pelvic infections dated, where recorded in fourteen histories, from seven days to six weeks before abortion or birth.

Comment on Pyelitis and Pyelonephritis.

The frequent association of puerperal septicemia and septic abortion with pyelitis, which is 66 percent of this series of 21 cases, suggests that a more than casual coincidence was present. In one of the articles on maternal mortality published in the *Roster* in 1932, Dr. Charles Wachs made the following statement: "Such cases (pyelitis in pregnancy) should be considered as potentially infected and in those cases at least in which operative interference may be required, an effort should be made to sterilize the urinary tract and thus destroy a focus from which possible future bacterial invasions may occur."[9]

---

[9] "Infections of the Urinary Tract in Pregnancy and Puerperium." Dr. Charles Wachs. Weekly Roster and Medical Digest, Phila. Co. Med. Soc., December 3, 1932.

DEATHS IN UNDELIVERED WOMEN

There were ninety-one women in this series of 717 who died undelivered or unoperated upon. Forty-one were under 28 weeks pregnant and 50 were over 28 weeks pregnant. Of the whole series, 12.6 percent died undelivered. Of the deaths in women over 28 weeks pregnant, 11.7 percent were in women undelivered. Of all the puerperal causes of death, 9.7 percent were undelivered women. There were approximately three white women to each negro and the same proportion in native and foreign born. Six women were illegitimately pregnant. Prenatal care was considered adequate for 22 women or 25 percent. A number of causes of death referred to cardiac conditions. It is noted that the heart was found abnormal in ten cases on physical examination, while a history of heart disease was found in fourteen records. A study of the age groups, gravidities and months of pregnancy showed nothing of value.

Forty-nine of these women had complications of pregnancy, 29 others had intercurrent diseases. Seventy-five died in the hospital, fourteen died at home. Of the 40 women over twenty-eight weeks pregnant who died undelivered in the hospital, 17 entered before labor. Of these, 4 were planned and 13 were emergency admissions.

Two deaths were listed under septic abortion, 2.2 percent. The sepsis caused death before expulsion of a four months fetus in each case. One death occurred from hemorrhage in a non-septic abortion, 1.1 percent, before the uterus was emptied in a five months pregnancy. Three deaths, 3.3 percent, were listed under placenta previa, and two, 2.2 percent, under premature separation of the placenta. Seven ectopic pregnancies, 7.7 percent, died unoperated upon. Twenty-two women died of albuminuria and convulsions, 24.2 percent. Ten died of vomiting of pregnancy, 10.9 percent; 6 of embolus and sudden death, 6.6 percent. Nine died of accidents of labor, 9.9 percent. Twenty-nine died of non-obstetrical causes, 31.9 percent, of whom nine were listed as some type of cardiac death.

In nineteen of this group of undelivered women, operation to deliver had been attempted prior to death as follows: forceps, 9; version, 3; breech extraction, 1; emergency Cesarean section, 9. In five instances the operative procedures were multiple. Twenty of the fifty women dying when over twenty-eight weeks pregnant had postmortem deliveries, as did one under twenty-eight weeks. Autopsies were performed in nineteen instances.

Spinal anesthesia was used once in this series. Death followed immediately after injection of the solution. In eight other cases the anesthesia was gas and ether, and in ten cases there was no anesthesia. The length of labor was noted in fourteen histories and was over twenty-four hours in nine of these.

The Analysis Committee regarded twenty-one causes of death, as certified, as not agreeing with the true cause of death. This was decided after a careful study of the records. In forty-seven cases the Analysis

Committee regarded death as non-preventable, in the remaining forty-four the death was considered preventable. Of this latter group, twenty-four were considered as instances where the responsibility should be assigned to a physician, and eighteen to the patient.

MULTIPLE PREGNANCIES

There were nineteen twin pregnancies among the 717 histories reviewed. If the normal proportion of twin pregnancies, two percent, had occurred in the 99,579 births in Philadelphia during the survey, there would have been 1,989. The incidence of maternal deaths among twin pregnancies was one percent. The causes of death in the five cases under twenty-eight weeks pregnant were: septic abortion, 2; pernicious vomiting, 1; encephalitis, 1; and heart disease, 1. In the fourteen deaths of women over twenty-eight weeks pregnant, the causes of death were: various accidents of labor, 5; toxemia, 4; septic infection, 3; embolus and sudden death, 1; and accidents of puerperium, 1.

Eight of the women were multiparas and eleven were primiparas. Eleven were delivered in hospitals, three at home, one of whom was referred to a hospital for further treatment. The hospital delivery was planned for nine of the women who died there, five were emergency admissions.

The delivery was accomplished by Cesarean section twice, one elective and one emergency. Forceps were used four times, version seven times, breech extraction three times. There were sixteen operations to deliver the twenty-eight babies. The placenta was extracted manually three times. The duration of labor was recorded in thirteen cases. It was over twenty-four hours in two, under twenty-four hours in eight, and there was no labor in three. Labor was induced twice, three times it was followed by a postpartum hemorrhage. A physician was the attendant in nine and an interne in five of the fourteen deaths in women over twenty-eight weeks pregnant. Twelve sets of twins were born alive, five sets dead, and one succumbed in each of the other two. Complications occurred in fourteen pregnancies, twice convulsive toxemias were present. It is not without interest to note that sepsis following elective version to deliver the second twin caused two deaths in this group.

PUERPERAL MORTALITY IN RELATION TO STILLBIRTHS

During the period of the survey, 4,185 stillbirths were registered in a total of 99,579 births in Philadelphia, making a stillbirth rate of 42 per 1,000 total births. The death rate among women who had stillbirths, 230 to 4,185, was 55 per 1,000 births, as contrasted with a general maternal mortality rate during the survey of 7 per 1,000 births—almost eight times as great. In the 84,470 white births there were 3,198 stillbirths, a rate of 37.8 per 1,000. In the 15,109 negro births there were 987 stillbirths, a rate of 65.3 per 1,000. The ratio of negro to white stillbirth rate was as 1.7 to 1. In the 3,885 illegitimate births there were 234 stillbirths, a rate of 60 per 1,000. In the 95,694 legitimate pregnancies there were 3,951 stillbirths, a rate of 41.2 per 1,000. The ratio between illegitimate and legitimate was as 1.5 to 1.

In the ordinarily accepted sense a stillbirth is one in which the fetus does not breathe or show other evidence of life. There is no one factor in maternal mortality statistics which varies so greatly as the definition of this term. Although it is not entirely germane to the subject of this inquiry, the proper definition of a stillbirth is one which merits the attention of those who are concerned with the statistics of maternity practice. Miller[10] sums up the situation very well in stating that in measuring the quality of maternity care by the uneven standards of vital statistics, a step forward would be made in defining as a stillbirth, "the birth of a dead fetus which had reached at least the twenty-eighth week or which measures 13.8 inches (35 cm.)." From the standpoint of good or bad obstetric care more can be learned from a study of the results obtained after the period of viability of the fetus has been reached. From the standpoint of the stillborn child Gagnon[11] pointedly remarks: "What is important to know in the case of a stillbirth is, not the cause of death, but why the child was born dead." The certificate of birth for Pennsylvania (form V. S. No. 11) defines a stillborn child as one that neither breathes nor shows other evidence of life after birth. The State of Pennsylvania requires a certificate regarding the birth, live or stillborn, for every fetus born after the fourth month of pregnancy. Accepting this legal requirement by period of gestation in this survey, there were 202 women who either died before the birth of the fetus or bore a dead fetus after the fourth month. In examining the records of the women who died undelivered or bore a dead fetus, it was found that eighteen were in the fifth month, thirty-one in the sixth month, twenty-one in the seventh month, twenty-seven in the eighth month, and one hundred and five in the ninth month or at term. Dividing the figures for stillbirths by the twenty-eighth week of pregnancy, there were forty-nine under twenty-eight weeks and one hundred and fifty-three over twenty-eight weeks.

Of the stillbirths, 163 occurred in the 597 white women of the series. 39 in the 120 negroes. One hundred and fifty-nine were in the 565 native-born women and 43 in the 143 foreign-born. In the age groups, 27 were in women under 21 years; 34 in 146 women from 21 to 25 years; 35 in 169 women from 26 to 30 years; 43 in 154 women from 31 to 35 years; 43 in 135 women from 36 to 40 years; and 20 in 41 women over 40 years.

Seventy were in the 241 primiparas, 132 among the 476 multiparas of the whole series, 56 in the 155 primiparas over 28 weeks pregnant, and 97 among the 270 multiparas over 28 weeks pregnant. Among the 78 non-obstetrical causes of death, 30 had associated stillbirths. Syphilis was present in only four mothers of the 202 who had stillbirths.

---

[10] "Can Vital Statistics Be Used to Measure the Quality of Maternity Care?" J. R. Miller. Trans. Am. Assn. Obst. Gyn. and Ab. Surg., 1931, 287.
[11] "What Is a Stillbirth?" E. Gagnon. Can. Health Jour., 1931, xxii, 16.

One hundred and nine of the 375 women who died after being delivered alive after the twenty-eighth week had stillborn children. Twenty-three of the 133 women over 28 weeks pregnant, who died after spontaneous delivery, had stillborn children; as did 85 of the 242 who were delivered by operation while alive. Of the 96 Cesarean sections in women who died, 25 had associated stillbirths; of the 112 forceps deaths there were 42 stillbirths; of the 65 version deaths, 34 stillbirths; of the 13 breech extraction or decomposition and extraction deaths, 10 stillbirths; of the 36 deaths associated with multiple operations to deliver 19 stillbirths. Of the two cases of hysterectomy to deliver, one was associated with a stillbirth; one case of abdominal section to deliver, ruptured uterus was associated with a stillbirth.

Physicians were associated in the origin of the delivery (pregnancies of over 28 weeks duration) of 127 stillbirths, internes in 17, students in 2, midwives in 4, other attendants in 1, and no attendant in 2.

In the deaths of the mothers of these 153 stillborn children, the Analysis Committee regarded a physician responsible in 66 cases, the patient in 28, and found 59 deaths to have been non-preventable. Only 56 of the 153 mothers whose deaths were associated with stillbirths had had adequate prenatal care, while lack of prenatal care was considered the avoidable factor by the Analysis Committee in but 11 of the other 97. These deaths were all associated with pregnancies of over 28 weeks duration.

Comment on Stillbirths.

The maternal mortality in women with stillbirths is excessively high. In the negro race and in the illegitimately pregnant women the stillbirth rate is much higher than in the white women and the married women. The majority of stillbirths occur at term. Operative delivery, which is followed by maternal death, carried a tremendous risk for the fetus. The theoretical preventability of the maternal deaths associated with stillbirths was 61 percent. Although but one-third of the cases had had adequate prenatal care, inadequate prenatal care was an almost negligible avoidable factor in the death of the mother. It must therefore be considered that operative interference, often the cause of stillbirths, was of considerable influence in the maternal mortality associated with them.

DEFORMED PELVES

Forty-seven (11%) of the 425 women over 28 weeks pregnant who died during the survey had contracted pelves. In over 100 of these 425 patients the measurements were either not taken or not recorded (30 "unknown," 74 "not done"). The contracted pelves occurred in the following proportions: 12 were in negroes, or 10 percent of the negro deaths of the whole series; 11 in foreign-born women; 21 in primiparas and 26 in multiparas. Among the multiparas sixteen had had previous operative deliveries ranging from one to six forceps deliveries in some cases, to two previous Cesareans in one case. Of these sixteen cases with previous operative deliveries, the majority had had inadequate prenatal care and died of sepsis.

Prenatal care was reported as adequate for 25 women with contracted pelves; 11 of whom died of sepsis, and 5 of accidents of labor. The incidence of sepsis was practically the same in cases with adequate prenatal care (44%) and in cases with inadequate or no prenatal care (40%). The attendant at delivery was a practicing physician in 42 cases of the 47 with contracted pelves; internes attended four and a student one. Forty-three patients were delivered and died in hospitals; three were delivered at home and died in hospitals; and one woman was delivered at home and died at home. Thirty-eight women had planned hospital admissions and five were emergencies.

The presentation of the fetus was vertex in 37 cases; breech in 7; and transverse in 3. Labor was under 24 hours in 12 patients; over 24 hours in 17; in 8 the duration of labor was not recorded; and in 10 there was no labor. Five women died undelivered and there were three postmortem deliveries.

Forty-two women with contracted pelves were delivered while alive, 37 by operation and 5 spontaneously. Of the 37 operative deliveries, 16 died of sepsis. Twenty-seven of the operative deliveries were Cesarean sections, 16 elective and 11 emergency.• Forceps were used 12 times, version five times, craniotomy but once, and in five cases the operations were multiple. Eleven of the infants or 24 percent in this group were born dead.

The principal cause of death, where contracted pelvis was a complication, was sepsis. Of the 47 deaths in this group, 20 or 42.5 percent were due to septicemia. The Analysis Committee felt that the infection arose in the hospital in 17 of these 20 cases. In nine of the 19 certificates that were incorrectly made out the cause of death was changed to sepsis.

The Analysis Committee considered 32 of the 47 deaths in this group as preventable. Of these, 29 were regarded as having been due to 17 errors in judgment and 12 errors in technic on the part of a physician.

ABNORMAL PRESENTATIONS OF FETUS

In the obstetrical histories of the deaths reviewed during this survey the position or presentation of the fetus was vertex in 377 cases, breech in 37, transverse in 14, face in 3, and unknown in 8; a total of 439 in the 425 deaths of women over 28 weeks pregnant. This total includes 14 twin pregnancies. It was observed by the Analysis Committee that in 93 of the 377 vertex presentations, almost 25 percent, that the avoidability of the death rested with the physician.

In the group of 37 breech presentations, 19 of the deaths of women were considered as non-preventable.. The remaining number, 18, were regarded as preventable, with the responsibility assigned to a physician in 14 and to the patient in 4. In the former group the determining factors were considered: nine errors in judgment, four errors in technic, and in one case lack of prenatal care. In the latter group, the patient's lack of co-operation in two and lack of prenatal care in two made up the elements of avoidability.

In regard to the 14 transverse presentations, 10 were considered as preventable and 4 as non-preventable. To the physician was assigned the responsibility for nine of these deaths, in five due to errors in judgment, in four because of undoubted errors in technic. Lack of co-operation on the part of the patient became the factor of avoidability in the last one of this group of ten preventable deaths.

All three of the deaths connected with face presentations were regarded by the Analysis Committee as preventable and due to errors in judgment on the part of a physician in two instances, and to an error in technic in one instance.

POST-MORTEM EXAMINATIONS

Autopsies were performed after 228 or 31.7 percent of all the deaths in this survey. Nine autopsies were done on patients who died at home, the remaining 219 on patients who died in hospitals. Two hundred and thirty-nine or 33.3 percent of the 717 deaths were coroner's cases. In this group, 123 had no autopsies; 88 had autopsies performed by the coroner's physicians and 28 had autopsies done by hospital pathologists.

The proportion of autopsies to the various causes of death is shown in Table No. 34. The Analysis Committee felt that the cause of death was incorrectly stated in 51 of the 228 cases having postmortem examinations. In other words, in spite of the autopsy examinations, 22.3 per-

TABLE 34

AUTOPSIES AND ERRORS ON DEATH CERTIFICATES BY CAUSE OF DEATH

	Number Deaths	Autopsies		Errors on Death Certificate*	
		Number	Percent	Number	Percent
TOTAL	717	228	31.8	51	22.4
Septic Abortion	162	95	58.6	15	15.8
Abortion Without Sepsis	26	7	26.9	2	28.6
Ectopic Gestation	33	11	33.3	4	36.4
Premature Separation of Placenta	12	2	16.7	0	....
Placenta Prævia	12	3	25.0	2	66.7
Postpartum Hemorrhage	27	6	22.2	3	50.0
Puerperal Sepsis	119	36	30.2	11	30.6
Albuminuria and Convulsions	85	19	22.4	1	5.3
Vomiting of Pregnancy	24	4	16.6	1	25.0
Embolus and Sudden Death	44	4	9.1	2	50.0
Accidents of Labor	79	19	24.1	4	21.0
Accidents of Puerperium	5	2	40.0	1	50.0
Non-Obstetrical	78	20	25.6	5	23.8

*Autopsied Cases.

cent of these death certificates failed to express the correct cause of death. As had been stated previously, acute yellow atrophy of the liver was not proven at autopsy in any case, although the condition had been so diagnosed and recorded on the death certificate in some instances.. In the 44 cases listed under 148 as embolus and sudden death, there were only four autopsies performed to substantiate the clinical diagnosis.' Four postmortem examinations were made on the 30 women who died undelivered, and four on the 20 women who were delivered after death.

CORONER'S CASES

There were 239 deaths in this series in which the death certificates were signed by the Coroner of Philadelphia. In the terminology of the record room, they were Coroner's cases as defined by law. Of these deaths, 71 were in pregnancies of 28 weeks duration, or over, and 168 were in pregnancies under 28 weeks. As the Coroner's office has the privilege of performing autopsies on such cases to determine the cause of death, the cases were reviewed as regards autopsies.

There were no autopsies in 123 of the 239 deaths. In 88 cases an autopsy was done at the City Morgue and in 28 the autopsy was done at the hospital. As many of the 168 cases under 28 weeks were septic abortions, it is of note that 63 had had no autopsy. In 85 an autopsy was done at the City Morgue, and in 20 the autopsy was done at the hospital.

In the 71 deaths in pregnancies over 28 weeks which became Coroner's cases, there were no autopsies in 55. In 8 instances the autopsies were done at the City Morgue and 8 more were done in the hospital. The autopsies done at the City Morgue were performed by physicians attached to the Coroner's office. In no instance was there a record of a report having been returned to the hospital where the death occurred. It is within the province and privilege of the Coroner's office to permit, by release, an autopsy by the staff pathologist at the hospital where the death occurs. Until this becomes a well-established custom in puerperal deaths, little of scientific value will be learned of the great majority of the puerperal deaths in Philadelphia hospitals which become the subject of the interest of the Coroner's office.

CHILDREN WHO SURVIVED THE DEATHS OF MOTHERS OVER TWENTY-EIGHT WEEKS PREGNANT

The death of a mother is more than a serious personal loss and frequently develops into a family catastrophe. How serious the results will be depends in a large measure on the background of a family. The effect on the husbands and surviving children presents an appalling thought.

Of the 425 women with pregnancies of 28 weeks duration or over, 335 left living children, 69 left no children, and for 21 no facts were available. There were 947 surviving children of these mothers, an average of 2.83. Of these, 272, 28.7 percent, were new-born infants, 103 being left by primiparas (Tables Nos. 35 and 36).

These orphaned children in almost all instances were from normal families and practically all of the new-born children were legitimate.

TABLE 35

NUMBER OF CHILDREN SURVIVING AT DEATH OF MOTHER

(Pregnancies of 28 Weeks and Over)

Surviving Children	Families	Total Children
TOTAL	425	947
Unknown	21	...
None	69	...
One	128	128
Two	69	138
Three	36	108
Four	30	120
Five	28	140
Six	19	114
Seven	11	77
Eight	9	72
Nine and Over*	5	50

*Three mothers left 9 children; one left 10; and one left 13.

TABLE 36

SURVIVING CHILDREN BY AGE GROUPS OF MOTHERS

(Pregnancies of 28 Weeks and Over)

Age Group	Total Deaths	Number Leaving Children	Children Left
TOTAL	425	335	947
TOTAL 35 YEARS AND UNDER	308	235	529
UNDER 21	41	25	29
21-25	79	57	87
26-30	98	79	162
31-35	90	74	251
TOTAL OVER 35 YEARS	117	100	418
36-40	94	80	310
Over 40	23	20	108

Three hundred and nineteen of the 335 mothers who died leaving children were married; 16, 4.8 percent, were "single" (including divorced and widowed). The children of these single women number only 29, 3.1 percent of the total 947 living children.

No figures are available as to the age of these children. The conclusion that a large percentage were young can be drawn from the age of the mothers at the time of death. Seventy percent of the women leaving children were under 36 years of age. These women left 526, 55.8 percent of the children. It is probable, in view of the size of the families left by the older women, that a large percentage of the children were also young. The effect of these deaths on the families and on the community cannot be measured. The above tables give the number of deaths, the number of deaths of women leaving children, and the number of surviving children. It is impossible to tell in how many families community help, either in solving the problem or in the care of the children, will become necessary. Certainly in 335 cases, more than 100 each year in which living children were left, a serious readjustment of plans was necessary if a family catastrophe was to be avoided. It is difficult to estimate the effects on the home life of these children who will grow up without a mother.

PLACE OF DELIVERY AND PLACE OF DEATH

Of the 717 deaths reviewed, 647 occurred in hospitals and 70 at home. There were 425 deaths in women over 28 weeks pregnant, of which number 320 were delivered in hospitals, 55 at home, and 50 died undelivered. Of these 320 hospital deliveries, 317 women died in hospitals and 3 at home. Of the 55 deaths following home deliveries, 32 occurred at home and 23 in hospitals. The classfication of the causes of death to the place of delivery appears in Table No. 37.

TABLE 37

CAUSE OF DEATH BY PLACE OF DELIVERY
(PREGNANCIES OF 28 WEEKS AND OVER)

CAUSE OF DEATH	TOTAL DELIVERED	DELIVERED WHILE ALIVE		POST MORTEM DELIVERY	
		Home	Hospital	Home	Hospital
TOTAL	395	55	320	2	18
Premature Separation of Placenta	9	..	9	...	..
Placenta Prævia	20	..	19	...	1
Postpartum Hemorrhage ...	27	5	22	...	..
Sepsis	119	21	98	...	..
Albuminuria and Eclampsia .	59	6	49	...	4
Vomiting of Pregnancy	5	..	5	...	..
Embolus and Sudden Death.	38	8	26	2	2
Accidents of Labor	75	7	61	...	7
Accidents of Puerperium ...	5	1	4	...	..
Non-Obstetrical	38	7	27	...	4

The 55 deaths which followed home delivery represent 12.9 percent of the 425 deaths in pregnancies over 28 weeks duration. The 320 deaths which followed hospital delivery represent 75 percent of the 425 deaths in pregnancies over 28 weeks duration. The 50 deaths in undelivered women represent 12.1 percent.

There were then 55 deaths following 29,154 home live births in the three years, a rate of 1.88 per 1,000 live births. There were 320 deaths following 65,626 hospital live births in the three years, a rate of 4.87 per 1,000 live births. If the hospital deliveries could be separated into planned or booked cases and emergency cases, a more impartial division of rates would be obtained. In view of the progressive increase in hospital deliveries, as shown in Graph No. 1, there can be little doubt that most of this increase is due to normal or planned admissions. Nevertheless, hospitals must continue to submit to the unfair criticism that the major proportion of maternal deaths occurs in institutions, regardless of the fact that many are emergency cases. Hospital maternal mortality rates could be corrected if it were possible to show the relation between the type of admission, whether planned or emergency, and the non-obstetrical deaths.

TABLE 38

CLASSIFICATION OF ATTENDANT AT DELIVERY IN
PREGNANCIES OF 28 WEEKS DURATION, OR OVER,
WHICH WERE FOLLOWED BY DEATH

ATTENDANT	TOTAL DELIVERIES	LIVE BIRTHS	STILL BIRTHS
General Practitioner	123	83	40
Obstetrician and Gynecologist	77	56	21
Obstetrician	65	40	25
Interne	55	43	12
Unattended (Self Delivered)	13	12	1
Surgeon	9	7	2
Gynecologist	8	6	2
Resident Obstetrician	8	3	5
Midwife	5	5	0
Osteopath	4	4	0
Healer	3	3	0
Student	2	1	1
Nurse	2	1	1
Pediatrician	1	1	0
	375	265	110

CLASSIFICATION OF ATTENDANT AT DELIVERY IN PREGNANCIES OF 28 WEEKS' DURATION, OR OVER, WHICH WERE FOLLOWED BY DEATH

In each maternal death a record was kept of the type of person actually in attendance at delivery, whether physician, nurse, midwife, healer, other or none. If the attendant was a physician, the classification of his specialty in practice was obtained from the directory of the American Medical Association. Some physicians held appointments as junior obstetricians in certain hospitals, yet if they were classified in the directory as general practitioners, they were so regarded and listed. This method of classification seemed to lead to more accuracy, because, if a physician was a very recent appointee, he might have had little more experience than an interne or resident physician. Table No. 38 shows the attendant for the 375 cases over 28 weeks pregnant, delivered prior to death.

Of the 50 women who died undelivered in pregnancies of 28 weeks duration or over, the attendant during the fatal illness was as follows:

Obstetrician and Gynecologist	24
Obstetrician	10
General Practitioner	10
Internist	2
Gynecologist	1
Surgeon	1
Dermatologist	1
Laryngologist	1

Postmortem deliveries were performed on 20 of these 50 patients who died undelivered.

CLASSIFICATION OF PHYSICIANS TO WHOM DEATHS WERE ASSIGNED

All of the deaths in pregnant women were assigned to specific physicians, regardless of whether these deaths were obstetrical or non-obstetrical, preventable or unavoidable. The attendant at delivery was not necessarily the person to whom the case was assigned. Some patients were undelivered, some had no attendant at delivery, and a few were delivered by healers, or at times a member of the family. For various reasons it was obviously impossible to make accurate assignment in each case, but the following is a list of the types of physicians who were responsible ultimately for the care of these patients or to whom the death was assigned:

Type of Physician	*No. of Physicians*	*No. of Patients*
General Practitioners	130	175
Obstetricians and Gynecologists	46	275
General Surgeons	29	55
Obstetricians	27	111
Internists	21	26

Type of Physician	No. of Physicians	No. of Patients
Gynecologists	12	45
Otolaryngologists	8	9
Osteopaths	3	4
Pediatricians	2	2
Neurologists	2	2
Dermatologists	2	2
Roentgenologists	2	3
Urologists	1	2
Proctologists	1	1
Pathologists	1	1

This classification of physicians was obtained from the Directory of the American Medical Association.

These figures are of no value unless they are carefully analyzed. For instance, the death attributed to a pathologist was due to arsphena-mine shock. The two cases assigned to neurologists were non-obstetrical cases. The relation of the attendant at delivery in pregnancies of 28 weeks duration or over, to the causes of death are shown in Table No. 39.

TABLE 39

ATTENDANT AT DELIVERY BY CAUSE OF DEATH
(PREGNANCIES OF 28 WEEKS AND OVER)

	TOTAL	PHYSICIAN	INTERNE	STUDENT	MIDWIFE CONTACT	OTHERS NONE AND UNKNOWN
TOTAL	395	306	58	2	10	19
Premature Separation of Placenta	9	7	2	...	..	..
Placenta Prævia	20	18	1	...	1	..
Postpartum Hemorrhage	27	17	7	...	3	..
Sepsis	119	92	15	2	2	8
Albuminuria and Eclampsia	59	44	7	...	1	7
Vomiting of Pregnancy	5	4	1	...	..	..
Embolus and Sudden Death	38	30	6	...	2	..
Accidents of Labor	75	65	8	...	1	1
Accidents of Puerperium	5	3	2	...	..	..
Non-Obstetrical	38	26	9	...	..	3

MIDWIVES

During the period of this survey midwives delivered a total of 3,818 women. These figures were obtained from the Bureau of Medical Education of the State of Pennsylvania. According to the Bureau of Vital Statistics, City Hall, Philadelphia, the midwives of the city cared for 3,182 of the live births of the survey period; in 1931, 1,410, or 4.2

percent of all live births; in 1932, 1,021, or 3.2 percent; and in 1933, 751, or 2.6 percent. It is unlikely that the difference of 636 births in the above two totals was entirely made up of stillbirths, and presumably some birth certificates were not filed with the local bureau during these three years.

During this period of three years, 42 women were delivered by a physician in consultation with the midwife. There were ten maternal deaths reported. This gives a maternal mortality rate of 2.6 per 1,000 births. This rate is exactly the same as that obtained in the student home delivery service. This gives an apparent advantage to the midwife, since her consultants are usually not the trained men who are called in to help the medical student.

The ten deaths considered here were all in multiparas, who left a total of sixty-nine living children at their deaths. No one of them had received any prenatal care. Three were native-born, seven foreign-born, all but one were white women. Six were delivered at home, four in hospitals, while one woman whose death occurred at home had been in a hospital for treatment for three days during a septic puerperium following home delivery.

The causes of death as certified after a critical review by the Analysis Committee were decided to have been inexactly stated in three instances. Changes were made to read shock in two, and postpartum hemorrhage in one. The causes of death for the group of ten were postpartum hemorrhage in three, placenta previa in one, puerperal sepsis in two, eclampsia in one, shock in two, and accident of labor in one. Physicians had been called to assist in the deliveries of the three postpartum hemorrhage deaths. In each instance the Analysis Committee felt the onus of the fatal outcome rested with the physician.

In the death from placenta previa, the patient's lack of co-operation was considered the determining factor in the disaster. She refused hospitalization until in a desperate condition. One of the septic deaths followed Cesarean section for placenta previa, where the woman had been promptly hospitalized, without examination at the onset of bleeding. The other followed the removal of an adherent placenta by a physician in the home, after the child had been delivered by a midwife. In both instances the Analysis Committee regarded the determining factor as within the responsibility of the physician through an error in technic.

The death from eclampsia was in a woman who had had a similar condition in the preceding pregnancy, for which she had been hospitalized. This time she refused hospitalization and died shortly after a forceps delivery, the convulsions occurring postpartum. Here lack of co-operation was regarded as the determining factor. In one of the shock cases three physicians had each attempted forceps before a successful version delivered the woman. Error in judgment on the part of the physicians was regarded as the avoidable factor by the Analysis Committee. In the second shock death the woman was hospitalized by a physician called by a midwife who recognized an abnormal presentation in labor. Unsuccessful high forceps on a face presentation was followed by version. The child was stillborn and the maternal death occurred twenty-seven hours later. Although the death certificate was certified as having a streptococcic septicemia contributory to a face presentation as the primary cause, the Analysis Committee considered the death one of shock due to trauma at delivery. In the final case, sudden death occurred shortly after a spontaneous delivery of a decipara by a midwife. There was no history of hemorrhage. The cause of death certified as myocardial insufficiency, by a physician who had attended the patient previously, was regarded as sufficient evidence for the Analysis Committee to consider the death non-preventable.

Study of the detailed histories obtained in connection with the deaths originating in midwife practice showed but one instance where the regulations governing them had been overstepped. This was in one of the cases of postpartum hemorrhage where the assistance of a physician was not called until the placenta had remained undelivered for seven hours.

Statistics show that the number of midwives in the Philadelphia district is diminishing.

> In 1926 there were 111 active midwives.
> In 1932 there were 77 active midwives.
> In 1933 there were 68 active midwives.

Of these 68, 26 were trained abroad; 3 were trained in American schools outside of Philadelphia, while 6 were trained in Philadelphia. The remaining 33 received their training by a method known in the Bureau as "Inheritance." This means that a midwife in active practice took a young woman, usually her daughter, and gave her practical training. This pernicious system has been abolished, and for many years past no woman has been admitted to practice in Philadelphia who has not had regular hospital training.

The control of midwives has been in force since January 1st, 1914, under the Bureau of Medical Education. The act upon which this control is based may be found in Bulletin 21M, 1929, of the State Board of Medical Education and Licensure.

It is to be noted further that these midwife cases have no care during their pregnancy. Midwives deal with a very ignorant class of people, who do not lend themselves to any supervision during pregnancy.

The Analysis Committee was of the opinion that the midwives played an unimportant part in the maternal mortality problem in Philadelphia.

STUDENT HOME DELIVERY SERVICE

During the period of the survey there were delivered at home 5,500 women, by the students of the five medical schools and one osteopathic school (Table No. 40). The total number of fourth or final year students engaged in this service was 1,589. If the students in osteopathy were eliminated, we would find that the medical student delivered an average of less than four women in the home delivery service. The

TABLE 40
STUDENT HOME DELIVERY SERVICES 1931-1933

SCHOOL	NUMBER OF GRADUATES	TOTAL DE-LIVERED AT HOME	CASES PER STUDENT	OPERATIVE DEL. AT HOME BY GRADUATE CON-SULTANT	REFERRED TO HOSPITAL	DEATHS	
						Home	Hospital
A	74	539	7.3	5	53	0	0
B	193	177	.9	7	5	0	0
C	212	263	1.2	0	0	0	1
D	283	547	1.9	6	27	0	1
E	403	2163	5.4	26	96	1	8
F	424	1811	4.3	15	72	1	3
TOTAL	1589	5500	3.5	59	253	2	13

total average for all students was even smaller. The requirement of the Pennsylvania State Board of Medical Education and Licensure, Bulletin 18M, 1932, states that every candidate for examination must have attended personally not less than six cases of obstetrics. There is no similar demand by regulation of graduates in osteopathy seeking license.

In these services a total of fifty-nine women were delivered at home by operation by a consultant graduate. This number is just over one percent. There were referred from these services to hospitals for operative intervention, 253 women, 4.5 percent. This figure is of importance in its possible reflection upon the number of emergency admissions to hospitals from the general domiciliary practice of the city as a whole.

There were two deaths among the 5,500 women delivered at home by the students or their graduate consultants, a mortality rate of 0.36 per 1,000 births. The two deaths in the student home delivery service resulted from puerperal septicemia. Of the 253 women referred to hospitals, 13 died, a mortality rate of 51 per 1,000 births. Of the total cases, 5,753, originating in the home practice of the students, there was a total of fifteen deaths, a mortality rate of 2.6 per 1,000 births.

RECOMMENDATIONS AND DISCUSSION

The problem of maternal deaths in Philadelphia is fourfold, namely:

1. Self-induced and criminal abortions.
2. Errors of judgment on the part of the medical profession.
3. Lack of appreciation of the need of prenatal care by the laity.
4. Failure of hospitals, organized medicine, and allied agencies, to grasp fully their responsibilities and opportunities.

With the present status of public opinion as indicated by existing laws in regard to the giving of contraceptive information, it is impossible to face the abortion situation frankly as has been done in some foreign countries. As an interim measure, the responsibility rests with the medical profession and interested lay groups under its direction. By every means available, the public should be informed of the perils of non-therapeutic abortion.

Errors of judgment may be summarized as being due to inexperience, to failure to note important danger signals, to undue faith in operative interference, and to a willingness to "take a chance." To overcome these conditions, there must be reorganization in the training of obstetricians, closer supervision of internes, and graduate instruction for physicians. An educational campaign for the entire medical profession is needed to make them fully aware of the dangers of ignoring symptoms requiring hospitalization or consultation with specialists.

The physician is responsible for educating the laity in regard to the necessity for adequate prenatal care in toxemias of pregnancy. Every expectant mother should realize the dangers not only to herself but also to her baby as a result of improper supervision in toxemias. A well-conducted educational campaign should tend toward eliminating "ignorance of the patient" as a factor in maternal deaths in these cases.

Hospitals, medical societies, and allied agencies should assume more responsibility regarding the factors tending to reduce maternal mortality in Philadelphia. Such organizations have wide influence both with the medical profession and with the lay public, and they should embrace every opportunity to advance the practice of obstetrics through co-operative education and legislation.

In order to meet the situation, changes are necessary in the attitude and procedure of various groups involved, therefore the following specific recommendations are made:

PHYSICIANS

The responsibility for the high maternal mortality rate in Philadelphia rests primarily with the medical profession, hence the problem of reducing it belongs to the physicians. They must assume leadership in the double role of raising the educational standards of physicians, nurses, and midwives, and of informing the laity of the need of adequate maternity care.

Physicians must instruct the lay public in the dangers of induced abortion. The simple and clear explanation of the infections following unclean abortions must be emphasized. Its dangers must be warned against if any progress is to be made in combatting this prevalent and increasing socio-medical problem.

Abortions—whether self-induced, criminal or spontaneous, with resulting septicemia—are the largest single puerperal cause of death in Philadelphia. For these deaths medical practitioners cannot hold themselves responsible, as patients come to them as a rule in a moribund condition. Nevertheless, any single factor resulting in an unnecessary death every week in this city requires medical leadership to meet the situation. In any educational program on prenatal and maternal care the danger of abortion should be stressed. Education will help, but it alone will not eliminate this cause of death.

The fact that the largest proportion of these deaths is among married women, many of whom have living children, would indicate that under present economic conditions the difficulty of providing for children and the desire to give them better opportunities may be the fundamental cause. A number of foreign countries have faced this problem either by allowing the free giving of contraceptive information, or by legalizing abortion.

The committee is not in agreement as to the desirability of changing the law in regard to either of these procedures. Concerning the legalization of abortion, the outstanding example is that of the U. S. S. R. The committee has considered a large amount of Russian material on this subject. The evidence on the advisability of this measure seems overwhelming, and it is hoped that within the near future an impartial analysis will be made of the results, especially in relation to the ability of those having undergone this operation to bear children. Such a study by qualified obstetricians, gynecologists and statisticians is suggested.

More opportunities should be offered to the physician who is desirous of advancing himself in the art and science of obstetrics. Unfortunately the material available for this purpose is poorly marshalled in this city. In some of the maternity services of the larger general hospitals the material appears sufficient to warrant a residency in obstetrics for the education of young specialists without seriously interfering with the training of internes.

There is a dearth of seminars and demonstrations in obstetrics open to the general practitioner. If such courses were arranged regularly and advertized sufficiently, possibly in connection with the current teaching of undergraduates, they might well serve as stimulating refresher courses to the general practitioner.

INTERNES

In certain institutions, internes apparently are allowed wide latitude in operative obstetrics without any supervision. This is injudicious and prejudicial to the best interests of the patient, to whom the attending obstetrician is fully responsible in the final analysis.

In the limited and constantly diminishing clinical material in this branch of medicine, opportunity should be sought to instruct internes and residents in the contra-indications as well as in the indications for operations in obstetrics; also in the selection and administration of anesthetics. Further, for the protection of the patient, a regulatory limitation of any interference by the interne is essential.

STUDENTS

This survey has shown that a large number of unsupervised deliveries are conducted by students in the out-patient departments of teaching institutions. How much more value might be derived from these cases if more than one student were assigned to each delivery is difficult to determine. From an educational standpoint absence of supervision of students would appear as inexcusable in obstetrical practice as in surgical procedures.

For students, the need for greater concentration on the elementary principles and the advocacy of conservative practice in obstetrics is apparent. Emphasis should be placed on the normal mechanism of labor, on proper antenatal hygiene, and on the essentials of postpartum care. A more rational and thorough training of students regarding the treatment of abortion should be considered.

NURSES

The teaching of nurses should fully ground them in the elements of practical obstetrics. Their education should include sufficient time in antenatal hygiene to enable them, if they become public health nurses, to recognize abnormal symptoms, and to act as liaison officers, ensuring co-operation of patients, and securing, when necessary, earlier hospitalization in potentially dangerous conditions. As in the case of physicians, facilities should be provided for the further education of the nurse who wishes to specialize in obstetrical nursing, whether institutional or private.

MIDWIVES

This survey has shown that the midwife is an almost negligible factor in mortality in Philadelphia. Perhaps nowhere in the United States is the midwife subject to closer regulation and supervision than in the Philadelphia district of this State. Should this standard be maintained, and should the progressive decline in midwife practice continue, she cannot be regarded as of importance in this problem.

LAITY

It is an evident fact that the number of seemingly preventable deaths from the standpoint of the responsibility of the patient is entirely too high. Certainly ignorance and lack of co-operation could be ruled out as avoidable factors through proper education. To the medical profession must be entrusted the task of teaching the lay public the need for adequate maternity care. Individually, with their own patients, and collectively, in groups, physicians must stress the relation of proper antenatal supervision to preventable catastrophies. The nature and importance of danger signals in pregnancy must be explained to each prospective mother, and her co-operation must be invited and insisted upon. All abnormal subjective or objective warnings must be talked over in sufficient detail to impress the patient with the need for immediately reporting any such condition to her medical adviser.

As surgical asepsis at delivery constitutes a part of adequate maternity care, women should be taught the need for the eradication of foci of infection in the cervico-vaginal tract, the avoidance of intercourse in late pregnancy, and the necessity for scrupulous personal hygiene. That a competent attendant and a suitable environment are of prime importance should merely need mention to be appreciated. It is necessary to explain also the changes that occur in the pelvic organs during convalescence and to stress the value of follow-up examinations as the final step in complete obstetrical supervision.

Group education of the lay public can be carried out opportunely through class meetings of prenatal clinic patients. Hygiene and other pertinent topics should be discussed either by a physician or a nurse, and questions should be encouraged. The education of husbands could be facilitated by periodic meetings for them. A response in better co-operation of the patient results when the husband is enlightened in regard to the necessity for co-operation. These plans are in successful operation in several hospitals at the present time.

There is a need, too, for educating the laity that maternity care should be remunerated sufficiently to encourage a physician to give his best professional efforts to his patient. The public should realize that the laborer is worthy of his hire.

ORGANIZED MEDICINE

Organized medicine must play an important part, too, if the maternal mortality rate is to be reduced.

First, medical societies should initiate and provide the means for studying the advances in obstetrical practice. This might be accomplished by case reports, clinical teaching, and demonstration.

Second, they should co-operate with the Bureau of Vital Statistics by insisting that practicing physicians carry out the regulations in regard to correct certification of births and deaths. That the profession in Philadelphia needs education in this respect was shown by the fact that one in every five maternal death certificates examined in this survey failed to give the correct cause of death.

Third, organized medicine should provide facilities for occasional surveys of this nature in order that the condition of obstetric practice in Philadelphia may be ascertained at intervals.

Fourth, organized medicine should be responsible for the distribution to the general medical public of manuals or bulletins, containing facts of timely importance in obstetrics, or discussions of particular phases of the subject. This would tend to awaken greater interest in the problem at hand.

OBSTETRICAL SOCIETY OF PHILADELPHIA

For the purpose of consolidating any gain which this survey may have made, it is recommended that the Obstetrical Society of Philadelphia conduct an annual review of the puerperal morbidity and mortality of the hospitals in the city. This could be carried out in the same manner in which the reviews of toxemias of pregnancy and of Cesarean sections have been conducted in recent years.

The adoption of a uniform record system in the maternity divisions of the hospitals of Philadelphia would be of great assistance in compiling an annual review of certain types of cases, and in making a comparison as to certain lines of treatment. As in the British system of annual reports, this should show the comparative results of planned or booked admissions and emergency admissions. A uniform hospital year regulated by the calendar would facilitate such a survey as the one just completed. To the same purpose is recommended a uniform system of nomenclature and classification of disease and procedure. The Obstetrical Society might well assume the responsibility for such a program.

HOSPITALS

Hospitals are intimately associated with maternal mortality, since it is, of necessity, in such institutions that the largest number of births and of maternal deaths occur. It is the duty and responsibility of the hospital staffs to investigate fully and frankly all the circumstances in relation to maternal deaths in order to prevent repetition of any avoidable errors.

The staff of an obstetrical department should insist that the directing authorities provide the minima of the standard for a maternity division as outlined by the American College of Surgeons.[a]

It is essential that they include at least facilities for isolation and segregation of potentially infected cases.

The maternity facilities of a hospital should offer all the conditions essential to the proper care of both public and private patients. An adequate allowance of antenatal beds is needed to provide proper care for cases requiring observation and treatment. This matter has been neglected in many hospitals. Some deaths recorded in this survey might have been avoided if patients suffering from toxemia, cardiac disease, and like conditions, had been cared for in prenatal wards instead of at home without adequate supervision.

Physicians in charge of prenatal clinics should have the support of an adequate staff of trained social workers to provide for complete follow-up of abnormal cases treated in hospitals and discharged before delivery. In this survey it was disclosed that a number of women who had had preliminary hospital treatment for toxemia were readmitted in convulsions. Many of these patients had not been seen for days and even weeks previously.

The maternity staff of a hospital should be composed of competent physicians sufficiently experienced to be able to handle difficult or complicated cases. Adequate training and operative ability should be required for such positions.

The courtesy privilege of the maternity division should be extended to all ethical practitioners wherever possible. The limited operative ability of some physicians as contrasted with the greater experience of

---

[a] American College of Surgeons. Twentieth Year Book, 1933, p. 68. Chicago, Ill.

others, should lead to certain intra-mural regulations as to restriction and supervision.

The immediate benefit of uniform regulations and limitations in all hospitals in regard to the courtesy staff is also apparent.

Hospital consultations should be obligatory in certain abnormalities as well as in certain operative procedures. The widespread adoption of such practice would tend to lessen the apparently unnecessarily high operative incidence.

A definite plan should be in operation in maternity divisions of hospitals for the proper training, supervision and education of internes, residents and assistants. The mere tenure of such positions, however, should not lead to the assumption that further supervision and training are unnecessary. The benefit of mature judgment is needed at all times in caring for maternity cases.

Obstetrical Staff conferences are essential, and by the ruling of at least one medical organization, whose stamp of approval is a recognition of good hospital conduct, they are obligatory. Such conferences conducted in an impersonal manner, with frank discussion, serve as educational centers not only for the junior staff but also for the courtesy members.

The adoption of a uniform morbidity standard by hospitals is recommended. A review of the cases showing morbidity would provide the possibility of detecting unseen breaks in technic which at times prove fatal. Such standards show only a febrile morbidity, yet this is often intimately related to septic infection. A review of such morbid cases should be made regularly.

This survey revealed that prenatal clinics cannot always exercise proper supervision over antenatal cases because of the great distances between the patients' homes and the hospitals. This difficulty might be solved to some extent by zoning the areas from which prenatal clinic patients were accepted. This question might be considered by the Hospital Association or by the Association of Hospital Social Service Workers.

It was noted in the histories of some of the cases dying from postpartum hemorrhage that donors were unavailable. Of course, it cannot be proven that transfusions would have saved any of these lives, yet it is wise to recommend that a list of readily available donors be compiled for emergencies of the maternity service.

A standard technic for delivery room service in hospitals is recommended. Uniformity of practice could be arranged by staff conference with mutual satisfaction as to personal differences in detail. Such uniformity would lead to better co-operation among obstetricians, internes, and nurses, and would obviate breaks in technic to a large extent. The courtesy staff should be compelled to conform to such established routine. A closer approach to complete aseptic technic in the delivery room would result from rigid insistence on a fixed standard of procedure.

It is recommended that hospitals include a copy of the death certificate in each puerperal or associated puerperal death, and thus make it an integral part of the case history.

PRENATAL CARE IN MIDWIFE CASES

It is recommended that some provision be made for the prenatal care of women registering with midwives for delivery. If midwives would notify their inspectors when prospective patients first register, it might be possible to secure antenatal care through the nursing system of the Division of Child Hygiene, at least to the extent that a physical and pelvic examination be made in every case.

BUREAU OF VITAL STATISTICS

It is recommended that the Bureau of Vital Statistics prepare an annual table to show not only the puerperal causes of maternal deaths, but also the associated or contributory causes; and in addition a table to show all deaths in which the puerperal state was certified as an associated factor. The Obstetrical Society is urged to take this up with the Director of the Department of Public Health of Philadelphia.

It is further recommended that the standard death certificate of the Birth Registration area in use in Pennsylvania be altered, at least locally, to show any possible puerperal connection with a death. This would aid greatly in making statistical reviews more complete and more fully informative.

It is further recommended that the standard birth certificate of the Birth Registration area in use in Pennsylvania be altered, at least locally, to show the type of operation performed at delivery where interference was used.

It is further recommended that the regulations of the Department of Health of the Commonwealth of Pennsylvania be altered to define a stillbirth as: "The birth of a dead fetus which had reached at least 28 weeks gestation, or measures 13.8 inches (35 cm.) or over, from heel to crown."

STATISTICAL REPORTS OF PRENATAL CLINICS

It is recommended that the statistical records of the prenatal clinics of all hospitals be continued and improved, and that an annual resumé and report be made to a central organization, preferably the Philadelphia Child Health Society. The value of such reports has been proven definitely by this present survey.

In view of the fact that many of the autopsies performed by coroner's physicians revealed few if any facts tending to establish a more accurate diagnosis of the cause of death, it is recommended that postmortem examinations on coroner's cases in hospital puerperal deaths be performed by a staff pathologist in the presence, if necessary, of a representative of the coroner.

EDUCATIONAL CAMPAIGN

During the period of the survey an effort has been made to awaken the minds of both the medical profession and the laity to the significant importance of the problem of maternal welfare.

In the second year of the survey 836 lay organizations were sent an offer of a qualified medical speaker on the subject, *"What Constitutes Adequate Maternity Care?"* This list of lay organizations was made up of all types of societies, associations and clubs, social, political and religious. The speakers' list comprised members of the Obstetrical Society of Philadelphia who were also members of the County Medical Society. A synopsis was furnished so that the points which were considered of importance would be in the hands of each speaker. In 1933 it was decided to confine the work to women's organizations, and 257 societies were sent offers of speakers.. Over seventy organizations have been furnished speakers for their meetings during these two years.

In 1932 and 1933 letters were sent from the office of the County Medical Society to the ministers of all churches in Philadelphia asking them to include in the church program for Mother's Day some reference to the need of expectant women for adequate maternity care.

In 1932 and 1933 a series of 58 articles dealing with various phases of maternal mortality were published in the *Weekly Roster and Medical Digest* of the County Medical Society. These articles were written by Doctors B. C. Hirst, F. E. Keller, F. B. Block, E. Jones, J. I. Richards, J. O. Arnold, C. S. Barnes, C. J. Stamm, E. B. Piper, G. M. Boyd, A. W. Tallant, N. L. Knipe, J. S. Lawrence, D. Longaker, C. Foulkrod, H. L. Hartley, S. E. Tracy, W. E. Parke, O. J. Toland, H. A. Duncan, G. A. Ulrich, C. B. Reynolds, G. C. Hanna, C. Wachs, J. Cutler, W. B. Harer, R. D. Porter, H. J. Tumen, W. C. Ely, J. P. Lewis, E. P. Barnard, J. V. Klauder, G. C. Griffith, J. C. Hartman, J. M. Lafferty, W. J. Thudium, F. C. Hammond, S. M. Stern, L. Averett, A. First, B. Mann, J. F. Carrell, L. C. Sheffey, J. C. Hirst, R. W. Mohler, H. Stuckert, C. A. Behney, D. P. Murphy, T. L. Montgomery, A. P. Keegan, W. W. Van Dolsen, N. W. Vaux, C. B. Lull, E. A. Schumann, R. A. Kimbrough, P. B. Bland, and Mr. Alexander Fleisher and Miss Blanche Hamer.

The Committee wishes to express their thanks to these authors for their co-operation.

In 1932 and 1933 the hospital staff conferences of the city, the various clinical medical societies and the branch and affiliated organizations of the county societies, were sent a circular letter discussing the maternal mortality situation in Philadelphia. In this letter they were requested to place the subject of *"Maternal Mortality"* prominently before their membership during each of the two years. A very hearty response followed this request, as noted by the number of meetings advertised in the *Roster* in which this item formed the whole or part of the program.

It is believed by the Committee that the subject of *"Maternal Mortality"* has been brought to the attention of a large number of physicians, and that the subject of *"Adequate Maternity Care"* has been properly presented by medical speakers to a large number of lay people, both men and women.

CONTINUANCE OF THE SURVEY

Feeling that any gain made by the survey could be held and a further improvement in the maternal mortality rate made, the Committee decided to continue the survey. Through a grant of $200 made by the Directors of the County Medical Society to cover necessary expenditures, a voluntary survey of hospital puerperal deaths is continuing. An auxiliary committee has been formed and the following hospitals are represented by a member of the staff: Broad Street, Dr. Newlin F. Paxson; Chestnut Hill, Dr. E. A. Schumann; Episcopal, Dr. Owen J. Toland; Frankford, Dr. John Laferty; Germantown, Dr. J. C. Hartman; Hahnemann, Dr. Newlin F. Paxson; Jefferson, Dr. J. F. Carrell; Jewish, Dr. J. M. Alesbury; Kensington, Dr. S. M. Stern; Lankenau, Dr. J. C. Hartman; Lying-In, Dr. R. A. Kimbrough; Methodist, Dr. J. C. Hirst; Misericordia, Dr. J. V. Missett; Mt. Sinai, Dr. Jacob Walker; Northeastern, Dr. F. E. Keller; Osteopathic, H. Walter Evans, D.O.; Philadelphia General, Dr. Albert Brown, Jr.; Presbyterian, Dr. W. C. Ely; Preston Retreat, Dr. J. C. Hirst; St. Agnes, Dr. H. J. Sangmeister; St. Joseph's, Dr. J. F. Carrell; St. Luke's and Children's, Dr. H. D. Lafferty; St. Mary's, Dr. John Laferty; St. Vincent's, Dr. H. J. Sangmeister; Temple, Dr. J. M. Alesbury; University, Dr. J. V. Missett; Woman's College, Dr. L. S. Cogill; Woman's Homeopathic, Dr. B. F. Biscoe; Woman's Hospital, Dr. D. E. Mieldazis; and Mercy, Dr. L. T. Sewell.

These physicians bring to a monthly meeting a copy of the record of any maternal death which may have occurred during the previous month. These records are discussed in an impersonal manner and the case or death is then classed in accordance with the following recapitulation:

1. Puerperal or extra-puerperal death?
2. No mention of true cause of death.
3. Certified cause found incorrect or non-existent.
4. Was the death preventable?
5. To whom should responsibility be assigned?

    (a) Physician.
    (b) Patient.
    (c) Midwife.

6. Primary avoidable factor.

    (a) Lack of prenatal care.
    (b) Negligence of patient or her friends.
    (c) Induction of abortion.
    (d) Error in judgment.
    (e) Error in technic.
    (f) Intercurrent disease.
    (g) Unavoidable disaster.

434

7. By what means might the death have been prevented?
8. Did sepsis arise in hospital?
9. Was case admitted as a normal case?
10. Was pathology known or recognized on admission?
11. Was pregnancy and labor responsible for the death?
    (a) Directly?
    (b) Contributory, with another primary cause?
    (c) No connection?

It is the intention of this Committee to continue the survey for three years, during which time the members of the Committee on Maternal Welfare and the Auxiliary Analysis Committee may have time to bring before the hospital staffs and medical societies their findings and recommendations.

FINANCIAL STATEMENT

The expenses of this survey amounted to $5,990.28.

(Signed)

> PHILIP F. WILLIAMS, M.D., *Chairman*
> T. RUTH H. WEAVER, M.D., *Recorder*
> JESSE O. ARNOLD, M.D.
> CHARLES S. BARNES, M.D.
> P. BROOKE BLAND, M.D.
> GEORGE M. BOYD, M.D.
> COLLIN FOULKROD, M.D.
> HARRIET HARTLEY, M.D.
> BARTON C. HIRST, M.D.
> J. K. JAFFE, M.D.
> CLIFFORD B. LULL, M.D.
> WILLIAM R. NICHOLSON, M.D.
> RICHARD C. NORRIS, M.D.
> EDMUND B. PIPER, M.D.
> JAMES L. RICHARDS, M.D.
> E. A. SCHUMANN, M.D.
> ALICE W. TALLANT, M.D.
> NORRIS W. VAUX, M.D.

> *The Philadelphia County Medical Society*
> *Committee on Maternal Welfare*

THE PHILADELPHIA COUNTY MEDICAL SOCIETY
MATERNAL MORTALITY STUDY

1. Serial No.   2. Reg. No.

MOTHER (information from death certificate)

3. PLACE OF DEATH:

    County   City

    Died at _____
    (Write word HOME or name of hospital)

4. Full name

    Address

PERSONAL AND STATISTICAL DATA

5. Age	6. Color	7. Marital status

8. Occupation of deceased—Housewife, Other (specify)

9. Birthplace of deceased

10. Interval between birth and mother's death:

    days   hours   mins.—Not reported, Not delivered (truly) (ectopic)

11. Number of children of this mother including this birth (or births)

    (a) Born alive and now living

    (b) Born alive and now dead

    (c) Stillborn   Not born

12. Date of final hospital admission

17. INTERNATIONAL CODE CAUSE OF DEATH:

    (a) Health Dept.

    (b) Study

18. No birth certificate—(a) Not required

    (b) Required but not registered

    Date of search and notes

19. Postmortem deliveries (counted under 24 as "not delivered")—State here the result: Postmortem alive, Postmortem stillborn. Type of postmortem delivery

BABY (information from birth certificate)

20. PLACE OF BIRTH:

    County   City

    Born at _____
    (write word HOME or name of hospital)

MEDICAL CERTIFICATE OF DEATH

13. Date of death (month, day, year)   , 19

14. I HEREBY CERTIFY, that I attended deceased from

    , 19   , to   , 19

    that I last saw her alive on   , 19

    and that death occurred on the above date

    at   m.

The CAUSE OF DEATH or DIAGNOSIS DURING THE LAST ILLNESS was as follows:

duration   years   mos.   days

Contributory (secondary) duration   years   mos.   days

    Signed

    Address

15. Autopsy—Examination, None

16. AUTOPSY REPORT:

21. Sex of child (or children if plural birth)— Male, Female, Not reported, Not determined (because of immaturity, etc.), Not delivered

22. Plural births—Twins, Triplets, Other (specify)

23. Legitimate, N.

CERTIFICATE OF ATTENDING PHYSICIAN OR MIDWIFE

24. I HEREBY CERTIFY, that I attended the birth of this child who was born on

    19   , at   m. o'clock. Alive, Stillborn, Not delivered

    Signed

    Address

25. CONDITIONS IN MOTHER, NONE, NOT KNOWN
   (a) Cardiac
   (b) Chronic nephritis
   (c) Tuberculosis
   (d) Tumors, etc.
   (e) Uterine displ.
   (f) Syphilis (specify)
   (g) Others (specify)
26. PAST MEDICAL OR SURGICAL HISTORY, NONE, NOT KNOWN
   Specify

27. INTERCURRENT DISEASES, OPERATIONS, ABNORMALITIES, ETC., NONE, NOT REPORTED
   Specify
28. Treatment by physician, None. Specify and describe

29. COMPLICATIONS OF PREGNANCY, NONE, NR
30. Albuminuria, N. Began or first noted ___ wk.
31. Convulsions, N. Began ___ wk.
32. Oedema, N. Where and when began or noted
33. High blood pressure, N. Began or first noted ___ wk.
   Normal ___ Lowest ___ Highest ___
34. Prolonged headache, N. Began or first noted ___ wk.
   Duration
35. Pernicious vomiting, N. Began ___ wk.
   Duration
36. Bleeding during pregnancy, N. Began ___ wk. Scanty, Moderate, Profuse, Once only, Recurred: daily, monthly, irregular
37. Treatment by physician, N. Specify

38. Abnormal conditions at onset of labor (not otherwise stated), N. Specify

39. PRENATAL CARE: Given by
40. Summary—Adequate, Inadequate, None, Excluded, NR
41. Visits

	Month of pregnancy											
	1	2	3	4	5	6	7	8	9			
									1	2	3	4
(a) Saw patient, N.												
(b) Urine exam., N.												
(c) Abdom. exam., N.												
(d) Blood pressure, N.												

42. Physical examination during pregnancy, N.
   (a) Heart, N — Normal, Abnormal (specify)
   (b) Lungs, N — Normal, Abnormal (specify)
   (c) Pelvis, N — Normal, Abnormal (specify)
   (d) Wassermann or Kahn, N — Negative, Positive +, NR
43. Abnormalities not observed by examining physician, N. Specify

44. Abnormalities affecting delivery and third stage, N
   (a) Placenta—Adherent, Retained, Praevia, Premature separation,
   (b) Hemorrhages — Antepartum, Intrapartum, Postpartum, Amount (estimate)
   (c) Ruptured uterus—Spontaneous, Instrumental, During labor, During delivery, Before labor, Not known. Describe
   (d) Others (specify)
   (e) Treatment

45. ABORTION—Complete, Incomplete, Missed Spontaneous, Induced (self), Questionable Therapeutic, N, Consultation, N, Indications for
46. ECTOPIC— Delivered, Not delivered (attempted) Notes

47. NOT DELIVERED:
   (a) In labor, N, No attempt at delivery
   (b) Attempted delivery
      1. Attempt to induce labor (a) Medical
         (b) Packing, etc.
      2. Attempted operative delivery

DELIVERY DATA:

48. Attendant at actual delivery—Physician, Interne, Midwife, Student, Other, None, NR, Not delivered
49. Assisted, N (specify by whom)
50. Technique—(a) Vaginal examinations, N, Number
      (b) Rectal examinations, N, Number
      (c) Gloves, N (d) Shaved, N
         (e) Sterile goods, N (f) Preparation method and agents used

51. Others attempting delivery (specify)
   Technique (a) (b) (c) (d) (e) (f)
52. Presentation—Vertex (ROA) (ROP) (LOA) (LOP)
      Transverse (specify)
      Face (specify)
      Other (specify)
      Breech (specify)
      Prolapsed (cord) (arm) (arms) (leg) (legs) etc.

53. Membranes—Ruptured, Not ruptured, Excluded (a) Spontaneous, Artificial (b) Length of time before delivery ___ hours
54. Labor—In labor, N, Excluded, Spontaneous, Induced (method used for induction)
      Describe labor Duration ___ hours ___ mins.
55. Delivery—Spontaneous, Operative (specify) (indications) Operative attempts (specify)
56. Third Stage—None, Normal, Abnormal (specify) Management of third stage (if abnormal) and how long after delivery
57. Tears—N (a) Episiotomy, N
      (b) Perineal, N, Degree
      (c) Repaired, N
      (d) Cervical, N, NR
      (e) Repaired, N
58. Anaesthetic—N (specify kind used)
      Given by M.D. or R.N.

59. MATERNAL HISTORY:
Times pregnant   Para   Gravida

№	Time between	Uterogestation (weeks)	Alive or stillborn (write the word)	Abnormalities that would affect pregnancy	Delivery (if operative, specify)
1					
2					
3					
4					
5					
6					
7					
8					
9					
10					

60. Operation preceding death (only if other than shown under 55), N. Specify (State how long after delivery or if not delivered how long before death.)

61. HOSPITAL CASE N: Delivered in hospital N Planned, Emergency

62. Entered hospital — Before labor, During labor, After delivery   days

63. Total hospital days
Days in hospital of delivery
Days in hospital of death
Days in other hospitals
Home   days
(These refer only to hospitals connected with delivery and puerperium.)

64. If septic—(a) Developed in hospital, N
    (b) Others in hospital at time, N

PRIMARY AND CONTRIBUTING CAUSES OF DEATH

140: Abortion with Septic Condition
Specify:

(Enter details under 45)

141: Abortion without mention of Septic Condition
Specify:

(Enter details under 45)

142: Ectopic Gestation
(a) Symptoms began   week. Describe
(b) Interval between recognition of first symptom and operation
(c) No operation   (d) Sepsis

(Enter details under 46)

143: Other Accidents of Pregnancy (not to include hemorrhages)
Specify:

144: Puerperal Hemorrhages
1. Placenta praevia—Premature separation of the placenta
   (a) When recognized
   (b) Specify method of control
   (c) Method of delivery (enter details under 55)

2. Ante, Intra, Postpartum hemorrhages, N. See entries under 44, 55, 56
   Inspection of placenta at delivery, N
   Left patient after delivery, N,   hours
   Patient's condition satisfactory with dropping pulse, N

3. Other causes under 144 (specify)
TREATMENT (describe fully)

TRANSFUSION (state definitely the time given, etc., in relation to hemorrhage, delivery, operative interference)

145: Puerperal Septicaemia not due to abortion
1. Operative delivery (enter the details under 55)
2. Spontaneous
3. Not delivered
4. Care after delivery:
   (a) First call   hours after,   days after
   (b) Nursing care   5. Symptoms appeared   hours before delivery,   hours after delivery (describe)
6. Intra-uterine manipulation, N—Before symptoms, After symptoms
7. Duration of sepsis: days
8. Spreading peritonitis, N
9. Blood culture, Smear, etc., N—Negative, Positive (give organism)
10. Specify treatment, transfusion, etc.

146: Puerperal Albuminuria and Eclampsia
(See prenatal care)
1. Medical supervision before convulsions, N, Duration   2. Condition when first seen
3. Symptoms began   before death Convulsions, N. Began   hours Before labor, During labor,   hours After delivery
4. Cooperation of patient—Good, Poor, None (reason)
5. Home case: Bed at first symptoms
6. Hospital case: Hospital at first symptoms or when in a serious condition

147: Other Toxaemias of Pregnancy
1. Pernicious vomiting (a) Duration
   (b) Operation, N.   Refused by patient, N
2. Others (specify)

*148: Phlegmasia Alba Dolens, Embolus,
Sudden Death (not specified as septic)*

1. Embolus (specify)
   (a) Respiratory distress, N
   (b) Cyanosis, N (c) Cough, N (d) Pain, N
   (e) Other (specify)
2. Other causes, under 148, Remarks

Remarks:

149: Other Accidents of Childbirth

1. Cesarean section:
   (a) Specify type of operation
   (b) Indications for
   (c) Elective, Emergency
   (d) Vaginal examination immediately be-
       fore, N
   (e) Membranes ruptured, N (hours)
   (f) Patient in labor, N (hours). Type
   (g) Temperature (specify)
   (h) Operative interference before Cesa-
       rean, N
2. Instrumental delivery and other operative
   procedures (enter the details under 55)

3. Ruptured uterus, N (a) Spontaneous, Instrumental
   (b) Treatment
4. Operative shock
5. Other causes under 149, Remarks, Treatment

---

*150: Other and Unspecified Conditions of the
Puerperal State*

Specify:

NON-PUERPERAL CAUSES OF DEATH *either*

Primary or Contributing

Give number as coded in the Manual of the
International List of Causes of Death with the
cause written after (as 121-Appendicitis)

A + Primary:

B + Contributory:

Informant

Agent

Date of Visit

In presenting this folder, the spacing has been condensed for convenience, and in reproducing it for practical use, the spacing must be rearranged. The following directions are of value in filling out the folders:

RETAIN FOR FUTURE USE

The Philadelphia County Medical Society

Maternal Welfare Study

Directions for filling in schedule

General: If item is applicable to the case, check it; if not, check *N* or *None;*
if information is not available, check *NR* or *Not known.*

1. Enter number assigned to the case in this study.

2. Enter number from death certificate.

3. If patient died at home, write "Home"; if she died in hospital, give name of institution.

4. As given on death certificate.

5. Age at death.

6. Enter "White," "Black," or "Yellow."

7. Enter "Married," "Single," "Widowed," or "Divorced."

8. Specify if other than housewife.

9. Copy from death certificate. Give state in addition to city.

10. In undelivered cases of 28 weeks gestation or over, check *Not delivered;* in undelivered cases of less than 28 weeks gestation, check also (*truly*) or (*ectopic*).

11. Enter postmortem deliveries under *Not born.*

12. Enter date patient was admitted to hospital in which she died. If she died at home, enter "None."

13. Copy from death certificate.

14. Copy from death certificate.

15. Check proper item.

16. Enter autopsy report in detail.

17. (a) As given on death certificate.
    (b) As determined by Advisory Committee or director of study.

18. Check proper item.

19. Check proper item and enter type of postmortem delivery.

20. Copy from birth certificate.

21. In case of plural births, check for each child.

22. Check proper item.

23. Check proper item.

24. Enter time and check proper item. In case of plural births of different sexes, indicate by numerals the order of delivery. Postmortem deliveries should be entered as not delivered.

25. Check proper item. Where history is vague, check probable conditions and write "Doubtful" in space beside *Not known.*

26. Check proper item.

27. Include here any conditions arising during pregnancy, except those properly considered complications of pregnancy.

28. Specify in some detail.

29. If any complications were present, check *Complications of pregnancy;* if none were present, check *None;* if there is no record, check *NR.*

30-36. If *None* or *NR* is checked in item 29, no further entries are required. Check proper items and make entries called for. Give date of onset or time it was first noted if condition was present at first examination. In item 31, give part affected.

37. Give treatment in detail.

38. This item calls for conditions which appeared at onset or during the course of labor, not those present during pregnancy.

39. Give name of physician, midwife, or clinic to whom patient went for prenatal care.

40. Check proper item according to classification as follows: Adequate, Inadequate; Excluded, all cases in which death occurred at or prior to fifteenth week of gestation.

41. Enter check in proper monthly column for each item if examination was made. If examination was not made at any time, check *N.*

(OVER)

42. Check proper items and enter data asked for, for all grades including "excluded" where such is available. If no examinations were made until admission or visit during labor, check examinations made at that time and write "On admission" across findings.

43. Specify conditions such as contracted pelvis, etc., not discovered by physician during prenatal period.

44. Check proper item and specify where necesary.

45. Check proper item. If abortion was self-induced, check both (*self*) and *Induced*; if it was induced by another, cross out (*self*).

46. Check proper item. If operation was attempted, give details.

47. This item applies only to cases of 28 weeks gestation or over. Check proper items. Items 48 through 58 are to be filled in for all cases. If information is not available, check *NR*.

48. Check proper item.

49. Check proper item. Specify as physician, interne, nurse, midwife, or other. Do not include anæsthetist.

50. Check proper items. Under (f) give antiseptic or antiseptics used on field.

51. Specify. Check proper items as for *Technique.*

52. Check proper items.

53. Check proper items and enter time. If membranes were ruptured in the course of actual delivery, write in "At delivery."

54. Check proper items. Give type as normal, slow, ineffective, or intermittent.

55. Check proper item. Enter after *Operative attempts*, delivery manœuvres aimed at delivery but failing to effect it. In case of plural births, enter procedure used for each child, numbering procedure according to baby. Two consecutive manœuvres resulting in delivery are to be counted as one e., version and extraction with forceps. For version and extraction, give interval between the version and extraction or indicate that it was version and immediate extraction. Enter after *Operative attempts* those performed on not delivered cases as well as attempts made prior to delivery.

56. Check and specify. In case of abortion, if D & C was done, enter here and in item 60. In cases of Cesarean where placenta was delivered through abdominal incision, check *None*.

57. Check proper item. Check *N* if there was episiotomy, unless there was an extension, then check *Tears, Episiotomy,* and *Perineal* and give degree.

58. Check proper item; give tpye or types and administrator.

59. After *Para,* enter number of viable births; after *Gravida,* enter number of viable and non-viable births. If gravidity is not known, write "NR" or "NR multigravida."

60. Enter any operation after delivery, or, in undelivered case, prior to death. Give interval between delivery and death.

61. Check proper items. If delivery had been arranged for, check *Planned* even if admission was an emergency.

62. Check proper items.

63. Give total time in days, including all admissions to any hospital relative to this delivery.

64. Check proper items.

Numbers 140 through 150 are the code numbers of puerperal causes of death as given in the *Manual of the International List of Causes of Death.* Check all conditions which were present, whether primary or contributory cause of death. The condition determined on by the Advisory Committee as the true cause of death will be checked in red and entered in item 17 (b) when decision is made. Answer all questions here whether or not they have been answered before..

Under *Non-puerperal causes of death,* enter name of condition and code number. Include all conditions not specified in items 140 through 150. Indicate whether the condition was considered primary or contributory cause of death.

Under *Remarks,* give an inclusive summary of the case, including any relevant data not properly included in the schedule itself. Also include range of temperature, pulse and respiration, and laboratory work.

Informant. Enter name of the person giving information. In case of a hospital, give chief of staff and name of the responsible visiting physician, not name of interne.

Dates of visits. Check proper items and give dates of all visits.

"Endless accumulation of observations leads nowhere."

Galen

"To benefit from reading we must ponder what we read."

Feather

Printed by James M. Armstrong, Inc., at 2116 Locust Street, Philadelphia, Pa.

TITLES IN THIS SERIES

10 *Risks for the Single Woman in the City, An Anthology of Studies by Late Nineteenth-Century Reformers*. David J. and Sheila M. Rothman, eds. New York, 1986

11 *Saving Babies: Children's Bureau Studies of Infant Mortality, 1913–1917*. David J. and Sheila M. Rothman, eds. New York, 1986

12 *The Sheppard-Towner Act, the Record of the Hearings*. David J. and Sheila M. Rothman, eds. New York, 1986

13 *Women in Prison, 1834–1928, An Anthology of Pamphlets from the Progressive Movement*. David J. and Sheila M. Rothman, eds. New York, 1986

14 Azel Ames, Jr., *Sex in Industry: A Plea for the Working Girl*, Boston, 1875

15 Robert South Barrett, *The Care of the Unmarried Mother*, Alexandria, 1929

16 Elizabeth Blackwell, M.D., *The Laws of Life, with Special Reference to the Physical Education of Girls*, New York, 1852

17 Alida C. Bower and Ruth S. Bloodgood, *Institutional Treatment of Delinquent Boys*, Washington, D.C., 1935–36

18 New York Assembly, *The Girls of the Department Store*, New York, 1895

19 Committee on the Infant and Preschool Child, *Nursery Education*, New York, 1931

20 Robert Latou Dickinson and Lura Beam, *The Single Woman: A Medical Study in Sex Education*, Baltimore, 1934

21 G. V. Hamilton, M.D., *A Research in Marriage*, New York, 1929

22 Elizabeth Harrison, *A Study of Child Nature from the Kindergarten Standpoint*, Chicago, 1909

23 Orie Latham Hatcher, *Rural Girls in the City for Work*, Richmond, 1930

24 William Healy, Augusta F. Bronner, et al., *Reconstructing Behavior in Youth*, New York, 1929

25 Henry H. Hibbs, Jr., *Infant Mortality: Its Relation to Social and Industrial Conditions*, New York, 1916

26 *The Juvenile Court Record*, Chicago, 1900, 1901

27 Mary A. Livermore, *What Shall We Do With Our Daughters?* Boston, 1883

28 *Massachusetts Society for the Prevention of Cruelty to Children: First Ten Annual Reports*, Boston, 1882

29 Maude E. Miner, *Slavery of Prostitution: A Plea for Emancipation*, New York, 1916

30 Maud Nathan, *The Story of an Epoch-Making Movement*, New York, 1926

31 National Florence Crittenton Mission, *Fourteen Years' Work Among "Erring Girls,"* Washington, D.C., 1897

32 New York Milk Committee, *Reducing Infant Mortality in the Ten Largest Cities in the United States*, New York, 1912

33 James Orton, ed., *The Liberal Education of Women: The Demand and the Method*, New York, 1873

34 Margaret Reeves, *Training Schools for Delinquent Girls*, New York, 1929

35 Ben L. Reitman, M.D., *The Second Oldest Profession*, New York, 1931

36 John Dale Russell and Associates, *Vocational Education*, Washington, D.C., 1938

37 William H. Slingerland, *Child Welfare Work in California*, New York, 1916

38 William H. Slingerland, *Child Welfare Work in Pennsylvania*, New York, 1917

39 *Documents Relative to the House of Refuge, Instituted by the Society for the Reformation of Juvenile Delinquents in the City of New York, in 1824*, New York, 1832

40 George S. Stevenson, M.D., and Geddes Smith, *Child Guidance Clinics*, New York, 1934

41 Henry Winfred Thurston, *Delinquency and Spare Time*, New York, 1918

42 U.S. National Commission on Law Observance and Enforcement, *Report on Penal Institutions, Probation and Parole*, Washington, D.C., 1931

43 Miriam Van Waters, *Parents on Probation*, 1927

44 Ira S. Wile, M.D., *The Sex Life of the Unmarried Adult*, New York, 1934

45 Helen Leland Witmer, *Psychiatric Clinics for Children*, New York, 1940

46 Young Women's Christian Association, *First Ten Annual Reports, 1871–1880*, New York, 1871–1880